McArdle Library APH

B10427·

KU-289-417

PASS
FINALS

A COMPANION TO KUMAR & CLARK'S
CLINICAL MEDICINE

SECOND EDITION

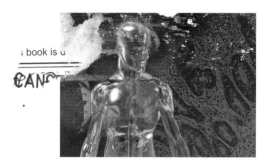

; book is u

CANC

For Elsevier:
Commissioning Editor: Pauline Graham
Project Development Manager: Ailsa Laing
Project Manager: Jess Thompson
Designer: George Ajayi
Illustrator: Richard Prime
Illustration Manager: Merlyn Harvey

PASS
FINALS
A COMPANION TO KUMAR & CLARK'S
CLINICAL MEDICINE

SECOND EDITION

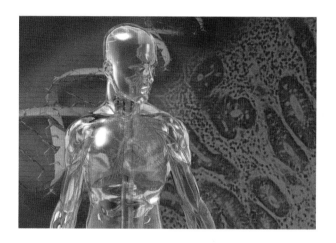

Geoff Smith MD MRCP

Consultant Physician and Gastroenterologist, Hammersmith Hospitals
NHS Trust, London

Elizabeth Carty BMedSci BMBS MD FRCP

Consultant Physician and Gastroenterologist, Whipps
Cross University Hospital, London

Louise Langmead MD MRCP

Consultant Physician and Gastroenterologist, University College
London Hospitals NHS Trust, London

Edinburgh London New York Oxford Philadelphia St Louis Sydney Toronto 2008

SAUNDERS
ELSEVIER

© 2008, Elsevier Limited. All rights reserved.
© Elsevier Limited 2004

No part of this publication may be reproduced, stored in a retrieval system, or
transmitted in any form or by any means, electronic, mechanical, photocopying,
recording or otherwise, without the prior permission of the Publishers. Permissions
may be sought directly from Elsevier's Health Sciences Rights Department, 1600 John
F. Kennedy Boulevard, Suite 1800, Philadelphia, PA 19103-2899, USA: phone: (+1) 215
239 3804; fax: (+1) 215 239 3805; or, e-mail: *healthpermissions@elsevier.com*. You may
also complete your request on-line via the Elsevier homepage (*http://www.elsevier.com*),
by selecting 'Support and contact' and then 'Copyright and Permission'.

First edition 2004
Second edition 2008

ISBN-13: 978-0-7020-2877-9

British Library Cataloguing in Publication Data
A catalogue record for this book is available from the British Library

Library of Congress Cataloging in Publication Data
A catalog record for this book is available from the Library of Congress

Knowledge and best practice in this field are constantly changing. As new research and
experience broaden our knowledge, changes in practice, treatment and drug therapy
may become necessary or appropriate. Readers are advised to check the most current
information provided (i) on procedures featured or (ii) by the manufacturer of each
product to be administered, to verify the recommended dose or formula, the method
and duration of administration, and contraindications. It is the responsibility of the
practitioner, relying on their own experience and knowledge of the patient, to make
diagnoses, to determine dosages and the best treatment for each individual patient, and
to take all appropriate safety precautions. To the fullest extent of the law, neither the
publisher nor the authors assume any liability for any injury and/or damage to persons
or property arising out or related to any use of the material contained in this book.

The Publisher

For information on all Elsevier publications visit our
web site at http://books.elsevier.com

your source for books,
journals and multimedia
in the health sciences
www.elsevierhealth.com

Working together to grow
libraries in developing countries
www.elsevier.com | www.bookaid.org | www.sabre.org
ELSEVIER   BOOK AID International   Sabre Foundation

The
Publisher's
policy is to use
**paper manufactured
from sustainable forests**

Printed in China

Preface to the First Edition

The range and depth of knowledge that medical students seem to be expected to retain grows continuously. This is despite the stated policy of many medical schools that the 'information load' should be reduced in undergraduate teaching. Over the last decade many traditional styles of examination have become less common, replaced by multiple-choice style examinations based on clinical scenarios and OSCE examinations, in place of long and short cases.

The advance of molecular medicine and the increasing links between basic sciences and clinical medicine have led us to include these topics in the text. Common radiological investigations are also included as they are becoming a key part of many examinations. The use of evidence-based medicine demands an understanding of statistics and trial design and these topics are, as a result, also included.

In this book we have tried to distil a core dataset in general and speciality medicine. The information is provided as bulleted lists and is supported by diagrams and self-assessment questions. By its nature, therefore, this is not a definitive textbook of clinical medicine and the page references to the 6th edition of Kumar and Clark's *Clinical Medicine* are designed to point the reader towards a more in-depth explanation of the subject. We hope, however, that it will act as a source of rapid access information for the important disease processes and thereby act as a useful revision aid.

Finally we would like to thank those individuals that have supported our efforts – notably Ellen Green and Siân Jarman at Elsevier for their efforts and Sarah Russell for the design work. Also to Parveen Kumar and Michael Clark for their critique of the text and for writing *Clinical Medicine* in the first place, and to our families for support and coffee during the writing. Finally, we should thank the Good Samaritan for ongoing inspiration.

Good Luck!

G.S.
E.C.
L.L.

ACKNOWLEDGEMENTS

Our thanks go to Dr Nick Reading (Consultant Radiologist, Whipps Cross University Hospital) for supplying images for the radiology chapter.

Preface to the Second Edition

We have, since the first edition, seen the rise of the OSCE as the key practical clinical assessment. As a result we have dedicated a chapter to this type of examination and, although it can never hope to outline all the possible stations that you would face, it should give you some idea as to what to expect.

We have updated the text extensively to bring it up to date and maintain the links to the latest edition of *Clinical Medicine*, as well as taking out some of the basic sciences information that appears less and less in clinical examinations in medicine.

We are, as ever, indebted to our families for their patience as we hammered away at keyboards, to Parveen Kumar and Michael Clark for allowing the use of material from *Clinical Medicine*, 6th Edn, and to Ailsa Laing and Andy Baxter for their calm approach as deadlines came (and went!)

G.S.
E.C.
L.L.

McARDLE LIBRARY
0151 604 7223

Contents

1. How to pass medical finals   1

2. Question types in medical finals   9

3. Objective Structured Clinical Examinations (OSCEs)   21

4. Clinical pharmacology   45

5. Radiology   71

6. Clinical chemistry   105

7. Infectious diseases   129

8. Respiratory medicine   161

9. Cardiology   195

10. Gastroenterology and hepatology   247

11. Rheumatology   305

12. Dermatology   333

13. Endocrinology   347

14. Renal medicine   381

15. Haematology   411

16. Oncology and genetic disease   451

17. Neurology   471

18. Psychological medicine   525

19. Statistics and evidence-based medicine   553

Appendix A. Answers to multiple choice questions   567

Appendix B. Answers to extended matching questions   571

Appendix C. Normal reference ranges Normal values for laboratory tests   577

Appendix D. Bibliography and further reading   579

Index   581

How to pass medical finals 1

There are, and always have been, several truisms about sitting final exams in medicine. At the end of the day, the vast majority of students pass their final exams and earn the right to call themselves 'Doctor'. There are, however, tactics and techniques that you can use to make the process less painful.

WRITTEN EXAMS

Much of this sounds obvious, but 'schoolchild errors' are commonly made in the stress of final exams.

Be prepared

▌ Exam technique is a learned skill
▌ Know the distribution of marks for the paper
▌ Make sure you know the format of the exam
▌ Practise questions from past papers
▌ Practise keeping to time

Directed learning

▌ The vast majority of questions are about common and important areas of medicine
▌ Rare syndromes are very unlikely to come up
▌ Medical emergencies are often asked about
▌ Remember the classic pitfalls in medicine (Table 1.1)

Read the instructions

▌ Make sure you are quite clear on how many questions you have to answer and how much time you have for each one
▌ If need be, write the start and finish times for each section on the top of the paper and stick to them

Table 1.1 The structured answer

For any disease, outline:
Incidence – common → rare
Distribution:
   Age
   Sex
   Geographical
   Racial
Pathology
Aetiology
Clinical features
Associated conditions
Investigations
Therapeutic options
Outcome or prognosis
Complications

Answer the question asked

- Read the question carefully – preferably twice
- Answer the question asked, not the one you want to answer – don't just write down everything that you remember about the topic

Answer all the questions

- Attempt the correct number of questions
- If you are running out of time, try to put something down on paper, even if it is only an essay plan – you may get some credit

Presentation

- Clear, neat handwriting is easier to mark
- Structure your answer: headings and subheadings speed up marking
- Spell accurately

Anonymous papers

- Many exams require you to put a name or candidate number on each page – make sure you do

MULTIPLE CHOICE PAPERS

- Several different formats exist: see Chapter 2
- Make sure that you know what question type is used

- Keep to time and answer all of the questions
- Do not spend long on a question you have no idea about – you can always go back to it
- Most questions have some obvious wrong answers – shortening the odds
- Practise as many questions as you can
- Questions are often re-used – do as many past papers as you can

Negative marking

- Rarely used
- Mark deducted for a wrong answer
- Aims to deter 'wild guesses'
- Informed guesses are risky but on balance worth it

CLINICAL EXAMS

Clinical exams can be more nerve-racking than written papers. The 'performance' in front of examiners is stressful. Again, basic tactics will help you out.

Dress code

- Go for smart, conservative and comfortable dress. Loud waistcoats and cartoon ties will not help

Equipment

- The vast majority of the equipment you will need for a clinical examination will be provided
- You will need:
  - A stethoscope – make sure it is clean and working
  - A pen – most important for long cases!
- Ophthalmoscopes should be provided, but if you have your own and are comfortable using it, take it with you. Make sure the batteries are fresh
- Everything else is a luxury. Pockets bulging with equipment are uncomfortable and heavy

Three key aims

- Do not hurt or embarrass the patient
- Ensure the examiner sees you carry out all parts of the examination competently
- Synthesise a diagnosis, differential and management plan

The order of importance of the above depends upon the examiner and the case. If the diagnosis is straightforward, the examiner will want you to reach it without too much of a performance. If the diagnosis is difficult, he or she will want you to demonstrate your ability to elicit clinical signs, even if the underlying cause escapes you.

Examination technique

- Make sure that your examination technique is swift and professional
- Do what you are asked
  - 'Examine the cardiovascular system' means a full examination starting with the hands
  - 'Listen to the heart' means just auscultation
  - Examiners should make it clear what they want

Dignity

- *NEVER* hurt or embarrass the patient
- *ALWAYS* introduce yourself
- *ALWAYS* ask permission to examine
- *ALWAYS* ask whether the area you are going to examine is painful or tender
- *THANK* the patient at the end of the exam

Scoring points

- A professional introduction, followed by an examination technique that is fluent and clearly well practised, is as important as reaching a diagnosis
- Even if the diagnosis eludes you, describe your findings
- Outline the positive findings at examination and the important negatives
- If you can, come up with a diagnosis and differential
- The longer you can talk, the fewer questions can be asked (although talking rubbish does not help)

VIVA VOCE EXAMS

Vivas or oral examinations still make up a part of final examinations in some medical schools. They may be routine for all candidates or used specifically to re-examine a borderline candidate. If you are called for a viva in the latter situation, remember that honours students may be examined as well and that a selection of candidates across the whole range of marks will be examined to provide a standard range of scores.

In general it is difficult to fail the whole exam because of a poor performance in a viva.

Dress

▌ Be smart and conservative

Format

▌ There are usually two examiners – one may be external
▌ You may be:

Asked questions

▌ e.g. What classes of drug are useful in the management of hypertension?

Given a case scenario

▌ e.g. Outline the management options for a 74-year-old woman who comes to see you with rheumatoid arthritis.

Asked about medical emergencies

▌ e.g. A 55-year-old man is admitted with haematemesis and a blood pressure of 90/50. What would you do?

Asked to report the results of an investigation

▌ e.g. A chest X-ray, ECG or blood test results

Identify an object

▌ Pathological specimen
▌ Piece of equipment (e.g. nasogastric tube, urinary catheter)

Tactics

▌ 'Engage your brain before your mouth'
▌ Structure your answer (Tables 1.1 and 1.2)
▌ Do not dig holes; if you realise that you are completely wrong, apologise and start again – the examiners expect you to be nervous

Table 1.2 Disease aetiology

For any clinical symptom or sign (e.g. diarrhoea*), classify the causes into:

Infective
Viruses
   Rotavirus
   Adenovirus
Bacteria
   Staphylococcus aureus
   Salmonella
   Cholera
Parasites
   Giardiasis
   Ascaris

Inflammatory
Inflammatory bowel disease

Neoplastic
Colorectal cancer

Autoimmune
Coeliac disease

Metabolic
Hypercalcaemia

Endocrine
Thyrotoxicosis

Neurological
Autonomic neuropathy

Trauma/surgery
Post-gastrectomy

Iatrogenic
Drugs, e.g. laxatives

Idiopathic

* List is not complete.

∎ When giving lists of causes, start with the commonest first
∎ When giving lists of investigations, start with the least invasive and explain how they help with the diagnosis
∎ Make sure the tests are appropriate; if you are going to mention a blood count, chest X-ray and so on, make sure you state why you are discussing them

LAST-MINUTE REVISION

What to revise

▌ Revising facts you already know is easier than learning new information in the weeks prior to the exam. Consistent learning throughout the course is the best preparation

▌ Target the revision to the exam. Base revision around past papers and the type of exam you are sitting

▌ In the last week, go over notes and take timed practice exams rather than trying to learn new data

How to revise

▌ Practise MCQs in a group. It is more fun and you will remember more

▌ Outline essay plans and fill in the essential facts. You do not need to write out complete essays except to check timings

▌ If your university offers mock or prize exams, sit them. They are good practice and will highlight weak areas

▌ Use tools such as mind maps and revision aids. The more senses you use, the better the chance of the information sinking in. Jotting down lists and notes will help you absorb what you read

▌ Remember to give yourself time to relax. Play sport, go out or meet your friends rather than burning the midnight oil. Learning when you are half-comatose is ineffective
Sleep and eat properly and avoid stimulants such as caffeine tablets

▌ The night before the exam, do as little as possible. Find a way of relaxing and get a good (and sober) night's sleep

▌ And finally, do you really learn anything by frantically flicking through a book as you walk into the exam?

Question types in medical finals 2

The ideal exam question, from the examiners' point of view, is one that discriminates between different levels of knowledge or ability. A question that everybody gets right or wrong says little about an individual and is therefore a poor discriminator. OSCE examinations are discussed in detail in Chapter 3.

QUESTION TYPES IN WRITTEN EXAMS

Multiple choice questions (Table 2.1)

❚ Questions usually comprise a stem that introduces the question, and five branches or options

---

Table 2.1 MCQ styles

1. Which of the following are true of aspirin?
   A. It may cause gastric ulceration
   B. It is associated with an increased risk of transient ischaemic attacks
   C. It is associated with renal dysfunction
   D. Its use is never indicated in acute myocardial infarction
   E. It may exacerbate inflammatory bowel disease

2. Which of the following are not true of paracetamol?
   A. It is an anti-inflammatory drug
   B. It results in hepatic necrosis in severe overdose
   C. It is metabolised in the liver
   D. It is usually given intravenously
   E. It is a non-steroidal anti-inflammatory drug

3. The following drugs are associated with the stated complication:
   A. Flucloxacillin: jaundice
   B. Loperamide: diarrhoea
   C. Enalapril: cough
   D. Prednisolone: weight loss
   E. Metronidazole: nausea

Answers: **1.** A, C, E
        2. A, D, E
        3. T, F, T, F, T

Best answer questions

▌ Choose the branch that provides the correct or best answer

Example

Which *one* of the following is a cause of liver cirrhosis?
A. Cigarette smoking
B. Alcohol
C. Heroin
D. Cannabis
E. Methadone
Answer: B

True or false?

▌ For each branch, decide whether the statement is true or false

Example

The following are recognised causes of cirrhosis:
A. Alcohol
B. Autoimmune hepatitis
C. Hepatitis C
D. Haemochromatosis
E. Cystic fibrosis
Answer: All are true

Negative marking

▌ A point is given for each correct answer, but a point is deducted for an incorrect answer. This system is designed to discourage blind guessing, however educated guessing should, on average, improve your score. This system is rarely used any longer

Tips and tactics

▌ Always ensure that you know how to complete the question paper – read the instructions carefully
▌ For computer-scored papers, make sure that the marks you make on the paper are clear and confined to the correct part of the paper. Always use the pencil provided. Pens may not be detected properly by the computerised reader
▌ Keep an eye on the time. You may only have 2–3 minutes per question
▌ Going through the whole paper once, answering the questions you are sure of, then going back to

those that need more time may ensure that you don't miss any easy points

▌ Look for obvious incorrect answers. *Always* and *never* are rarely correct. Read the stem very carefully.

▌ Check for negatives in the stem: e.g. Which of the following are *not* causes of abdominal pain? Getting this wrong could cost you five marks

▌ 'Educated guesses' are usually correct; however, 'blind guesses' are risky if the paper is negatively marked

▌ Even if you have no idea about the subject of a question, read the possible answers – there may be sections for which no specialist knowledge is required

Extended matching questions

▌ For a small set of questions, a common list of 15–30 options provides the list of possible answers

Example
Question 1   Theme: Jaundice

A. Alcohol-related cirrhosis
B. Carcinoma of the pancreas
C. Hepatitis A
D. Hepatitis B
E. Hepatitis C
F. Haemochromatosis
G. Wilson's disease
H. Acute haemolysis
I. Gilbert's syndrome
J. Primary sclerosing cholangitis
K. Primary biliary cirrhosis
L. Autoimmune hepatitis
M. Budd–Chiari syndrome
N. Cystic fibrosis
O. Gallstone in the common bile duct

For each of the following questions, select the best answer from the list above:

I. A 28-year-old man notices that his eyes have a yellow tinge following a bad cough and cold. His liver function tests are normal apart from a bilirubin of 78 μmol/L.

II. A 76-year-old woman presents with jaundice and weight loss. She denies any abdominal pain.

Table 2.2 Picking out key facts

'A 76-year-old woman presents with *jaundice* and *weight loss*. *She denies any abdominal pain*. Her bilirubin is 280 μmol/L and the alkaline phosphatase 590 IU/L. The alanine aminotransferase is 87 IU/L. She has a family history of ischaemic heart disease. An ultrasound of her abdomen reveals a *dilated common bile duct*.'

Here, the classical combination of painless jaundice and weight loss gives you the diagnosis of carcinoma of the pancreas

---

Her bilirubin is 280 μmol/L and the alkaline phosphatase 590 IU. The alanine amino-transferase is 87 IU. She has a family history of ischaemic heart disease. An ultrasound of her abdomen reveals a dilated common bile duct (Table 2.2).

III. A 45-year-old man with known diabetes presents with jaundice. He is noted to have a deep tan and hepatomegaly. His ferritin is 1201 μg/L.

Answers
I. I
II. B
III. F

Example Question 2

A. Haemoglobin
B. Myoglobin
C. Albumin
D. Ferritin
E. Transferrin
F. Alanine aminotransferase
G. Collagen
H. Fibrinogen
I. Factor VIII
J. Immunoglobulin
K. Serotonin (5-hydroxytryptamine, 5HT)
L. Niacin
M. Intrinsic factor
N. Glucose-6-phosphatase
O. Lactate dehydrogenase

For each of the following questions, select the best answer from the list above:

I. A peptide important in the absorption of vitamin B_{12} *(M)*

II. An iron-containing protein derived from muscle *(B)*

III. A neurotransmitter released by carcinoid tumours *(K)*

IV. A helical structural connective tissue protein *(G)*

V. A protein to which bilirubin is bound in the blood *(C)*

VI. A protein capable of carrying oxygen in the circulation *(A)*

VII. A substance the deficiency of which results in pellagra *(L)*

VIII. A protein precursor of bilirubin *(A)*

IX. A protein released by injured hepatocytes *(F)*

X. A protein that exists in five subclasses *(J)*

▌ Note that any answer from the list may be appropriate for more than one question

A second type of EMQ

▌ This asks for more than one answer for each question

Example

XI. State two molecules capable of carrying oxygen *(A, B)*

XII. State two proteins secreted into the intestine *(J, M)*

XIII. State three proteins found in erythrocytes or leucocytes *(A, N, O)*

Tips and tactics

▌ The examiner is usually looking for the best answer to the question; however, there may be other possible answers that will gain some marks

▌ Make an attempt at each part if you can, for the reasons given above. For each part of the question, underline the key facts and investigation results that may help you reach the correct answer

▌ Don't be put off by diseases on the list of options that you know little about. They may well not be the answer to any of the questions posed

Short answers

▌ These questions ask you to write notes or a short summary on three or four related topics

Example

1. Write short notes on each of the following:
   A. Thrombolysis in myocardial infarction
   B. Risk factors for ischaemic heart disease
   C. Aspirin in ischaemic heart disease

Tips and tactics

▌ These require short, structured answers
▌ If time is short, consider bulleted points or headings and lists
▌ Do not attempt to put down everything you know about the subject – stick to answering the question being asked
▌ Keep a close eye on the time – it is easy to get carried away and spend far too much time on a single part of a question
▌ There are only a limited number of marks. Writing excessive amounts will not get you extra points

Patient management problems

▌ A description of a patient history and examination is given, followed by two or three questions. For each question there is a list of options and you are asked to grade the correctness of each option

Example

A 55-year-old man, who works for a building company, is referred complaining of a cough. The cough has been present for 3 months and on four occasions he has coughed up some blood. He now feels breathless after mild exertion. His wife has rheumatoid arthritis and he is her main carer. He has had a previous admission for angina and attends a diabetes clinic at his local GP's. He is a smoker who drinks about 40 units of alcohol a week as beer.

He is 180 cm tall and weighs 70 kg. He has some crackles at left midzone of his lungs but no other findings on examination.

Which four of the following would be most useful in making an immediate diagnosis?
   1. ECG
   2. Exercise ECG
   3. CT of the chest
   4. MRI of the lungs
   5. Peak flow measurements

6. Lung function tests
7. Full blood count
8. Blood cultures
9. Arterial blood gases
10. Chest X-ray

Answer: 1, 5, 8, 10

A chest X-ray reveals calcified pleural lesions and increased lung markings, most notably in the bases. Based on this, what is the most likely diagnosis?

A. Carcinoma of the bronchus
B. Chronic congestive cardiac failure
C. Streptococcal pneumonia
D. Asbestosis
E. Rheumatoid lung disease

Answer: D

▌ The second variation of this question type asks for one-line answers to a series of questions about a case

Example

A 66-year-old man presents with chest pain. This started suddenly 2 hours ago. The pain is central and radiates to both shoulders. He is sweaty and feels very unwell. On examination he is apyrexial and tachycardic with a blood pressure of 110/60.

1. What is the most likely diagnosis?
   Answer: Acute myocardial infarction
2. What two investigations would be of immediate use?
   Answer: ECG and troponin
3. State four immediate therapeutic steps you would institute.
   Answer: High-flow oxygen, i.v. diamorphine, morphine, aspirin and consider thrombolysis or angioplasty
4. Suggest three possible complications of the therapies you suggest.
   Answer: Haemorrhage, gastrointestinal ulceration, respiratory depression

When answering these questions, remember that although your answers may be correct, there may be a better way of answering in order to show off your knowledge.

▌ Give a full answer – *Acute myocardial infarction* rather than *Heart attack*

- Give investigations of different modalities – *ECG and troponin* rather than *Troponin and creatine kinase*
- Give specific rather than general treatments with differing aims – *High flow oxygen* rather than *Oxygen or i.v. access*, *Diamorphine and aspirin* rather than *Aspirin and clopidogrel*
- Give complications specific to each treatment you have mentioned – *Haemorrhage, GI ulceration, respiratory depression* rather than *GI haemorraghe, intracerebral haemorrhage and retinal haemorrhage*

Essay questions

- These provide a title and sometimes some specific requirements for an essay

Example

Outline the important considerations in palliation of a patient with an inoperable lung carcinoma. In your answer outline the important therapies you would consider using.

Tips and tactics

- Read the question carefully and underline any 'riders' or specific instructions
- Spend a minute sketching an essay plan with section headings. This allows you to order your thoughts before committing them to paper
- Headings help the examiner as they speed up marking
- Answer the specific questions being asked; do not write a general essay on the subject in the hope of getting credit
- Always include the basics. The examiner may not assume that you know something even if it seems obvious
- Time the paper carefully. Writing two 30-minute essays instead of three 20-minute essays makes passing much harder
- Read through your answer
  - Does it all make sense?
  - Does it answer the question?
  - Is the spelling correct?
  - Is it structured and easy to read?
- If you are running out of time, write out a structured essay plan with key facts about the

subject. Most marking schemes will give you some credit for this
▌ If the examiners cannot read your writing, they cannot mark the essay!

CLINICAL EXAMS

Short cases

▌ A series of patients are seen with the examiners who give you specific instructions
  – 'Look at this patient – what is the diagnosis?'
  – 'Examine this man's chest'
  – 'Listen to this woman's heart'
▌ You will then be expected to:
  – Introduce yourself
  – Carry out the appropriate examination
  – Present your findings and give a diagnosis, differential and management plan

Tips and tactics

▌ Be professional
▌ Do not embarrass or hurt the patient
▌ Follow the instructions you are given
▌ Answer the questions you are asked
▌ Remember, very unwell patients are unlikely to be in a clinical exam. Chronic conditions are more common. You may be given tips or a brief introduction
  – 'This gentleman gets breathless on exertion – examine the heart'
    → Think about heart valve murmurs and cardiac failure

Common topics for short cases
Cardiac

▌ Heart sounds and murmurs
▌ Cardiomegaly
▌ Dextrocardia (rare)
▌ Hypertensive retinopathy

Respiratory

▌ Chronic obstructive pulmonary disease
▌ Surgery for tuberculosis
▌ Pulmonary fibrosis

- Pleural effusions
- Chest infections
- Cystic fibrosis

Gastrointestinal

- Chronic liver disease
- Ileostomy/colostomy
- Fistulating Crohn's disease
- Hepatosplenomegaly

Urinary

- Transplanted kidney (right iliac fossa)
- Arteriovenous shunt for dialysis (left arm)
- Ileal urinary conduit (urine in the bag)
- Palpable kidneys (often polycystic kidney)

Neurological

- Multiple sclerosis
- Ophthalmoplegia
- Facial palsy
- Brachial plexus injury
- Ulnar or radial nerve damage
- Carpal tunnel syndrome
- Hemiparesis or paraparesis
- Charcot–Marie–Tooth
- Friedreich's ataxia (check speech)
- Parkinson's disease
- Cerebellar ataxia

Endocrine

- Thyroid status (Table 2.3)
- Acromegaly
- Diabetic retinopathy
- Diabetic sensory loss
- Hypopituitarism
- Cushing's syndrome

Table 2.3 'Examine this patient and assess her thyroid gland'	
Hypothyroidism	**Hyperthyroidism**
Thick, rough, dry skin	Thin patient
Obesity	Sweaty
Bradycardia	Tachycardia $\pm$ atrial fibrillation
Slow relaxing reflexes	Exophthalmos with lid lag
Loss of outer third of the eyebrow	Tremor

Rheumatological

- Systemic sclerosis
- Rheumatoid arthritis
- Osteoarthritis
- Ankylosing spondylitis
- Paget's disease of bone

Long cases

- A prolonged period with a patient prior to presenting the case to an examiner. You may be taken back to the patient in order to assess a specific part of the examination technique
- Take a detailed history
- With chronic disabling conditions, the social history is very important
- Perform a thorough clinical examination
- Keep an eye on the time and make legible notes. Divide the time into:
  - History-taking
  - Examination
  - Reviewing your findings
  - Going back to ask further questions
- When presenting, adhere to the preferred format for your medical school
- Give the positive and important negative findings
- Outline a diagnosis and a differential
- Outline the investigations that are appropriate
- Outline treatment options, including long-term care needs if appropriate

Objective Structured Clinical Examinations (OSCEs) 3

In the last 15 years OSCEs have gradually taken over as the most common form of clinical examination. They allow for standardisation of the examination for all candidates and a formalised marking system. They are relatively expensive in terms of the number of examiners needed, but allow a large number of candidates to be assessed in a relatively short period of time. They are also fairer as every candidate does the same stations.

Structure

- There is a 'round robin' of test stations
- The examiner stays at the station
- Each station lasts 5–10 minutes
- Stations may be paired, e.g. a clinical examination at one station and questions about the examination and diagnosis at the next
- Each station has a strict marking sheet – Fig. 3.1
- A wide variety of stations can be included, allowing broad testing of skills and knowledge

TYPES OF STATION

General

- Taking a targeted history for a clinical scenario
- Examining a 'patient' (often an actor!) – see speciality chapters
- Patient photographs
- X-rays – see radiology chapter 5
- ECGs – see cardiology chapter 9
- Laboratory test interpretation – see *Clinical Chemistry*, Chapter 6

Candidate Name: Examination number:

Candidate instructions: Mrs Lewis has been referred having noticed blood in her stools. You have been asked by the consultant to take a focussed history of the presenting complaint. You do not need to ask about the past medical or social history, the drug history or to carry out a systems review. You do not need to present your findings to the examiner.

Examiner instructions: Please assess the candidate using the criteria listed.

		adequate	inadequate
1	Introduces self to patient, using own name, patient's name, role and a greeting		
2	States reason for the interview		
3	Obtains consent to proceed		
4	Asks patient's age		
5	Asks about occupation		
6	Obtains history of PR bleeding		
Specific information points elicited			
7	Nature of bleeding (bright red, mixed with stool) both to score		
8	Duration of symptoms		
9	Frequency of bleeding		
10	Previous episodes		
11	Recent change in bowel habit		
12	Normal bowel habit		
13	Weight loss or anorexia (both to score)		
14	Dietary changes		
15	Shortness of breath		
16	Medication history		
17	Family history		
18	Associated symptoms		
Approach to patient			
19	Active listening (verbal and non-verbal)		
20	Clarifies and reviews		
21	Avoids leading question		
22	Avoids multiple questions		
23	Does not use jargon or gives explanations		
24	Patient's rating of the candidate		

Examiner's rating

4 good	3 pass	2 borderline	1 fail

Fig. 3.1 Each station has a strict marking sheet.

Practical skills

- Measuring blood pressure
- Inserting a cannula
- Inserting a urinary catheter
- Taking blood
- Checking a blood transfusion
- Cardiopulmonary resuscitation

Management questions

- Medical emergencies
- Writing a fluid chart
- Writing a prescription
- Reviewing a drug chart

Communication

- Explaining a prescription to a patient
- Discussing a diagnosis to a patient
- Obtaining consent
- Describing a practical procedure
- Breaking bad news

Tips and tactics

- Make sure you are comfortable with the common procedures that crop up in OSCEs
- Practise the commonly needed practical skills in a clinical skills lab if possible. These are easy marks to get
- At stations with a 'patient' ALWAYS introduce yourself, explain who you are and ask permission. NEVER embarrass or hurt the 'patient'
- Follow the (usually written) instructions
- At 'patient-based' stations, the examiner will have no verbal role. If you are expected to present findings the instruction sheet will specifically tell you
- Even if a station has gone badly, you may have picked up some marks for professionalism, communication or rapport with the patient
- At the end of the station, forget it and clear your mind ready for the next one. Remember each station is a fresh start

EXAMPLE STATIONS

For each of the following stations, the key 'point-scoring' things that you should do are highlighted. There are general points for each type of station that are outlined at the beginning of each category. Don't forget to confirm your examination number and name with the examiner before you start.

Clinical history
Remember to

▌ Introduce yourself (to the patient) using your and their name
▌ Read the instructions and follow them exactly
▌ Ignore the examiner unless specifically instructed to present to them
▌ Explain who you are and ask permission to proceed
    – This doesn't have to be too formal: 'Would you mind if I asked you a few questions?'
▌ Ask a couple of general questions then rapidly target in on the key facts pertinent to the case
▌ Try not to lead the patient – 'So where do you get the pain' rather than 'So you have chest pain?'
▌ Give the patient a chance to expand on the answer
▌ Ask if there is anything else they want to tell you
▌ Avoid going into a long discussion about your diagnosis – these stations are about you getting the appropriate history, not explaining the diagnosis to the patient
▌ Once the bell goes, thank the patient and leave

Chest pain

Mr Davis is a 57-year-old man who has attended accident and emergency with chest pain. Take an appropriate history from him. The 'patient' will have some specific pain features indicating the cause of the pain. This is most commonly acute myocardial infarction or angina. Less commonly gastro-oesophageal reflux disease (p. 256). Your history needs to elicit these. The key facts that you should ask about are:

▌ Duration of the pain
▌ Previous episodes
▌ Character of pain
    – Heavy/crushing in acute MI

- Dull/tight in angina
- Continuous or varying

❚ Intensity (on a range from 1–10)

❚ Site

❚ Radiation – to neck or left arm in cardiac ischaemia

Associated features

❚ Nausea

❚ Sweating

❚ Dizziness/faintness

❚ Shortness of breath

❚ Inducing activities
- Exercise
- Cold windy days

❚ Relieving activities
- Rest
- Taking glyceryl trinitrate

❚ Risk factors for ischaemic heart disease
- Family history of heart disease, stroke, hypertension of diabetes
- Smoking history
- Diabetes mellitus
- Hypertension
- Previous history of ischaemic heart disease
- Elevated cholesterol

❚ Treatment history
- Cardiovascular drugs

❚ Allergies to medication

❚ Risk factors for treatment

❚ Recent GI bleeding

❚ Recent major surgery

❚ Recent cerebrovascular accident

❚ Blood coagulopathy

❚ Diabetic eye disease

Shortness of breath without chest pain

Mrs Jones is a 78-year-old woman with increasing shortness of breath. Take an appropriate history from her.

The initial differential is

❚ Congestive cardiac failure/acute pulmonary oedema

❚ 'Silent' ischaemic heart disease

❚ Pneumonia/lower respiratory tract infection

- Exacerbation of chronic obstructive pulmonary disease/asthma
- Bronchogenic carcinoma

Initial questions to determine the most likely cause

- New symptom or recurrence of previous symptom
- Duration and whether getting worse
- Associated symptoms
  - Cough
  - Sputum production and type – purulent/non-purulent/frothy
  - Presence of orthopnoea and paroxysmal nocturnal dyspnoea
- History of ischaemic heart disease
- Risk factors for ischaemic heart disease or COPD

Once the underlying cause is clear, you should target your history to the appropriate disease.

Silent ischaemic heart disease

- As for chest pain above

Congestive cardiac failure/pulmonary oedema

- Onset and severity
- Initiating, exacerbating and relieving factors
- Orthopnoea and paroxysmal nocturnal dyspnoea
- Cough/frothy sputum
- Ankle swelling
- Palpitations
- Chest pain
- Past history
  - Ischaemic heart disease
- Risk factors as for cardiac chest pain
- Medication history

Pneumonia/lower respiratory tract infection

- Cough
- Purulent sputum/colour of sputum
- Pleuritic chest pain
- Sweats/fevers
- Associated diarrhoea (atypical pneumonia)
- Peri-oral herpes simplex (*Strep. pneumoniae*)
- Risk factors
  - Smoking
  - Occupational exposure (dust/asbestos)
  - Animal exposure (birds)

Chronic obstructive pulmonary disease/asthma

- Cough
- Sputum production
- Wheeze
- Acute or insidious onset
- Exposure to precipitant
- Usual peak flow
- Usual exercise tolerance
- Exercise tolerance at present
- previous admissions
- previous admissions to ITU
- Smoking history
- Use of steroids
- Domicilliary oxygen cylinders/concentrator
- Home nebuliser
- Indicators of infection
  - Fevers
  - Purulent sputum

Shortness of breath with chest pain

Peter Smith is a 25-year-old man who presents with severe left-sided chest pain and shortness of breath.

Differential diagnosis

- Pneumonia (see above)
- Pleurisy
- Ischaemic heart disease (see above)
- Pulmonary embolus
- Pneumothorax

Pleurisy
- Preceding cough/sputum
- Fever
- Flu like illness
- Pleuritic chest pain (worse on deep breathing)

Pulmonary embolus
- Sudden onset
- Pleuritic chest pain
- Shortness of breath
- Haemoptysis
- Swollen calf
- Risk factors
  - Immobility (travel/surgery/other illness)
  - Smoking
  - Oral contraceptive pill

           – Pro-coagulapathy (family history)
           – Previous miscarriages
           – Inflammatory disease
           – Malignant disease
           – Previous DVT/PE

Pneumothorax
- Classically tall thin young man
- Sudden onset
- Chest wall injury
- Short of breath with or without pain
- No fever
- No prodrome
- Risk factors
  – Asthma
  – COPD
  – Pulmonary fibrosis

Abdominal pain

Mr Flintoff is a 65-year-old man with abdominal pain. Take a history to ascertain the cause.

Basic questions

Site
- Epigastric – gastro-oesophageal reflux or dyspepsia
- Right subcostal – liver/biliary tree (e.g. gallstones)
- Left sided – diverticulosis/IBS/constipation
- Supra-pubic – bladder/pelvis
- Renal angles – renal stones/pyelonephritis

Character
- Constant
- Spasms
- Colicky

Associated symptoms
- Nausea
- Vomiting
- Diarrhoea
- Constipation
- Abdominal distension

Exacerbating features
- Eating
- Posture changes
- Deep breaths
- Specific foods

Relieving features
- Eating
- Vomiting
- Defaecation
- Antacids

Gastro-oesophageal reflux

- Central epigastric and retrosternal pain
- Burning/acidic in nature
- Induced by alcohol/caffeine/spicy foods
- Relieved by antacids
- Wakes from sleep at night
- Better when lying on left side
- Worse when bending over

Biliary colic

- Colicky pain (comes in waves)
- Right subcostal region
- Associated nausea/vomiting
- Associated jaundice
- Dark urine
- Pale stools

Renal colic

- Loin pain radiating to iliac fossa/testes/labia
- Vomiting
- Very severe colicky pain
- Associated symptoms
  - Haematuria
  - Anuria
- Risk factors
  - Hot weather
  - Previous stones
  - Gout
  - Vitamin D intake
  - Crohn's disease
  - Urinary tract infections
  - Diuretics

Interpretation of results stations
Radiology

Radiology images in OSCEs tend to be simple investigations (chest X-rays, abdominal films, rarely CT scans of the head) with gross abnormalities and a short clinical history giving clues as to the diagnosis. They may also ask about the management of the abnormality. Chapter 5 covers all of the important films.

Chest X-rays
- Pneumothorax
- Tension pneumothorax
- Air under the diaphragm
- Pneumonia
- Pulmonary oedema
- Bronchogenic carcinoma

Abdominal films
- Renal stones
- Small bowel obstruction
- Sigmoid volvulus
- Toxic megacolon
- Pancreatic calcification

CT head
- Subdural/extradural/sub-arachnoid haemorrhage
- Mass lesions with oedema and midline shift
- Acoustic neuroma

Example

A 67-year-old man is admitted with anorexia and a productive cough. He has been feeling unwell for about 2 weeks with a cough productive of blood-stained sputum. His chest X-ray is shown (Fig. 3.2).

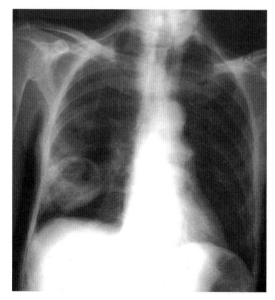

Fig. 3.2 Chest X-ray.

His temperature on admission is 36.7°C, oxygen saturation 93% on air.
1. Describe the abnormality seen.
   Cavitating lesion in right lung
2. Suggest three diagnoses in order of likelihood.
   Lung abscess
   Bronchogenic carcinoma
   Pulmonary metastasis
3. Name two further appropriate investigations.
   High resolution CT scan of the chest
   Sputum microscopy and culture

Example

A 58-year-old woman is admitted for a CT guided biopsy of a mass in the liver. List the important complications about which she should be advised and explain the procedure to her in order to gain informed consent.

Complications

▌ Pain
▌ Bleeding
▌ Perforation of bowel
▌ Injury to right kidney
▌ Perforated gallbladder
▌ Pneumothorax

Example

A 76-year-old man presents with right loin pain and haematuria. His abdominal X-ray is shown (Fig. 3.3).
1. Describe the abnormality seen.
   Calcified mass in the right lateral abdomen
2. Suggest two possible diagnoses
   Calcified (porcelain) gallbladder
   Renal calcification (nephrocalcinosis)
3. Suggest two useful radiological investigations
   Renal ultrasound
   CT abdomen

Laboratory investigations

Again, these tend to be simple investigations and ask for your interpretation and management (see Chapter 6).

Example

With reference to the following blood test results, answer the questions beneath:
▌ Hb 9.8 g/dL WCC 7.2 × 10^9/L platelets 198 MCV 101fl

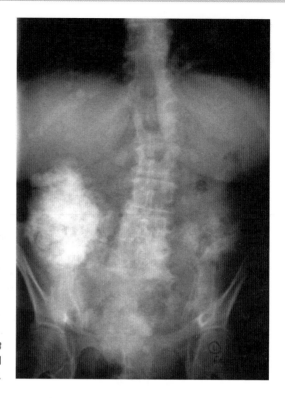

Fig. 3.3
Abdominal
X-ray.

▌ Blood film: hypersegmented neutrophils
    A. What is the haematological diagnosis?
       Macrocytic (megaloblastic) anaemia
    B. List 3 possible causes of your diagnosis.
       Vitamin B_{12} deficiency
       Folic acid deficiency
       Chronic liver disease
    C. Name two tests that would help you in
       determining the diagnosis.
       Liver biochemistry
       Serum haematinics

Practical procedure stations

As with clinical stations there will be a short clinical scenario followed by an instruction. As always, introduce yourself, explain the procedure, get verbal consent and give clear instructions to the patient. You may also be asked to list possible complications or comment on the result.

Measuring peak flow

Mrs Robinson has asthma and is breathless. Please measure the peak flow.

Instructions for patient
▌ Please follow the student's instructions as they are given. Do not try to help or hinder the student but do try to do as they say

Instructions to to examiner
▌ The student introduces his/herself using his/her name and gains verbal consent
▌ Ensures a new disposable mouthpiece is attached
▌ Explains to the patient what to do including
  – Asking the patient to take a deep breath in
  – Then blow out as hard and as fast as possible into the mouthpiece
▌ Ensures that the patient understands the lips should be tight around the mouthpiece
▌ Ensures that the patient can hold the meter without obstructing the linear scale
▌ Measures the Peak Flow reading using the linear scale
▌ Remembers to assess the best of three measurements
▌ Encourages and thanks the patient

Recording a 12 lead ECG
▌ Ensure the patient is comfortable at rest, ideally laying flat
▌ Turn the machine off

Limb leads
▌ Right leg – Black
▌ Right arm – Red
▌ Left leg – Green
▌ Left arm – Yellow

Chest leads
▌ V1 – 4th intercostal space, right of sternum
▌ V2 – 4th intercostal space left of sternum
▌ V3 – Half way between V2 and V 3
▌ V4 – Apex of the heart
▌ V5 – Same horizontal plane as V4, anterior axilliary line
▌ V6 – Same horizontal plane as V4, mid axilliary line

- Turn on ECG machine, choose: Gain 10 mm/mV, speed 25 mm/second
- Select 12 lead ECG and press start

Taking the blood pressure

- Ensure the patient is at rest and comfortable
- Explain procedure
- Choose appropriate sized cuff
- Palpate brachial artery
- Place cuff round upper right arm with the inflation bag over the brachial artery (precise location usually marked with an arrow on the cuff
- Inflate until the radial pulse is not palpable then increase by 20 mmHg
- Place diaphragm of stethoscope over brachial artery just below the cuff
- Gradually reduce pressure until first sound is head (Korotkoff I = systolic blood pressure)
- Continue to reduce until silence (Korotkoff V = diastolic pressure)
- Note: the sounds may disappear (Korotkoff II) then reappear (Korotkoff III) before becoming muffled (Korotkoff 4)

Urinary retention/catheterisation

Instructions to student
- This patient is complaining of difficulty passing urine and excruciating lower abdominal pain. He is unable to keep still easily because of pain. Please take a brief history and proceed as appropriate

Instructions to examiner
- The student is presented with male in acute urinary retention. No complicating features. Needs urgent catheterisation
- The student introduces his/herself
- Obtains hx of urinary retention
- Explains procedure of urethral catheter and gains consent
- Administers prophylactic antibiotics after checking for allergies
- Uses sterile technique
- Uses local anaesthetic gel
- Chooses appropriate size catheter
- Inserts catheter
- Obtains specimen of urine for analysis

■ Attaches bag
■ Documents procedure and leaves appropriate instructions for care of catheter

Taking blood cultures

■ An aseptic technique is vital to avoid skin contaminants
■ Repeat cultures from different sites at different times
■ Wear gloves for the procedure
■ Select an appropriate vein
■ Thoroughly clean the overlying skin
■ Do not touch the skin
■ Take 15–20 ml of blood
■ Open the tops of the culture bottles
■ Clean the top of the bottle with a sterile wipe
■ Place a fresh needle on the syringe and insert through the seal of each bottle, placing 8–10 ml of blood in each bottle
■ Clearly label the samples
■ Send to laboratory or place in incubator

Completion of microbiology request forms

In order to make an accurate diagnosis, the following information is vital:

■ Patient details
■ Clinical details: duration and type of illness, other related features
■ Antibiotic therapy: duration and type of treatment
■ History of foreign travel
■ Type of specimen
■ Requested investigation
■ Clinical risks – viral hepatitis/HIV

Specific clinical examination stations

Sometimes you will be asked to demonstrate a specific piece of history taking or examination such as those below.

Examination of a patient with Parkinson's disease

Instructions to student   ■ Please examine this patient, paying particular attention to the power and tone of upper limbs. Do not examine sensation. You may undertake any further examination of the neurological system you consider appropriate. You have 5 minutes after

which you will be asked to summarise the findings
and come up with a diagnosis.

Instructions to
examiner

▌ The student introduces themselves and makes sure
patient is comfortable
▌ Observation (tremor, muscle bulk, fasciculation,
bradykinesia, mask-like facies, lack of blinking)
▌ Asks about pain
▌ Moves arms demonstrating cogwheel rigidity
▌ Examines arms for power
▌ Tests reflexes
▌ Extra mark for: asking the patient to walk,
glabellar tap, asking for example of handwriting,
assessing function, e.g. buttons, knife and fork
▌ Presentation of main features
▌ Diagnosis

Examination of the thyroid gland and thyroid status

▌ Mrs White has had palpitations and weight loss.
Examine her thyroid gland.
▌ General inspection – look for signs of thyroid disease
▌ Examine the neck
▌ Look for a goitre
▌ Ask patient to take a sip of water and hold it in the
mouth, then ask them to swallow while you watch
the neck – look for movement of goitre with
swallowing
▌ Stand behind the patient and gently feel the
thyroid with both hands starting in the centre
below the thyroid cartilage over the trachea,
moving laterally to the two lobes which extend
behind the sternomastoid muscle. Ask the patient
to swallow again while you palpate. Assess the
goitre for size, nodularity or diffuse enlargement,
discrete nodules and firmness
▌ Palpate for lymph nodes
▌ Auscultate – listen over the thyroid for a bruit
▌ Assess thyroid status
▌ Pulse – count the rate and note presence or absence
of atrial fibrillation
▌ Palms – warm and sweaty
▌ Tremor of fingers on outstretched arms
▌ Reflexes – slow relaxing in hypothyroidism, brisk
in hyperthyroidism
▌ Examine the eyes for exopthalmus, lid retraction,
lid lag

■ Examine the reflexes for slow relaxation of in hypothyroidism

The mini-mental state examination

Instructions for student
■ This patient's wife has noticed that he is forgetting things. Please perform a mini-mental state exam

Instructions for patient
■ Please follow the student's instructions as they are given. For each student please try to make errors in three tasks

Instructions to examiner
■ The student introduces themselves and gains verbal consent
■ Explains to the patients what will happen
■ Performs Mini MSE:
'What day of the week is it?' [1 point]
'What is the date today?' day:month:year [1 point each]
'What season is it?' [1 point]
'What country are we in?' [1 point]
'What is the name of this town?' [1 point]
'What are two main streets nearby?' [1 point]
'What floor of the building are we on?' [1 point]
'What is the name of this place?' [1 point]
Say the following then give the patient a piece of paper: 'I am going to give you a piece of paper. When I do, take it in your right hand. Fold the paper in half with both hands and put the paper down on your lap' [1 point for each of three actions]
Show a pencil and ask what it is called [1 point]
Show a wristwatch and ask what it is called [1 point]
Say the following: 'I am going to say something and I would like you to repeat it after me: No ifs and buts' [1 point]
Say: 'Please read what is written here and do what it says' then show a card with 'Close your eyes' written on it [1 point if correct action carried out]
Say: 'Write a complete sentence on this sheet of paper' [1 point if sentence contains a verb and makes sense]

Say: 'Copy this drawing'
[1 point if angles are preserved and if the two figures intersect to form a four-sided figure]

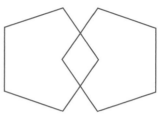

Say: 'I am going to name three objects. After I have finished saying all three I want you to repeat them, e.g. apple, table, penny' [1 point each for first try]

Say: 'Now I would like you to take 7 away from 100. Now take 7 away from the number you get and repeat until I tell you to stop' [Score 1 point each time the difference is 7 – continue until five subtractions done]

Say: 'Now name those three objects I told you earlier' [1 point each]

▌ Student calculates the mini MSE score remembering that a score < 23 will pick up 90% of patients with cognitive impairment

▌ Student also knows that there are 10% false positives and considers depression or acute confusional state

▌ Encourages and thanks the patient

Deliberate self-harm assessment

Instructions for student	▌ This patient is recovering from a paracetamol overdose. Please assess her risk factors for suicide
Instructions for patient	▌ Please answer the student's instructions as they are asked. You have a previous history of depression and your brother killed himself by hanging. Your husband has recently left home and your daughter has an incurable cancer. Please act withdrawn and give answers slowly. Please ensure it is clear that you did not expect your suicide plan to be discovered
Instructions to examiner	▌ The student introduces his/herself and gains verbal consent
	▌ Performs suicide assessment:
	▌ Questions to ask:
	– Was there a clear precipitant/cause for the attempt?

- Was the act premeditated?
- Did the patient leave a suicide note?
- Had the patient taken pains not to be discovered?
- Did the patient make the attempt in strange surroundings (i.e. away from home)?
- Would the patient do it again?
- Be concerned if any answer to the above is positive

▌ Also establish:
  - Has the precipitant/cause for the attempt resolved?
  - Is there continuing suicidal intent?
  - Does the patient have psychiatric symptoms?
  - What is the patient's social support system?
  - Has the patient inflected self harm before?
  - Has anyone in the family ever taken their life?
  - Does the patient have a physical illness?

Communication with patients

▌ This may involve explaining a diagnosis, prescription or procedure, taking consent or breaking bad news

▌ Always use lay language rather than medical jargon, allow the patient time to speak and specifically ask if there are any questions

Explanation of the diagnosis of epilepsy

Instructions to student
▌ This 30 year old mother of two has been referred by her GP with new tonic clonic seizures due to grand mal epilepsy. Please explain the diagnosis to the patient and give them appropriate advice on living with epilepsy and include suggestion to start therapy with any one of the first line single agent therapies available. You have 10 minutes

Instructions to the patient
▌ You have been referred to the hospital after having had two seizures which your GP thinks are epilepsy. Tests have confirmed the diagnosis. This doctor is going to explain the diagnosis and how to live with the condition and suggest treatment with tablets to reduce the number of fits

Instructions to examiner
▌ The student introduces his/herself and makes su[...] patient is comfortable

- Explains diagnosis using lay terms and medical terms
- Checks understanding
- Explains options for treatment
- Explains likely benefits of drug therapy
- Gives information on side effects of drugs
- Discusses driving regulations
- Makes time to listen to patients questions.
- Gives extra back up information to take home (e.g. leaflet, website address of epilepsy foundation, nurse specialist number, secretary's number)

Corticosteroid prescription and dispensing

Instructions to student
- You are giving this patient a 6 week course of prednisolone, starting at 40 mg to treat polymyalgia rheumatica. You are aiming to reduce the dose to half or less over 6 weeks. Please write a prescription and give it to the patient with appropriate advice

Instructions to examiner
- The student introduces themselves
- Checks patient's details
- Asks about drug allergies
- Issues accurate prescription: date, address, name, contact number, patient's name and address and GP, legible accurate prescription and signature
- Gives patient steroid card
- Explains to patient that they must show this to any medical professional they see
- Advice about side effects (psychiatric symptoms, skin changes, weight changes and fat distribution, diabetes, bone loss, immunosuppression)
- Warns patient not to stop drug suddenly
- Issues prescription for bone protection (calcium and vitamin D or a bisphosphonate)

Diabetes: starting insulin

Mr Coleman is a 21-year-old man recently diagnosed as having insulin requiring diabetes mellitus. Explain to him how to use insulin and self administration.

Marking sheet
- Explanation of insulin regime
- Explains and demonstrates 'stix' testing of blood glucose using a pinprick
- Instruction and demonstration of sub-cut injection, watch patient attempt to give injection, give feedback on technique
- Explain importance of varying site of injection

- Warn about hypoglycaemic episodes
- Warn about other side effects
- Warn about failure to take insulin increasing risk of keto-acidosis
- Explain importance of taking insulin when ill
- Check understanding, listen to questions
- Arrange follow up appointment
- Give contact detail of responsible health professional (e.g. diabetes clinical nurse specialist)

Controlled drug prescriptions

Miss Maddon is a 65-year-old woman with meta-static breast carcinoma who is taking morphine. Write a prescription for 10 mg of oral liquid morphine (oramorph) four times a day for one month.

- Name/address/date of birth of patient
- Write out name of drug, dose regimen and total amount to be dispensed in words and numbers in indelible ink:
  - Morphine sulphate suspension ten (10) milligrams four (4) times a day for twenty-eight (28) days, total prescribed one thousand, one hundred and twenty (1120) milligrams)
- Sign, print your name and date the prescription

Completion of death certificates

Personal details of the deceased
- Name
- Age – in completed years or if less than 1 year in completed months
- Place of death – for hospital patients this is the name of the hospital
- For patients at home it is the private address
- For deaths elsewhere the locality is recorded

Circumstances of certification
- Last seen alive by me – record the date that you last saw the patient alive

Information from post-mortem
- You should indicate here if the information you give takes account of a post-mortem.
  - Ring option 1 if a post-mortem has been done
  - Ring option 2 if information from post-mortem may be available later
  - Ring option 3 if a post-mortem is not being held

Table 3.1 Referral decisions

A death should be referred to the coroner/procurator fiscal for investigation if:
The cause of death is unknown
The deceased was not seen by the certifying doctor either after death or within 14 days before death
The death was violent or unnatural or suspicious
The death may be due to an accident
The death may be due to self-neglect or neglect by others
The death may be due to industrial disease or related to the deceased's employment
The death may be due to an abortion
The death occurred during an operation or before recovery from the effects of an anaesthetic
The death may be a suicide
The death occurred during or shortly after detention in police or prison custody

Seen after death ▌ Ring one option (a, b or c) only to indicate whether you or another medical practitioner saw the deceased after death

Cases reported to the coroner Some cases are discussed with the coroner/procurator fiscal and a certificate is completed by the attending doctor after agreement with the coroner/procurator fiscal, e.g. patients dying within 24 hours of arrival at hospital but for whom the cause of death is known. If this is the case then ring option 4 and tick box A on the back of the certificate. Remember for cases referred to the coroner for investigation a certificate is not completed by the attending doctor (see Table 3.1).

Cause of death statement ▌ Remember always avoid abbreviations
▌ This section of the certificate is divided into 2 parts

Part I ▌ Here the immediate cause of death and any underlying cause(s) are recorded
▌ It is vital that this section is completed accurately and fully with as specific details as possible e.g. histological cell types for malignancies if known

Example

A patient died from an intracerebral haemorrhage caused by cerebral metastases from a primary malignant neoplasm of the left main bronchus.
  This should be entered as follows:

▌ Disease or condition that led directly to death
  I (a) Intracerebral haemorrhage

Table 3.2 Terms implying a mode of death rather than a cause of death

Asphyxia	Debility	Respiratory arrest
Asthenia	Exhaustion	Shock
Brain failure	Heart failure	Syncope
Cachexia	Hepatic failure	Uraemia
Cardiac arrest	Hepatorenal failure	Vagal inhibition
Cardiac failure	Kidney failure	Vasovagal attack
Coma	Renal failure	Ventricular failure
	Liver failure	

▌ Intermediate cause of death
  (b) Cerebral metastases
▌ Underlying cause of death
  (c) Squamous cell carcinoma of the left main bronchus

Occasionally there are apparently two distinct conditions leading to death. If there is no way of choosing between them they should be entered on the same line and it should be indicated that they are joint causes of death.

Do not use terms that imply a mode of dying rather than a cause of death (Table 3.2).

Part II Any significant condition/disease that contributed to the death but which is not part of the sequence leading directly to death is recorded. Do not list all conditions present at the time of death. Do list any that may have hastened the death.

Example

A diabetic patient died from an intracerebral haemorrhage caused by cerebral metastases from a primary malignant neoplasm of the left main bronchus.

This should be entered as follows:
▌ Disease or condition that led directly to death
  I (a) Intracerebral haemorrhage
▌ Intermediate cause of death
  (b) Cerebral metastases
▌ Underlying cause of death
  (c) Squamous cell carcinoma of the left main bronchus
▌ Other conditions contributing to death
  II Diabetes mellitus

Employment-related death

- If you believe that the death may have been due (or contributed to by) the employment followed at any time by the deceased, you should indicate this by ticking the appropriate box on the front of the certificate and report the death to the coroner/ procurator fiscal
- Signature of certifying doctor and name of the consultant
- Sign the certificate and add your qualifications, address and the date
- Print your name in block capitals also
- If the death occurred in hospital, the name of the consultant responsible for the care of the patient must also be recorded
- Finally complete the Notice to Informant section and the counterfoil of the certificate

SUMMARY

OSCE examinations can include any practical aspect of day-to-day medical practice. Use textbooks of clinical skills and clinical skills labs to get an idea of the techniques and procedures.

Remember the cardinal rules

- Use lay language
- Introduce yourself
- Seek consent
- Follow the instructions
- Develop a rapport with the patient
- Clear your mind between stations

Clinical pharmacology 4

▌ The study of chemicals or drugs that interact with the human body

PRINCIPLES OF DRUG ACTION (K&C, P. 991)

Pharmacodynamics

▌ The study of biochemical and physiological effects of drugs and their mechanism of action

Pharmacokinetics

▌ The study of the way the body handles a drug

Pharmacodynamics (K&C, P. 995)

Non-specific actions

▌ Drugs act by virtue of their physicochemical properties
 – Osmotic diuretic (mannitol)
 – Antacids (sodium bicarbonate)

Inhibitors of transport systems

▌ Drugs act by blocking or facilitating transport mechanisms in tissue or cells
 – Calcium channel blockers (amlodipine)
 – Na/K-ATPase inhibitor (digoxin)
 – Neurotransmitter reuptake inhibitors (sertraline)

Enzyme inhibitors

▌ Drugs act by competitively or irreversibly altering enzyme function
 – Angiotensin-converting enzyme (ACE) inhibitor (captopril)

- Cyclo-oxygenase (COX) inhibitor (aspirin)
- Phosphodiesterase inhibitor (sildenafil)

Hormones

▌ Drugs may act by inhibiting or enhancing hormone production and/or release
- Oral contraceptive pill (inhibits FSH/LH production)
- Sulphonylureas (enhance insulin secretion eg, gliclazide)

▌ Or hormone may be replaced if production is deficient
- Insulin in type 1 diabetes mellitus
- Thyroxine in primary hypothyroidism

Receptor agonists and antagonists

▌ The majority of drugs act by interacting with target receptors either to activate them (agonists) or to inactivate and block them (antagonists)
- β_2-adrenergic agonists (salbutamol)
- H_2-receptor antagonists (ranitidine)

Drug–receptor interactions

The biological effects of a drug which acts via a receptor will depend on several factors. Important terms and their definitions are listed below.

Affinity

▌ Capacity of drug to bind to receptor

Efficacy

▌ Pharmacological response resulting from drug–receptor interaction

Potency

▌ Dose of drug required to produce a given effect

Dose-response

▌ Biological response measured with increasing doses of a drug

LD_{50}

▌ Lethal dose of a drug in 50% of population

ED_{50}

▌ Effective dose of a drug in 50% of population

Therapeutic index

▌ LD_{50}/ED_{50}

Agonists

▌ Drugs that bind to receptors to elicit a dose-response effect, e.g. salbutamol is a β_2-agonist

Partial agonists ▌ Drugs that competitively bind and activate receptor, but cannot elicit same maximal response as full agonist
▌ Antagonise effects of full agonist
– buprenorphine is an opiate receptor partial agonist

Antagonists

▌ Drugs that bind to receptors but do not activate them; they may be competitive or irreversible

Competitive antagonists ▌ Drugs that compete with agonist for receptor-binding
▌ Effect can be reversed by agonist in adequate concentration
– propranolol is a competitive β-antagonist

Irreversible antagonists ▌ Drugs that bind irreversibly with receptors so that any amount of agonist cannot reverse effect
– phenoxybenzamine is an irreversible antagonist

Pharmacokinetics (*K&C*, p. 993)
Routes of administration

Oral ▌ Drug enters body by gastrointestinal absorption via the portal venous system, before entering systemic circulation

Intravenous ▌ Drug enters directly into systemic bloodstream

Intramuscular or subcutaneous injection ▌ Drug enters systemic circulation rapidly via absorption through muscle or subcutaneous capillaries

Topical ▮ Drug acts locally to application
- ointments, eye drops
- usually minimally absorbed into circulation

Inhalation ▮ Drug may be absorbed or act locally
- volatile anaesthetics
- asthma drugs

Sublingual ▮ Drug is absorbed directly into systemic circulation,
and rectal bypassing portal system

Absorption

▮ The mechanism by which a drug enters the
systemic circulation from the site of administration

Dependent on ▮ Route of administration
▮ Lipid solubility of drug
▮ Stability in acid and digestive enzymes
▮ Food in the stomach
▮ Gut motility
▮ Degree of first-pass metabolism (see below)

Distribution

▮ Distribution of a drug around the body tissues
after it has reached the circulation

Dependent on ▮ Lipid solubility
▮ Plasma protein-binding

Volume of distribution (V_D)

▮ The apparent volume into which a drug is
distributed

Low V_D (<5 L) ▮ Drug is retained in vascular compartment

Medium V_D (<15 L) ▮ Drug is restricted to extracellular space

High V_D (>15 L) ▮ Drug is distributed throughout total body water

$t_{1/2}$ (half-life)

▮ Time taken for the concentration of drug in the
blood to fall by half its original value

Dependent on	▌ Elimination in urine
	▌ Elimination in bile
	▌ Metabolism (usually by the liver)

Elimination kinetics

▌ The fall in plasma concentration of drug with time

First-order	▌ Most drugs
kinetics	▌ Exponential fall in plasma concentration
(K&C, p. 993)	▌ Elimination is dependent on drug concentration

Zero-order kinetics	▌ Rate of elimination is constant and not affected by increased concentration of drug
	▌ Usually due to saturation of enzyme responsible for metabolism
	– phenytoin

Excretion

▌ Most drugs/metabolites are excreted by the kidneys

Renal excretion	▌ Glomerular filtration rate
dependent on	▌ Lipid solubility
	▌ Reabsorption in renal tubules

Biliary excretion	▌ Some drugs are concentrated in the bile
	– morphine after conjugation with glucuronide
	▌ May be reabsorbed from the intestine (enterohepatic circulation)

Drug metabolism

▌ Drug is made more hydrophilic, therefore is more rapidly excreted by the kidney
▌ Metabolites are usually less active than the parent drug

Phase I

▌ Transformation of drug into more polar metabolite

Oxidation
▌ Most common
▌ Cytochrome P450-dependent mixed function oxidases
  – Warfarin

Reduction – Methadone

Hydrolysis – Aspirin

Phase II

▌ Drugs or phase I metabolites that are not sufficiently polar to be excreted by the kidneys are conjugated with endogenous compounds to facilitate renal elimination

Types of conjugation
▌ Acetylation
▌ Glucuronidation
▌ Methylation
▌ Sulphation
▌ Glutathione conjugation
▌ Glycine conjugation

Enzyme induction/inhibition

▌ Some drugs increase or inhibit cytochrome P450 activity. This may affect their own and other drug metabolism

Inducers

▌ Phenytoin
▌ Carbamazepine
▌ Barbiturates
▌ Rifampicin
▌ Alcohol
▌ Griseofulvin

Inhibitors

▌ Omeprazole
▌ Diltiazem
▌ Erythromycin
▌ Valproate and verapamil
▌ Isoniazid

- Cimetidine and ciprofloxacin
- Sulphonamides

Pharmacogenetics
- How genetic determinants affect drug metabolism

Slow acetylation
- Half the population acetylate isoniazid slowly due to autosomal recessive gene
- Causes accumulation of drug and adverse reactions
- Similar polymorphisms exist for other drug acetylation

Plasma pseudocholinesterase
- 1:2500 have inactive enzyme
- Causes grossly prolonged action of suxamethonium

Thiopurine methyl transferase (TPMT)
- 1:300 are homozygote deficient in the gene responsible for TPMT
- Causes significant leucopenia with azathioprine

ADVERSE DRUG REACTIONS (K&C, P. 996)

Types
- Dose-dependent
- Often result from known pharmacological effects of drugs
  - Gout and thiazide diuretics
- Dose-independent (idiosyncratic)

Type I Hypersensitivity (anaphylactic reaction)
- Common in atopic individuals
- Occurs on second or third exposure to drug

Pathology
- IgE-mediated mast cell degranulation with release of histamine and other inflammatory mediators

Clinical features
- Penicillin

Type II Hypersensitivity
Pathology

- Humoral type response
- Production of antibody to drug protein complex, causing complement activation
  - Coombs' positive haemolytic anaemia with methyldopa

Type III Hypersensitivity
Pathology

- Formation of antigen-antibody complex, which lodge in small vessels
- Eosinophilia
  - Lupus-type reaction with hydralazine

Type IV Hypersensitivity
Pathology

- Cell-mediated response to antigen
  - Contact dermatitis to topical antibiotic

Long-term adverse effects

- Occur after long-standing exposure to a drug
  - Osteoporosis with corticosteroids
  - Pulmonary fibrosis with amiodarone

Reporting adverse events

Doctors and pharmacists are urged to report adverse drug reactions to the appropriate control agency.

United Kingdom yellow cards

- Prepaid yellow cards for reporting adverse events are available at the back of the British National Formulary (BNF) and from the Medicines and Healthcare Regulatory Authority (MHRA)

DRUG INTERACTIONS

Types

- Pharmacokinetic
- Pharmacodynamic

Examples of pharmacokinetic interactions

Absorption

▌ Impaired absorption of iron with coadministration of calcium salts

Distribution

▌ Displacement from plasma proteins and tissue-binding sites of digoxin by quinidine

Metabolism

▌ Induction of P450 enzymes (see above)
▌ Inhibition of an enzyme used to metabolise another drug
  – Allopurinol (xanthine oxidase inhibitor)
  – Azathioprine (metabolised via xanthine oxidase)

Elimination

▌ Impaired excretion of lithium by thiazide diuretics

Examples of pharmacodynamic interactions

▌ ACE inhibitors and loop diuretics cause hypotension
▌ Verapamil and β-blockers cause bradycardia
▌ Digoxin toxicity precipitating hypokalaemia caused by thiazide diuretics

Common important drug interactions

See Table 4.1.

Table 4.1 Common important drug interactions

Drug	Interacting drugs	Effect
Warfarin	P450 inhibitors	Increased INR Bleeding
Theophylline	P450 inhibitors	Arrhythmias
Digoxin	Amiodarone	Arrhythmias
	Verapamil	Heart block
	Quinidine	
	Diuretics	
β-blockers	Verapamil	Bradycardia
	Diltiazem	Asystole
Lithium	Thiazides	Ataxia
		Fits
Oral contraceptive pill	Antibiotics	Failure of contraception
Azathioprine	Allopurinol	Bone marrow failure

POISONING (*K&C*, P. 1002)

Causes

- Deliberate self-harm
- Substance abuse
- Accidental
- Criminal
- Iatrogenic

General management

- Supportive care
  - Airways, breathing, circulation
- Decrease drug absorption (within 4 hours of ingestion)
  - Gastric lavage
  - Absorbent, e.g. activated charcoal
  - Induced vomiting (in children)
  - Whole bowel lavage
- Antagonise effects of poisoning (Table 4.2)

Aspirin poisoning (*K&C*, p. 1009)

Pathology

- Salicylate stimulates respiratory centre → Hyperventilation → respiratory alkalosis with renal compensation
- Salicylate → metabolic acidosis
  Lactate, ketones and pyruvate

Clinical features

- Tinnitus
- Nausea and vomiting
- Hyperventilation
- Hyperpyrexia
- Sweating
- Tachycardia

Table 4.2 Antidotes of common poisons

Poison	Antidote	Mechanism
Iron	Desferrioxamine	Formation of inert complex
Paracetamol	N-acetylcysteine	Accelerates detoxification
Methanol	Ethanol	Competes with metabolic enzymes
Organophosphates	Atropine	Blocks receptors which mediate toxic effect
Opiates	Naloxone	Drug receptor antagonist

- Confusion
- Fits
- Coma
- Cerebral oedema
- Pulmonary oedema

Management

- Gastric lavage (up to 12 hours due to delayed gastric emptying)
- Activated charcoal

Salicylate levels > 500 mg/L

- Forced alkaline diuresis (use with care)

Salicylate levels > 700 mg/L

- Haemodialysis

Paracetamol poisoning (*K&C*, p. 1017)

- Most common form of poisoning; 45% of cases in UK

Pathology (see Fig. 10.9)

- Paracetamol converted to toxic metabolite
- Metabolite is normally inactivated by reduction of glutathione
- Glutathione reduced by large doses of paracetamol
- Toxic metabolites
- Hepatic necrosis

Clinical features

- Malaise
- Nausea and vomiting
- Abdominal pain
- Jaundice
- Bleeding
- Delirium

Management (Fig. 4.1)

- Blood for paracetamol level
- Gastric lavage (for large amounts)
- Activated charcoal (within 4 hours of ingestion)
- N-acetylcysteine (Table 4.3)
- Treatment is given if plasma paracetamol concentration is on or above the treatment line

High-risk groups

- Malnourished
- Concomitant or chronic alcohol ingestion
- Use of P450 enzyme-inducing drugs
- AIDS

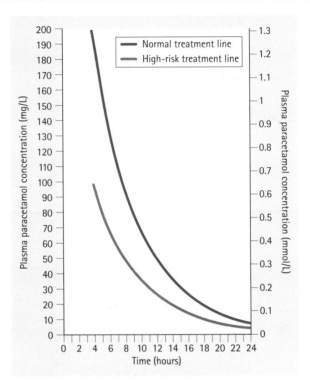

Fig. 4.1 Normogram for the treatment of paracetamol overdose. From: British National Formulary (1988) with permission.

Table 4.3 N-acetylcysteine (NAC) treatment regime
150 mg/kg NAC in 200 mL 5% dextrose over 15 minutes 50 mg/kg NAC in 500 mL 5% dextrose over 4 hours 100 mg/kg NAC in 1000 mL 5% dextrose over 16 hours

Treatment is given stat if a potentially toxic dose is known to have been taken – no need to wait 4 hours for levels (Table 4.3). Treatment is continued while paracetamol level >10mg/L or patient symptomatic.

Monitoring for liver damage
- INR
- Creatinine
- Arterial pH

Refer to specialist liver unit
- INR >3
- Creatinine >normal (or rising)

▌pH <7.3
▌Encephalopathy

Benzodiazepines (*K&C*, p. 1010)

▌40% of drug overdoses

Clinical features

▌Drowsiness
▌Ataxia
▌Dysarthria
▌Nystagmus
▌Coma
▌Respiratory depression

Management

▌Supportive
▌Ventilate if necessary

Tricyclic antidepressants (*K&C*, p. 1019)

Clinical features

▌Reduced level of consciousness
▌Fits
▌Increased muscle tone
▌Hyperreflexia
▌Fixed dilated pupils
▌Urine retention
▌Hypotension
▌Sinus tachycardia
▌Ventricular arrhythmias
▌Cardiac arrest (PEA)

Management

▌Gastric lavage
▌Activated charcoal
▌ITU with assisted ventilation if necessary
▌Correct acid–base disturbances
▌Cardiac monitoring

Opiate poisoning

Clinical features

▌Drowsiness
▌Vomiting
▌Respiratory depression
▌Aspiration
▌Pinpoint pupils

Management

- Naloxone infusion
- Respiratory support

Ethanol poisoning

Clinical features

- Depression of conscious level
- Vomiting
- Fits
- Hypoglycaemia
- Respiratory depression
- Aspiration of stomach contents

Management

- Gastric lavage
- Respiratory support

COMMON DRUG GROUPS

The following section lists the important features of many commonly used drugs.

British National Formulary (BNF)

There are many preparations and formulations of most of the commonly used drugs. The BNF lists all prescribable and over-the-counter medications licensed for use in the UK.

It is available paperback and electronically. It has sections on prescribing in liver disease, renal failure and pregnancy and a comprehensive list of drug–drug interactions. It is an invaluable reference for both revision and prescribing.

Gastroenterology (Tables 4.4 and 4.5)

Table 4.4 H$_2$-receptor antagonists

Examples
Cimetidine
Ranitidine

Indications
Dyspepsia
Reflux oesophagitis

Mechanism of action
Reduce gastric acid secretion by blocking H$_2$-receptors

Side-effects
Diarrhoea
Abnormal LFTs
Headache
Rash
Confusion in elderly
Gynaecomastia (cimetidine)

Cautions/contraindications
Renal failure

Interactions
Warfarin
Phenytoin   } Cimetidine
Theophylline

Table 4.5 Proton pump inhibitors

Examples
Omeprazole
Lansoprazole

Indications
Peptic ulcer healing
Reflux oesophagitis
H. pylori eradication

Mechanism of action
Reduce gastric acid secretion by blocking proton pumps

Side-effects
Diarrhoea
Headache
Rash
Nausea

Cautions/contraindications
Liver disease

Interactions
Omeprazole – Warfarin

Diuretics (Tables 4.6–4.8)

Table 4.6 Thiazide diuretics

Examples
Bendroflumethiazide (bendrofluazide)
Metolazone

Indications
Hypertension
Chronic heart failure

Mechanism of action
Inhibit sodium reabsorption in proximal tubule

Side-effects
Postural hypotension
Hypokalaemia
Hyponatraemia
Erectile dysfunction
Gout
Rash
Nausea

Cautions/contraindications
Severe renal impairment
Hypokalaemia
Hyponatraemia
Addison's disease

Table 4.7 Loop diuretics

Examples
Furosemide
Bumetanide

Indications
Pulmonary oedema
Chronic heart failure
Oliguria due to renal failure

Mechanism of action
Inhibit reabsorption in ascending limb of loop of Henle

Side-effects
Postural hypotension
Hypokalaemia
Hyponatraemia
Gout
Tinnitus and deafness

Cautions/contraindications
Anuric renal failure
Liver failure

Table 4.8 Potassium-sparing diuretics

Examples
Amiloride
Spironolactone

Indications
In addition to potassium-wasting diuretics
Chronic heart failure (spironolactone)
Ascites due to liver disease

Mechanism of action
Spironolactone inhibits aldosterone
Amiloride blocks renal sodium uptake

Side-effects
GI disturbance
Hyperkalaemia
Hyponatraemia
Erectile dysfunction
Gynaecomastia (spironolactone)
Rash

Cautions/contraindications
Severe renal impairment
Hyperkalaemia
Hyponatraemia

Cardiac drugs (Tables 4.9–4.14)

Table 4.9 Cardiac glycosides

Examples
Digoxin

Indications
Heart failure
Supraventricular arrhythmias, particularly atrial fibrillation

Mechanism of action
Increase contractility of heart and reduce conductivity

Side-effects
Associated with toxicity
Anorexia
Nausea and vomiting
Diarrhoea
Headache
Drowsiness
Confusion
Arrhythmias
Heart block

table continues

Table 4.9 Continued

Cautions/contraindications
Hypokalaemia
Renal impairment
Complete heart block
Wolff–Parkinson–White syndrome

Interactions
Potassium-wasting diuretics

Table 4.10 β-blockers

Examples
Propranolol (non-selective)
Atenolol (cardioselective)
Metoprolol (cardioselective)
Acebutolol (partial agonist)

Indications
Hypertension
Angina
Myocardial infarction
Arrhythmias
Thyrotoxicosis
Chronic heart failure

Mechanism of action
Block β-adrenergic receptors

Side-effects
Hypotension
Bradycardia
Bronchospasm
Peripheral vasoconstriction
Fatigue
Sleep disturbance
Erectile dysfunction
Rash

Cautions/contraindications
Asthma
Obstructive airways disease
Uncontrolled heart failure
Heart block
Cardiogenic shock

Interactions
Calcium channel blockers

Table 4.11 Angiotensin-converting enzyme (ACE) inhibitors

Examples
Captopril
Enalapril
Lisinopril

Indications
Hypertension
Diabetic nephropathy
Myocardial infarction
Chronic heart failure

Mechanism of action
Block conversion of angiotensin I to angiotensin II

Side-effects
Profound hypotension
Renal impairment
Hyperkalaemia
Dry cough
Tachycardia
Fatigue
Erectile dysfunction
Rash

Cautions/contraindications
Renovascular disease
Aortic stenosis

Interactions
Diuretics (hypotension)
Potassium salts

Table 4.12 Angiotensin II receptor antagonists

Examples
Losartan
Valsartan

Indications
Hypertension

Mechanism of action
Block angiotensin II receptors (do not effect breakdown of bradykinin)

Side-effects
Hypotension
Hyperkalaemia
Cough

Cautions/contraindications
Renovascular disease
Pregnancy

Interactions
Diuretics (hypotension)
Potassium salts

Table 4.13 Nitrates

Examples
Glyceryl trinitrate (GTN)
Isosorbide mononitrate

Indications
Acute angina (GTN)
Angina prophylaxis

Mechanism of action
Vasodilatation
Reduced cardiac preload
Coronary artery dilators

Side-effects
Throbbing headache
Postural hypotension
Tachycardia

Cautions/contraindications
Severe renal impairment
Severe liver disease
Hypotension
Aortic stenosis
Closed angle glaucoma

Table 4.14 Calcium channel blockers

Examples
Verapamil
Nifedipine
Amlodipine
Diltiazem

Indications
Hypertension
Angina prophylaxis
Supraventricular tachycardia (verapamil)

Mechanism of action
Smooth muscle relaxation
Peripheral vasodilatation
Reduce myocardial contractility
Coronary artery dilatation
Slow heart rate (verapamil, diltiazem)

Side-effects
Headache
Oedema hypotension
Worsen heart failure
Atrioventricular block (verapamil, diltiazem)

Cautions/contraindications
Severe renal impairment
Severe liver disease
Hypotension
Left ventricular failure

Interactions
β-blockers

Anticoagulants (Tables 4.15 and 4.16)

Table 4.15 Heparin

Examples
Unfractionated heparin
Low molecular weight heparin (LMWH) (enoxaparin, tinzaparin)

Indications
Unstable angina
Myocardial infarction
Deep venous thrombosis (DVT)/Pulmonary embolism (PE)
DVT prophylaxis

Side-effects
Bleeding
Thrombocytopenia (care for LMWH)

Cautions/contraindications
Severe liver disease

Monitoring
Requires monitoring of activated partial thromboplastin time
(not for LMWH)

Table 4.16 Warfarin

Indications
DVT/PE
Prophylaxis of thromboembolism
Prosthetic heart valves
Previous PE
Arrhythmias (especially atrial fibrillation)

Mechanism of action
Antagonises vitamin K

Side-effects
Bleeding
Teratogenic

Cautions/contraindications
Severe renal impairment
Severe liver disease
Pregnancy

Monitoring
Requires monitoring of INR (prothrombin ratio)

Interactions
P450 inhibitors

Lipid-modulating drugs (Tables 4.17–4.19)

Table 4.17 Anion exchange resins

Examples
Cholestyramine

Indications
Hyperlipidaemia

Mechanism of action
Prevents bile acid reabsorption and alters hepatic lipid metabolism

Side-effects
GI disturbance
Constipation

Cautions/contraindications
Severe renal impairment
Liver disease
Pregnancy
Breast-feeding

Table 4.18 Fibrates

Examples Bezafibrate	**Side-effects** Gallstones Pruritus Erectile dysfunction
Indications Hyperlipidaemia	
Mechanism of action Unknown	**Cautions/contraindications** Severe renal impairment Liver disease Pregnancy Breast-feeding

Table 4.19 Statins

Examples Simvastatin Atorvastatin	**Side-effects** Myositis Headache Abnormal LFTs
Indications Hypercholesterolaemia	**Cautions/contraindications** Severe renal impairment Liver disease Pregnancy Breast-feeding
Mechanism of action HMG CoA reductase inhibitors	

Others (Tables 4.20–4.22)

Table 4.20 Benzodiazepines

Examples
Diazepam
Nitrazepam
Temazepam

Indications
Insomnia
Anxiety

Mechanism of action
Potentiate action of GABA

Side-effects
Drowsiness
Dependence
Withdrawal syndrome
Ischaemic heart disease

Cautions/contraindications
Respiratory disease
Pregnancy
Severe liver disease

Table 4.21 Non-steroidal anti-inflammatory drugs (NSAIDs)

Examples
Non-selective COX inhibitors
Ibuprofen
Indometacin
Naproxen
Diclofenac

COX-2 inhibitors (fewer GI side-effects)
celecoxib

Indications
Inflammatory joint disease
Pain associated with inflammation (e.g. post-operative)
Musculoskeletal pain

Mechanism of action
Cyclo-oxygenase inhibitors

Side-effects
Dyspepsia
GI ulceration and bleeding
Hypersensitivity reactions
Renal impairment

Cautions/contraindications
Elderly
Peptic ulcer disease
Renal impairment
Asthma
Pregnancy
Increased risk of ischaemic heart disease with COX-2 inhibitors

Interactions
Warfarin (enhance anticoagulant effect)
Diuretics (increase risk of renal toxicity)

Table 4.22 Oxygen

Indications
Acute hypoxaemia (e.g. asthma)
− High-flow 60–100%
Chronic respiratory failure
− Low concentration 24–28%

Side-effects
Hypercapnia due to loss of hypoxic respiratory drive

BOX 4.1

Name: John Smith

Address: St Elsewhere's
London
AB1 2CD

Date of birth: 13.9.40

1 **Prescription**
Morphine sulphate tablets (MST Continus)
20 mg three times daily to be taken orally
5 days' supply
Total = 300 mg, three hundred milligrams

Signature: **Date:** 01.01.01

Name of prescriber: Dr I Hope
The Surgery
West Street
London
AB2 3EF

PRESCRIPTIONS

Writing prescriptions

I Write in ink/biro
I State full name and address or hospital number of patient
I State date of birth of patient
I State dose and frequency of drug
I State number of days drug is prescribed for
I Use generic name of drug
I Do not use abbreviations
I Sign and date prescription

Controlled drug prescriptions (Box 4.1)

- Must be written in prescriber's own handwriting
- State name and address of patient
- Name, preparation and strength of drug
- Total quantity of drug in words and figures
- Dose and frequency
- Repeat prescriptions are not permitted

MULTIPLE CHOICE QUESTIONS

Best of five multiple choice questions

1. The following drugs exert their effect by binding to receptors:
   A. Aspirin
   B. Propranolol
   C. Nifedipine
   D. Cimetidine
   E. Omeprazole

2. The following drugs are receptor agonists:
   A. Salbutamol
   B. Atenolol
   C. Pilocarpine
   D. Phenylephrine
   E. Captopril

3. The following drugs undergo extensive first-pass metabolism:
   A. Glyceryl trinitrate
   B. Lidocaine (lignocaine)
   C. Insulin
   D. Benzylpenicillin
   E. Probenecid

4. The following drugs induce P450 enzymes:
   A. Phenobarbital
   B. Rifampicin
   C. Cimetidine
   D. Paroxetine
   E. Carbamazepine

5. In paracetamol overdose:
   A. Paracetamol levels are essential in planning treatment
   B. Hepatic necrosis can occur up to 48 hours after ingestion
   C. N-acetylcysteine prevents paracetamol absorption from the stomach
   D. Rising INR is a poor prognostic indicator
   E. Coingestion of alcohol enhances paracetamol toxicity

6. In salicylate overdose:
   A. Aspirin delays gastric emptying
   B. Respiratory alkalosis occurs in conjunction with metabolic acidosis
   C. Acidifying the urine enhances aspirin excretion by the kidney
   D. Activated charcoal may be useful up to 12 hours after ingestion
   E. N-acetylcysteine improves prognosis in large overdoses

Radiology 5

Medical imaging remains a vital part of the diagnostic process. Diagnostic imaging is complemented by therapeutic procedures carried out by the radiologist. Interpretation of chest X-rays, abdominal X-rays and CT scans of the head, thorax and abdomen, combined with the role of imaging in diagnosis and the risks of radiological procedures are important subjects in examinations.

Many radiological procedures involve exposure to ionizing radiation. They should therefore only be used when a strong indication is present. Care must be taken in women of childbearing age in order to avoid exposing the foetus.

TYPES OF IMAGING

X-rays

- Utilise electromagnetic radiation
- Commonest form of medical imaging
- Image illustrates the variations in radiodensity of tissues to X-rays

Contrast studies

- Introduction of radio-opaque contrast
- Outlines hollow organs, e.g. Barium enema
- Water-soluble contrast substances allow
  - Examination of vasculature containing the agent, e.g. angiography
  - excretion of the contrast agent, e.g. intravenous urogram

Computerised axial tomography (CT)

- Utilises X-rays
- Integrates large quantities of data
- Allows computerised reconstruction of cross-sectional images

Ultrasound

- Utilises high-frequency sound
- Measures reflection of sound waves
- Non-invasive and no radiation exposure
  - Obstetric ultrasound
  - Hepatic and pancreatic imaging

Magnetic resonance imaging (MRI)

- Magnetic fields used to induce 'proton spin'
- Data reconstruction allows detailed images
- Signal depends on water content of tissue

Nuclear medicine

- Use of isotopes in imaging
  - $\dot{V}/\dot{Q}$ scan for pulmonary embolus
  - Renal function studies
  - White cell scans for occult infection
  - Bone scans for malignancy
  - PET scans

THE CHEST X-RAY (FIG. 5.1) (K&C, P. 741)

Order of analysis
Basic details

- State name and age of the patient
- Date of the X-ray
- Antero-posterior (AP) or postero-anterior (PA) (describes the direction of travel of the X-rays)
- Check left and right markers

Rotation of film

- Look at medial ends of the clavicle
- Symmetry either side of spinous processes
- Sternum and vertebral column should be in line

Pneumothorax

- Collapse of lung → free air in the pleural space

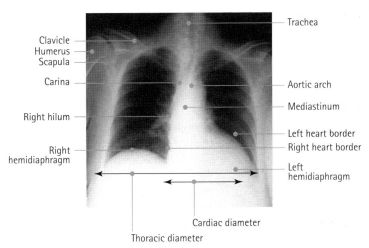

Clavicle
Humerus
Scapula
Carina
Right hilum
Right
hemidiaphragm

Trachea
Aortic arch
Mediastinum
Left heart border
Right heart border
Left
hemidiaphragm

Cardiac diameter
Thoracic diameter

Fig. 5.1 The normal chest X-ray.

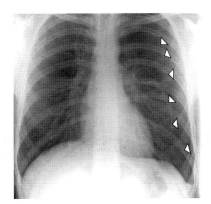

Fig. 5.2 A large left sided pneumothorax is seen.

Simple (Fig. 5.2)
❙ Lung collapse
❙ No mediastinal shift

Tension
❙ Mediastinal shift away from the side of the pneumothorax
❙ Usually due to penetrating chest wall injury (Fig. 5.3)

Is there air under the diaphragm?
❙ Black line immediately under diaphragm (Fig. 5.4)

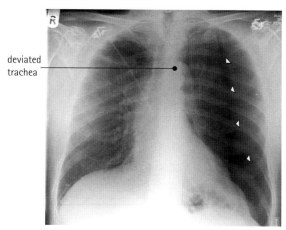

deviated
trachea

Fig. 5.3 A left sided pneumothorax is visible, with tracheal shift away from the left, suggesting a tension pneumothorax.

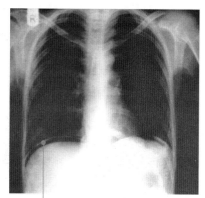

Fig. 5.4 Air under the diaphragm indicates an intra-abdominal perforation.

Right hemidiaphragm (thin white line) with air (black shadow) beneath it

Expansion

■ Count posterior ribs visible in the lung field
■ Normal is 6–7

Trachea

■ Is the trachea deviated? Mediastinal shift
■ Is the carina splayed? Right atrial enlargement

Hilar shadows

■ Look for mass lesions

Diaphragm

▌ Flattening – over-expansion
▌ Calcification – asbestosis

Lung fields

▌ Look at lung markings
▌ Dark areas
  – Loss of vascular markings (PE, emphysema)
  – Hyperinflation (chronic obstructive pulmonary disease, COPD – Fig. 5.5)
▌ White shadows
  – Collapse (loss of air volume)
  – Consolidation (infection) Figs 5.6–5.8
  – Mass lesion

Dark hyperinflated lung fields

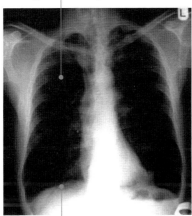

Flattened hemidiaphragm

Fig. 5.5 Chronic obstructive pulmonary disease. (K&C, p. 900)

Collapsed right upper lobe

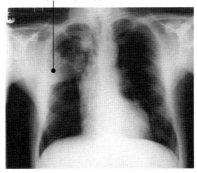

Fig. 5.6 Lobar collapse. (K&C, p. 886)

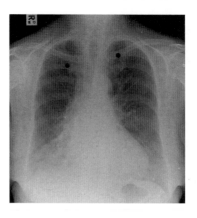

Fig. 5.7 There is shadowing adjacent to the right heart border suggesting a right middle lobe pneumonia.

Right bronchopneumonia

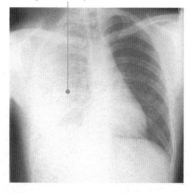

Fig. 5.8 Right bronchopneumonia. (K&C, p. 922)

- – Fluid in pleural space – pleural effusion
- – Alveolar fluid – pulmonary oedema
- – Calcification
- ▮ Check the lung apices – fibrosis suggests old tuberculosis

Cardiac shadow

- ▮ Look at heart size
  - – PA film only
  - – Normal <50% thoracic diameter
- ▮ Shape of cardiac outline
- ▮ Presence of mechanical valves
- ▮ Double right heart shadow – enlarged right atrium

Bones

- ▮ Look for rib fractures
- ▮ Bone lesions, e.g. metastases

Infections
Lobar pneumonia (Figs 5.6–5.7)
- White patches of consolidation in lung field
- Collapse of lobe → loss of lung volume
  → Local structures may be moved, e.g.
  - Elevated hemidiaphragm
  - Reduced rib spacing
- Bronchopneumonia (Fig. 5.8)
- Diffuse shadowing across more than one lobe

Lung abscess (Fig. 5.9)
- Circular lesion with air fluid level

Tuberculosis (Figs 5.10–5.11)
- Apical shadowing or discrete lesion
- May show calcification
- Chest wall deformity due to thoracoplasty (removal of ribs)

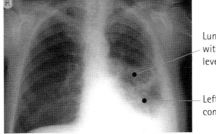

Lung abscess with air fluid level

Left base consolidation

Fig. 5.9 Left lung abscess. (K&C, p. 929)

Rib deformity

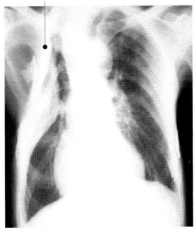

Fig. 5.10 Tuberculosis. Old sites of infection appear as apical shadows. Thoracoplasty was a surgical deflation of the infected lobe used prior to antituberculous therapy. (K&C, p. 930)

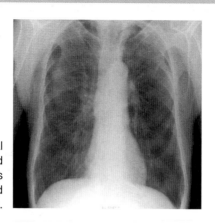

Fig. 5.11 Apical fibrosis and volume loss suggests old tuberculosis.

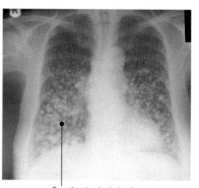

Fig. 5.12 Miliary shadowing. This is classically seen after chickenpox pneumonia or miliary tuberculosis; however, it can also occur due to lung metastases.

Small spherical shadows

Miliary shadows (Fig. 5.12)

- Miliary (blood-spread) tuberculosis
- Old chickenpox pneumonia
- Metastatic cancer, typically:
  - renal
  - prostatic
  - breast
  - bone
  - GI tract
  - cervix
  - ovary

Neoplasms
Bronchogenic carcinoma (Fig. 5.13)

- Dense white shadows in lung field
- Mediastinal lymphadenopathy
- Hilar enlargement

Mass arising from right hilum

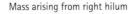

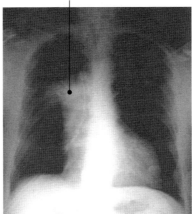

Fig. 5.13
Bronchogenic
carcinoma. (K&C,
p. 947)

Mediastinal mass

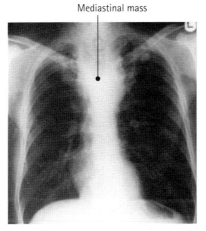

Fig. 5.14 Mediastinal mass. Masses may be due to lymphadenopathy (malignancy, lymphomas or tuberculosis), tumours (thymomas, germ cell tumours) or large retrosternal goitres.

Lymphoma (Fig. 5.14)
▮ Mediastinal masses

Metastases (Fig. 5.15)
▮ Cannonball lesions – discrete masses

Bony infiltration (Figs 5.16–5.17)
▮ Mottling or radiolucent areas in bones

Cardiac lesions
Mechanical valves
▮ Visible metal valve ring or cage

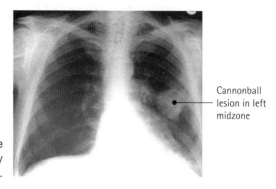

Cannonball lesion in left midzone

Fig. 5.15 A single pulmonary metastasis.

Mottled shadowing of humerus

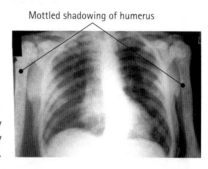

Fig. 5.16 Bony infiltration by tumour.

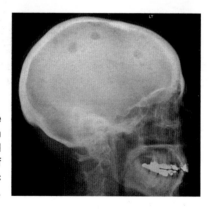

Fig. 5.17 Multiple lucent lesions in the skull suggestive of myloma lytic lesions.

Cardiac surgery (Fig. 5.18)

❚ Midline sternotomy wires

Enlarged heart (Fig. 5.19)

❚ Cardiac:thoracic ratio >50% (PA film)
❚ Loss of atrial appendage shadow
❚ Atrial enlargement
  – Splayed carina
  – Double right heart border

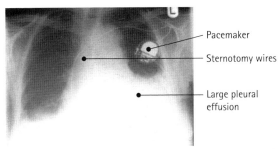

Fig. 5.18 Sternotomy wires from a previous coronary artery bypass graft are clearly visible. A large left pleural effusion can also be seen.

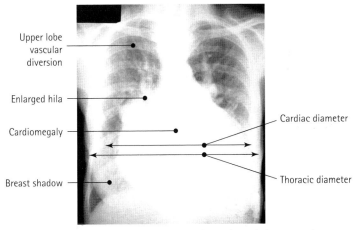

Fig. 5.19 Pulmonary oedema. The heart is enlarged, and the vascular engorgement is visible as increased upper zone vascular markings. The hila are also engorged. (K&C, p. 744)

Abnormal cardiac outline

- Boot-shaped heart – tetralogy of Fallot
- Globular heart – pericardial effusion

Pulmonary oedema (Figs 5.19–5.20)

- Enlarged heart
- Pleural effusions
- Enlarged hilum
- Fluid in the horizontal fissure
- Kerley B lines (interstitial oedema)
- Upper lobe pulmonary vascular filling
- Peribronchiolar cuffing

Thoracic aortic aneurysm (Fig. 5.21)

- Dilated aortic arch

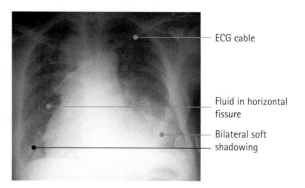

Fig. 5.20
Pulmonary
oedema. There
are bilateral fluffy
basal shadows
and fluid in the
horizontal fissure.

ECG cable

Fluid in horizontal
fissure

Bilateral soft
shadowing

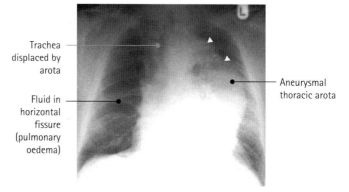

Trachea
displaced by
arota

Fluid in
horizontal
fissure
(pulmonary
oedema)

Aneurysmal
thoracic arota

Fig. 5.21 Aneurysm of the thoracic aorta.

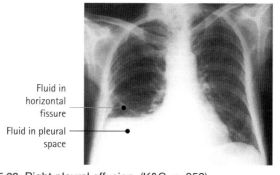

Fluid in
horizontal
fissure

Fluid in pleural
space

Fig. 5.22 Right pleural effusion. (K&C, p. 953)

Pleural effusions

▌ Loss of costophrenic angle
▌ Dense white shadow with no lung markings

Unilateral (Fig. 5.22)

▌ Pneumonia
▌ Malignancy

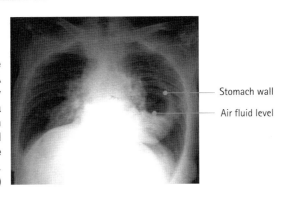

Fig. 5.23 Large hiatus hernia. A hiatus hernia may be seen as a hollow viscus with an air fluid level behind or to the left of the heart. (K&C, p. 274)

Stomach wall

Air fluid level

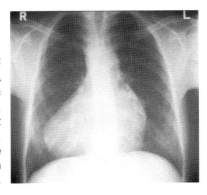

Fig. 5.24 Dextrocardia. A right-sided cardiac shadow, sometimes as part of situs inversus. Always check the side markers on an X-ray.

▌ Pulmonary embolus
▌ Cardiac failure

Bilateral

▌ Cardiac failure
▌ Vasculitis, e.g. rheumatoid arthritis
▌ Hypoalbuminaemia

Miscellaneous
Hiatus hernia (Fig. 5.23)

▌ Air fluid level in a viscus visible behind or to the left of the heart shadow

Dextrocardia (Fig. 5.24)

▌ A right-sided heart shadow may represent true dextrocardia or incorrectly placed side markers

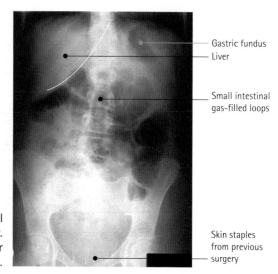

Gastric fundus
Liver

Small intestinal
gas-filled loops

Fig. 5.25 Normal abdominal X-ray. Dotted line = liver edge.

Skin staples from previous surgery

THE PLAIN ABDOMINAL X-RAY (FIG. 5.25)

Order of analysis
Introduction

▌ Patient's name, age, date of X-ray
▌ Erect or supine

Bones

▌ Thoracic and lumbar spine

Gas shadows

▌ Gastric shadow – under left hemidiaphragm
▌ Small bowel loops – fold lines extend across the full width of the bowel
▌ Colonic shadow – haustral pattern does not extend across the full width of bowel

Organ shadows

▌ Liver (right upper quadrant)
▌ Gallbladder (if calcified gallstones present)
▌ Kidneys (and presence of calcification)
▌ Pancreatic calcification (chronic pancreatitis)

Gastrointestinal abnormalities
Stomach (Fig. 5.26)

▌ Dilated stomach
  – Ileus
  – Pyloric stenosis
  – Diabetic gastroparesis

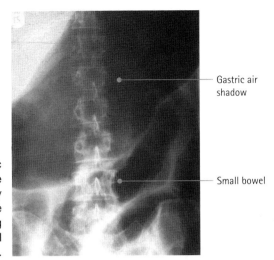

Fig. 5.26 Gastric dilatation. The stomach is grossly distended. There is accompanying small bowel distension.

Gastric air shadow

Small bowel

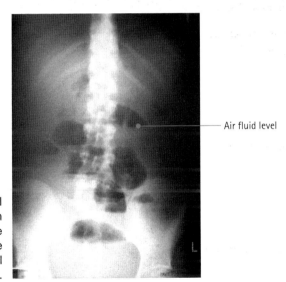

Fig. 5.27 Small bowel obstruction with ileus. Multiple air fluid levels are seen in the small bowel (erect film).

Air fluid level

Small intestine (Fig. 5.27)

▌ Obstruction
  – Multiple air fluid levels
  – Dilatation
▌ Inflammation – separated bowel loops (due to thickened bowel wall)

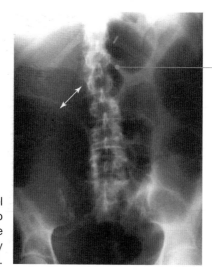

Small bowel, with folds extending across width of bowel

Fig. 5.28 Bowel distension due to obstruction. The loops are markedly dilated (arrow).

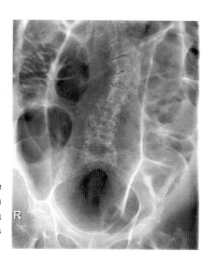

Fig. 5.29 The typical coffee bean shape shadow of a sigmoid volvulus on a plain film.

Colon (Figs 5.29–5.32)

▌ Faeces – speckled appearance
▌ Toxic megacolon – dilated colon
▌ Volvulus – sigmoid dilatation (coffee bean sign)
▌ Colitis
  – Featureless colon
  – Ulceration
  – Mucosal islands

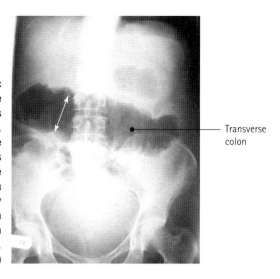

Fig. 5.30 Toxic megacolon. The transverse colon is dilated (arrow). Classically, the transverse colon is the site of the dilatation. This is a medical emergency as there is a high risk of perforation and peritonitis. (K&C, p. 309)

Transverse colon

Loss of haustral pattern in transverse colon

Dilated proximal colon

Featureless sigmoid colon

Fig. 5.31 Ulcerative colitis. The colon is smooth and featureless. (K&C, p. 309)

Liver

▌ Enlargement
▌ Gallstones
▌ Ascites – diffuse ground glass appearance

Pancreas

▌ Speckled calcification (chronic pancreatitis)

Urinary tract
Kidneys (Fig. 5.33)

▌ Calcification
▌ Staghorn calculi
▌ Stone in ureter

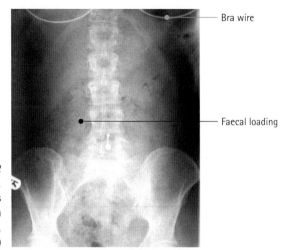

— Bra wire

— Faecal loading

Fig. 5.32
Constipation.
Faeces appear as
a speckled pattern
in the colon. (K&C,
p. 320)

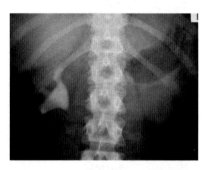

Fig. 5.33 Staghorn
renal calculus.
(K&C, p. 648)

Bladder

▌ Stones
  – Urinary catheter

CONTRAST STUDIES

Contrast (oral or rectal barium or intravenous water-soluble contrast) is used to define specific organs radiologically.

Barium studies
Barium swallow

▌ Visualises the pharynx and oesophagus
▌ Achalasia
  – Rat's tail appearance of narrowed lower oesophageal stricture (Fig. 5.34)

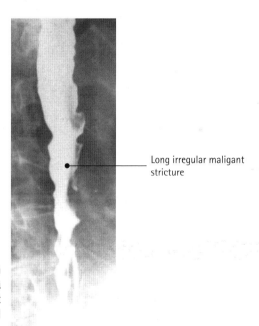

Fig. 5.34
Achalasia. This
barium swallow
shows the
classical rat's tail
appearance of the
distal oesophagus
in achalasia. (K&C,
p. 277)

Dilated oesophagus

Narrowed lower
oesophageal sphincter

Long irregular maligant
stricture

Fig. 5.35 Barium
swallow showing a
malignant
oesophageal
stricture. (K&C,
p. 279)

– Dilated oesophagus, often with food debris
❚ Strictures
– Benign – short and smooth
– Malignant – long and ragged (Fig. 5.35)

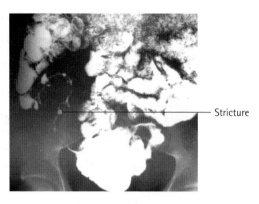

Fig. 5.36 Barium meal and follow-through showing a terminal ileal stricture (the string sign of Kantor) in Crohn's disease. (K&C, p. 313)

— Stricture

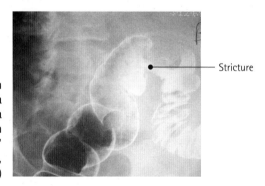

Fig. 5.37 Barium enema of a colonic carcinoma demonstrating an 'apple-core' stricture. (K&C, p. 330)

— Stricture

Barium meal

- Visualises the stomach and duodenum
- Ulcer – discrete collections of barium
- Cancers – filling defects

Barium follow-through (Fig. 5.36)

- Visualises small bowel
- Strictures ⎫
- Inflammation ⎬ Crohn's disease
- Tumours ⎭
- Diverticulae – Meckel's diverticulum

Barium enema (Figs 5.37–5.39)

- Visualises colon
- Malignancy – apple-core lesions
- Diverticular disease
- Inflammatory colitis
- Polyps

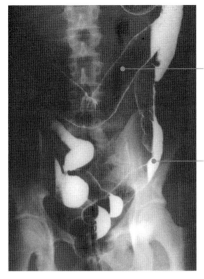

Transverse colon

Barium (patient lying on left side)

Fig. 5.38 Barium enema in ulcerative colitis. The colon is featureless with a loss of the normal haustral pattern. (K&C, p. 316)

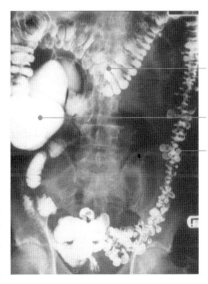

Normal transverse colon

Caecum

Diverticulae with stricturing in ascending colon

Fig. 5.39 Diverticular disease on a barium enema. (K&C, p. 325)

COMPUTED AXIAL TOMOGRAPHY (CT)

Computerised axial tomography (CT or CAT scans) utilise computer-generated images captured using an array of X-ray beams. They have a high radiation dose. Intravenous contrast can be given to enhance

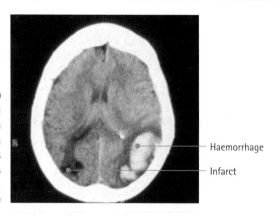

Fig. 5.40 Ischaemic and haemorrhagic stroke. Fresh blood appears white; infarcts appear dark. (K&C, p. 1209)

Haemorrhage

Infarct

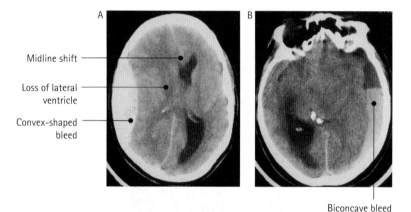

Midline shift

Loss of lateral ventricle

Convex-shaped bleed

Biconcave bleed

Fig. 5.41 Intracranial bleeds. A. Extradural haematoma. B. Subdural haematoma. (K&C, p. 1217)

vascular lesions. Oral contrast can be given to enhance the bowel.

CT scans of the head

Cerebrovascular accidents (Fig. 5.40) (*K&C*, p. 1209)

- Ischaemic strokes may not be apparent for 48 hours; they appear as dark areas
- Haemorrhagic strokes appear as white areas

Intracranial bleeds (Figs 5.41–5.42)

- Acutely blood appears white
- Extradural haemorrhages are biconvex
- Subdural haemorrhages are crescent-shaped

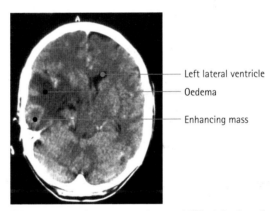

Fig. 5.42
Subarachnoid
haemorrhage.
Fresh blood
appears white and
is seen in the
cortex and
fissures. (K&C, p.
1217)

— Blood

— Left lateral ventricle
— Oedema

— Enhancing mass

Fig. 5.43 Intracerebral mass lesion (contrast-enhanced CT of the head).
There is an enhancing mass with surrounding oedema and obliteration of the
right lateral ventricle with midline shift. (K&C, p. 1243)

    ❚ Intracerebral bleeds are within the substance of the
      brain
    ❚ Subarachnoid bleeds appear as white areas in the
      ventricular system of the brain

Mass lesions (Fig. 5.43)
    ❚ Malignancies (primary or secondary)
    ❚ Local oedema appears black
    ❚ Look for midline shift

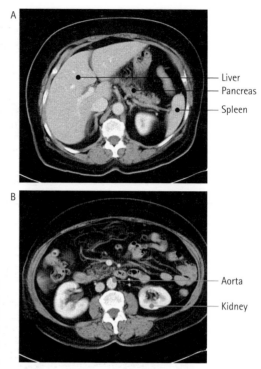

Fig. 5.44 Normal CT appearances of the abdomen at the level of (a) the liver and (b) the kidneys.

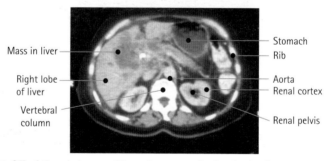

Fig. 5.45 CT of the abdomen. There is a mass lesion in the liver.

CT scans of the body (Figs 5.44–5.47)

CT scans of the body are useful for a very wide range of diseases. Staging of malignancy and location of occult malignancy are common uses. Variations in the scanning protocol allow for specific organs to be optimally imaged:

- CT pneumocolon for colonic cancer and polyps
- Pancreatic protocol for pancreatic tumours and pancreatitis

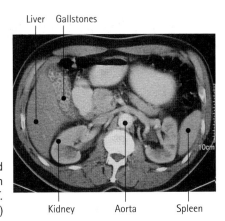

Fig. 5.46 Calcified gallstones on abdominal CT. (K&C, p. 398)

Liver   Gallstones

Kidney   Aorta   Spleen

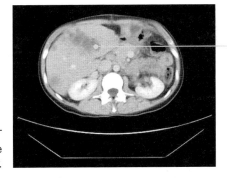

Metastatic cancer in the liver

Fig. 5.47 The CT shows a large mass in the liver.

- CT KUB for urinary tract stones
- CT pulmonary angiogram for pulmonary embolus

ULTRASOUND

Ultrasound utilises sound waves and their reflections in order to image structures. It is safe, quick and non-invasive. Boundaries between solids and fluids give strong signals, making ultrasound useful for identifying collections such as abscesses and pleural effusions.

Liver, pancreas and biliary tree (Fig. 5.48)
- Mass lesions in the liver
- Stones in the biliary tree
- Biliary obstruction

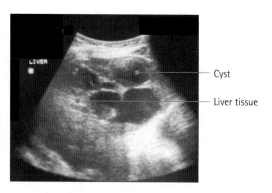

Cyst

Liver tissue

Fig. 5.48 Hepatic
ultrasound
showing liver
cysts. (K&C,
p. 395)

▌ Pancreatic cysts
▌ Carcinoma of the pancreas

Renal ultrasound

▌ Renal masses
▌ Hydronephrosis
▌ Renal stones
▌ Congenital renal abnormalities

Vascular tree

▌ Doppler ultrasound of leg veins for deep vein
thrombosis
▌ Carotid dopplers for stenosis in cerebrovascular
disease

MAGNETIC RESONANCE IMAGING (MRI) (FIG. 5.49)

MRI provides high-resolution imaging of internal
structures based on the water content of the tissue.
It is useful for accurate localisation of pathology and
its relationship to surrounding structures, notably in
the central nervous system.

INTRAVENOUS CONTRAST STUDIES

Angiograms

▌ Outline vascular tree (Fig. 5.50)
▌ Coronary arteries for ischaemic heart disease
▌ Renal arteries for hypertension
▌ Cerebral arteries for subarachnoid haemorrhage

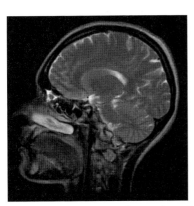

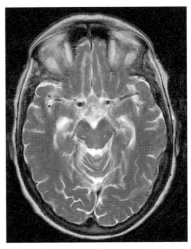

Fig. 5.49 Saggital and Coronal sections through a normal brain on MRI.

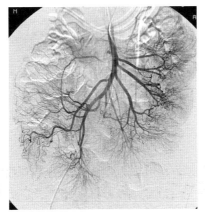

Fig. 5.50 Normal mesenteric angiogram.

Digital subtraction angiography

▌ The digitised image prior to contrast is electronically subtracted from that with contrast, leaving just the contrast-outlined vascular bed
▌ Removes any overlying anatomical features

Urograms

▌ Intravenous contrast excreted by kidneys
▌ Outlines the collecting ducts, renal pelvis, ureters and bladder
▌ Detects:
 – Non-functioning kidney
 – Hydronephrosis

– Tumours
– Calculi

NUCLEAR MEDICINE

Isotopes can be detected with photosensitive films or a gamma camera. The isotope is incorporated into a molecule designed to be picked up by a specific organ or excreted by the liver or kidney. Alternatively, blood cells can be labelled.

$\dot{V}/\dot{Q}$ scans (Fig. 5.51)

▮ Ventilation and perfusion scans of lung fields
▮ A well ventilated area with no perfusion suggests a pulmonary embolus

PET (Fig 5.52)

▮ Positron emission tomography
▮ Utilises labelled glucose to identify tissues with a high metabolic rate
▮ Used in cancer detection and stage assessment

Red cell scan

▮ The patient's erythrocytes are labelled and re-injected
▮ May detect a site of occult blood loss

White cell scan (Fig. 5.53)

▮ Labelled leucocytes are injected
▮ Localise at site of infection or inflammation, e.g. abscesses

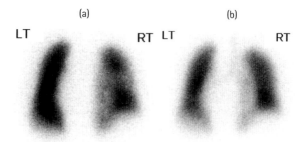

(a)   (b)

LT   RT LT   RT

Fig. 5.51 A $\dot{V}/\dot{Q}$ scan. The perfusion scan (a) shows a left mid-zone defect not seen on the ventilation scan (b), suggesting a pulmonary embolus.

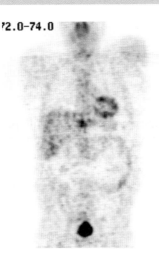

Fig. 5.52 A PET scan demonstrating normal cardiac activity and a high signal mass in the lower oesophagus.

'2.0-74.0

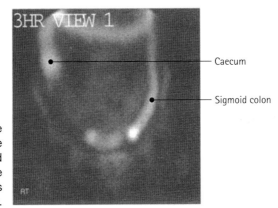

3HR VIEW 1

— Caecum

— Sigmoid colon

RT

Fig. 5.53 White cell scans. The colon is outlined due to an acute pancolitis (ulcerative colitis).

Bone scan (Fig. 5.54)

▮ Shows sites of high bone turnover, e.g. bone metastases

Renal function scans

[^{99}Tc]DTPA scans

▮ Technetium diethylenetriaminepentaacetic acid
▮ Measures glomerular filtration
▮ Each kidney measured separately

[^{99}Tc]DMSA scans

▮ Tc-labelled dimercaptosuccinic acid
▮ Measure renal tubular function

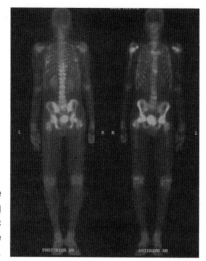

Fig. 5.54 A bone scan showing multiple metastatic deposits in the skeleton.

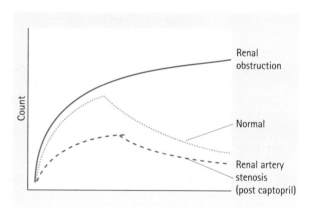

Fig. 5.55 Renal scintigraphy. The strength of signal over the kidney is measured. A normal kidney reaches a peak signal at 10–12 minutes. With an obstructed kidney the count reaches a plateau rather than reducing, as the technetium does not pass into the bladder. Renal artery stenosis results in a delay in reaching a signal peak, with a lower peak. This is most marked after captopril is given.

Captopril scans (Fig. 5.55)

I DTPA scan with captopril given
I May reveal renal artery stenosis
I Indicated by a delay in peak signal

INTERVENTIONAL RADIOLOGY

Interventional radiology allows therapeutic and diagnostic procedures to be carried out without the need for general anaesthetic and in a less invasive way than surgery, although haemorrhage and perforation of a viscus or a blood vessel are important risks. Vascular procedures carry the risk of arterial spasm or occlusion and therefore tissue ischaemia.

Directed biopsy

▌ Masses can be biopsied under CT or ultrasound control rather than requiring an open procedure under general anaesthetic

Vascular procedures

▌ Angioplasty of arterial stenosis
▌ Insertion of filters to prevent embolism
▌ Insertion of coils into berry aneurysms to prevent subarachnoid haemorrhage

Biliary stenting

▌ Insertion of a stent to overcome obstruction of the biliary tree, e.g. in cholangiocarcinoma
▌ Percutaneous transhepatic cholangiography (PTCA)

Drain insertion

▌ Nephrostomies to relieve hydronephrosis
▌ Insertion of drains into abscesses

SELF-ASSESSMENT QUESTIONS

Multiple choice questions

1. The following are accepted risks of CT-guided biopsy:
   A. Haemorrhage
   B. Secondary tumours along the path of the biopsy needle
   C. Radiation mucositis
   D. Intestinal perforation
   E. Abscess formation

2. The following are true of CT scans of the head:
   A. A CT scan carried out within 24 hours of an ischaemic stroke is often normal
   B. Fresh blood appears dark on an unenhanced CT scan
   C. Acoustic neuromas are seen as masses arising from the pituitary fossa
   D. Oedema around mass lesions appears black
   E. Intravenous contrast is useful in the diagnosis of intracerebral mass lesions

Best one of five questions

3. A 32-year-old man was admitted with severe colicky abdominal and loin pain and haematuria. Which of the following would be the most useful diagnostic test?
   A. Plain abdominal X-ray
   B. Ultrasound of the abdomen
   C. CT KUB
   D. MR cholangiogram
   E. Barium follow-through

4. A 54-year-old woman with a long history of alcohol misuse was seen following a fall. She was drowsy and incoherent. Which one of the following would be most appropriate?
   A. Plain skull X-ray
   B. CT brain
   C. Ultrasound of the portal vein
   D. CT pancreas
   E. Plain chest X-ray

5. A 76-year-old man was referred with deteriorating renal function on blood tests following the prescription of lisinopril. Which of the following would be most appropriate to confirm the diagnosis of renal artery stenosis?
   A. CT KUB
   B. Ultrasound of the renal tract
   C. Captopril renogram
   D. Renal angiogram
   E. MRI both kidneys

6. A 16-year-old asthmatic man was admitted with worsening shortness of breath and chest pain. Which one of the following indicates a tension pneumothorax?
   A. Visible pleural shadow
   B. Loss of peripheral lung markings
   C. Tracheal shift towards the affected lung
   D. Tracheal shift away from the affected lung
   E. Visible air-fluid level

7. A 43-year-old woman was admitted with abdominal pain and vomiting. An erect chest X-ray demonstrates air under

both hemidiaphragms. Which one of the following may result in this sign?

A. Liver haematoma
B. Splenic rupture
C. Duodenal ulcer
D. Acute pancreatitis
E. Ectopic tubal pregnancy

8. A 76-year-old man is admitted with back pain and pain in his left thigh. He has had previous treatment for a renal cell carcinoma. Which of the following tests would be appropriate in his further investigation?
   A. Plain X-rays of the thoracic and lumbar spine
   B. Nucleotide bone scan
   C. CT scan of the abdomen
   D. Venogram of the left leg
   E. MRI scan of the spine

Extended matching questions

For each of the following questions, select the best answer from the following list:

A. Plain PA chest X-ray
B. Plain AP chest X-ray
C. Plain abdominal X-ray
D. Plain skull X-ray
E. CT head
F. High resolution CT scan of the chest
G. CT pulmonary angiogram
H. CT abdomen
I. CT Chest abdomen and pelvis
J. Whole body PET scan
K. Ultrasound of the upper abdomen

1. Which investigation would give the most accurate assessment of cardiac size?

2. Which investigation is most useful in assessing the stage of an oesophageal tumour?

3. Which investigation is most useful to determine the nature of liver cysts?

4. Which investigation is most useful to detect multiple myeloma?

Clinical chemistry 6

Throughout this chapter the following simple abbreviations will be used:

▌ Sodium – Na^+
▌ Potassium – K^+

FLUID AND ELECTROLYTE BALANCE (*K&C*, P. 689)

If you need more detailed explanation refer to Kumar & Clark, Clinical Medicine, Chapter 12.

Water

Total body water

▌ 50–60% of lean body weight ♂
▌ 45–50% of lean body weight ♀
▌ In a 70 kg male total body water is 42 litres
  – 28 litres intracellular
  – 9.4 litres interstitial
  – 4.6 litres plasma

Distribution of water

▌ Osmotic pressure is the primary determinant of water distribution between compartments
▌ In each compartment the following are responsible for osmotic pressure
  – Intracellular compartment – K^+
  – Extracellular fluid compartment – Na^+
  – Vascular compartment – proteins

Distribution of 1 litre of standard intravenous replacement fluids

▌ 5% dextrose distributes equally across all three compartments

- 0.9% saline remains in the extracellular compartment
- Colloid stays in the vascular compartment

Normal fluid and electrolyte requirements

- Normal daily fluid requirement is 2–3 litres with 100 mmol Na^+ and 70 mmol K^+ which allows for urinary, faecal and insensible loss

Sodium content of standard intravenous replacement fluids

- 1 litre of 0.9% (physiological) saline contains 150 mmol Na^+
- 1 litre of 5% dextrose contains no Na^+
- 1 litre of dextrose saline contains 30 mmol Na^+

An example of a standard 24-hour fluid regime

- 1 litre 0.9% saline
- + 2 litres 5% dextrose
- Each with 20 mmol KCl added

When to decrease the above fluid regime

- Elderly patients – require less volume, particularly if in heart failure
- Acute renal failure – replace fluids as the previous day's urine output + 500 mL (remember these patients are often hyperkalaemic and may not require KCl supplements)
- Heart failure – reduce the volume
- Drugs – can alter water and electrolyte excretion, e.g. ACE inhibitors induce K^+ retention

When to increase the above fluid regime

- Dehydration
- Shock
- Increased GI losses – replace nasogastric losses with KCl supplemented 0.9% saline
- Increased insensible losses – fever/burns
- Pancreatitis
- Drugs – can alter water and electrolyte losses, e.g. diuretics increase Na^+ and water loss

Regulation of extracellular fluid volume (Fig. 6.1) (K&C, p. 691)

- Extracellular fluid volume is regulated by Na^+ excretion from the kidneys which is dependent on the circulating blood volume
- Circulating volume is determined by neurohumoral mechanisms via

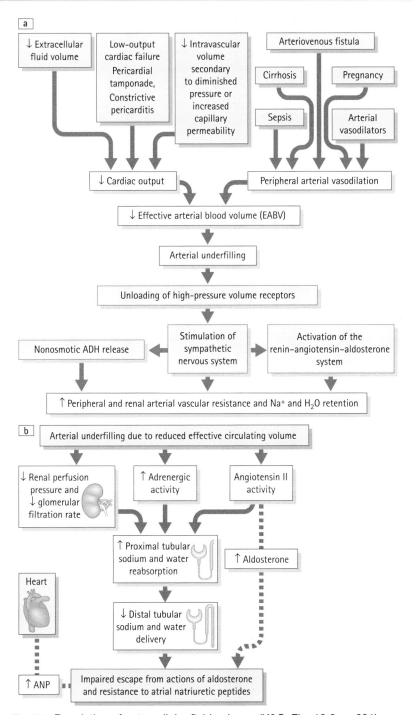

Fig. 6.1 Regulation of extracellular fluid volume. (K&C, Fig. 12.3, p. 691)

- Volume receptors
- Catecholamines
- Atrial natriuretic peptide
- Renin/angiotensin/aldosterone

Regulation of water homeostasis (*K&C*, p. 693)

▌ Water homeostasis is affected by thirst and the concentrating and diluting functions of the kidney via the effects of antidiuretic hormone (ADH)

Increased extracellular volume (*K&C*, p. 695)
Aetiology

▌ Heart failure
▌ Hypoalbuminaemia, e.g. Nephrotic syndrome
▌ Cirrhosis
▌ Renal sodium retention
  - Acute nephritis
  - Chronic renal failure
  - Oestrogens
  - Mineralocorticoids
  - NSAIDs

Clinical features

▌ Peripheral oedema
▌ Pulmonary oedema
▌ Pleural effusion
▌ Ascites
▌ Raised jugular venous pressure
▌ Raised blood pressure
▌ Third heart sound

Management

▌ Diuretics
▌ Treat underlying cause where possible

Decreased extracellular volume (*K&C*, p. 699)
Aetiology

▌ Haemorrhage
▌ Burns
▌ GI losses
  - Vomiting
  - Diarrhoea
  - Ileostomy
  - Ileus

- Renal losses
  - Polyuria
  - Diuretics
- Reduced renal tubular Na^+ conservation
  - Reflux nephropathy
  - Papillary necrosis – NSAIDs, diabetes mellitus, sickle cell disease

Clinical features

- Loss of skin turgor
- Postural hypotension – a fall in BP from lying to standing (normally the blood pressure rises on standing). May be due to reduced circulating volume, altered autonomic function or prolonged bed rest (Table 6.1)
- Low jugular venous pressure
- Peripheral vasoconstriction (cold skin and empty veins in the peripheries)
- Tachycardia
- Hypotension

Septicaemia

- Note that in septicaemia the physical signs listed above occur despite normal body water/Na^+ because of vasodilatation and increased capillary permeability

Management

- Replacement of fluid/electrolytes lost
- Treat underlying cause

Table 6.1 Causes of postural hypotension

Hypovolaemia

Autonomic failure
Diabetes mellitus
Shy–Drager syndrome
Systemic amyloidosis

Drugs altering autonomic function
Ganglion blockers
Tricyclic antidepressants

Drugs altering peripheral vasoconstriction
Nitrates
Calcium channel blockers
α-blockers

Prolonged bed rest

Sodium (*K&C*, p. 701)

▌ Disorders of Na^+ concentration are caused by disturbance of water balance

▌ In all disorders of Na^+ concentration treatment should aim for slow changes in Na^+ concentrations to avoid precipitating cerebral oedema

▌ Plasma and urine osmolality are often useful measures to investigate the cause of altered sodium concentrations

▌ Plasma osmolality can be estimated as:

$$2\,[Na^+] + [urea] + [glucose]$$

Hyponatraemia

▌ May be associated with normal extracellular volume and body Na^+ content, salt deficiency or water excess

Hyponatraemia with normal extracellular volume
Aetiology

▌ Abnormal ADH release
- Syndrome of inappropriate antidiuretic hormone (ADH) (see Ch. 13)
- Addison's disease
- Hypothyroidism
- Vagal neuropathy
- Stress
- Osmotically active substances causing ADH release, e.g. glucose, mannitol, alcohol, sickle cell syndrome

▌ Psychiatric illness
- Psychogenic polydipsia
- Tricyclic antidepressants

▌ Drugs
- DDAVP
- Oxytocin
- Tolbutamide/chlorpropamide

Clinical features

▌ Normovolaemia
▌ Signs of underlying cause

Management

▌ Treat underlying cause

Salt-deficient hyponatraemia
Aetiology

- GI losses
  - Vomiting
  - Diarrhoea
  - Haemorrhage
- Renal losses
  - Osmotic diuresis (e.g. hyperglycaemia)
  - Diuretics
  - Adrenocortical insufficiency
  - Tubulo-interstitial renal disease
  - Unilateral renal artery stenosis
  - Recovery phase of acute tubular necrosis

Clinical features

- Hypovolaemia (see above)

Management

- Replace lost fluid/electrolytes
- Treat underlying cause

Hyponatraemia due to water excess
Aetiology

- Heart failure
- Liver failure
- Oliguric renal failure
- Hypoalbuminaemia
- Excess fluids (iatrogenic)

Clinical features

- Volume overload (see above)
- If severe can cause drowsiness, convulsions and coma
- Signs of underlying disease

Management

- Fluid restriction
- Treat underlying cause
- 3% saline in severe cases

Pseudohyponatraemia

- Rarely hyperlipidaemia or hyperproteinaemia produces a spuriously low measured Na^+ concentration
- Plasma osmolality is normal

Hypernatraemia

- Hypernatraemia nearly always indicates water deficiency

- In normal individuals with an intact thirst axis and free access to water hypernatraemia is rare
- Thirst is frequently deficient in elderly patients which makes them more prone to hypernatraemia

Aetiology

- Inadequate water intake PLUS
- ADH deficiency
  - Diabetes insipidus
- Insensitivity to ADH (nephrogenic diabetes insipidus)
  - Drugs (e.g. lithium, tetracyclines, amphotericin B)
  - Acute tubular necrosis
- Osmotic diuresis
  - Hyperosmolar diabetic coma
  - Total parenteral nutrition

Clinical features

- Volume depletion (see above)
- Confusion/convulsions
- Fever
- Features of underlying cause

Investigations

- Plasma osmolality will be high
- A low urine osmolality indicates diabetes insipidus

Management

- Replace fluid
- Treat underlying cause

Potassium (*K&C*, p. 704)

Serum K^+ concentrations are determined by:

- Uptake of K^+ into cells (Fig. 6.2)
- Renal excretion (controlled by aldosterone)
- Extrarenal losses, e.g. gastrointestinal

Hypokalaemia
Aetiology

- See Table 6.2

Clinical features

- If severe, muscle paralysis
- Cardiac arrhythmias in abnormal hearts
- Potentiation of digoxin toxicity

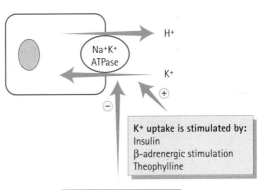

Fig. 6.2 Regulation of uptake of potassium into cells.

K+ uptake is stimulated by:
Insulin
β-adrenergic stimulation
Theophylline

K+ uptake is decreased by:
α-adrenergic stimulation
Acidosis
Cell damage or cell death

Management

■ Give supplements
■ Potassium-sparing drugs
■ Treat underlying cause

Hyperkalaemia
Aetiology

■ See Table 6.3

Clinical features

■ Cardiac arrhythmias
■ Hypotension/bradycardia if severe
■ Kussmaul breathing (associated acidosis)
■ Widened QRS/tented T waves on ECG

Management

■ See page 398 for emergency treatment
■ Calcium resonium – exchange resin given orally or rectally
■ Dialysis
■ Treat cause

Calcium

Disorders of calcium metabolism are discussed in Chapter 11 (p. 325)

Table 6.2 Causes of hypokalaemia

Increased renal excretion
Diuretics – thiazide and loop

Increased aldosterone secretion
Liver failure
Heart failure
Nephrotic syndrome
Cushing's syndrome
Conn's syndrome
Adrenocorticotrophic hormone (ACTH) producing tumours

Exogenous mineralocorticoid
Corticosteroids
Carbenoxolone
Liquorice

Renal disease
Renal tubular acidosis types 1 and 2
Renal tubular damage
Acute leukaemia
Cytotoxics
Nephrotoxic drugs, e.g. gentamicin
Release of urinary tract obstruction

Severe dietary deficiency
Redistribution into cells
β-adrenergic stimulation
acute myocardial infarct
β-agonists, e.g. salbutamol
Insulin, e.g. treatment of diabetic ketoacidosis
Correction of vitamin B_{12} deficiency
Alkalosis

GI losses
Vomiting
Diarrhoea
Purgative abuse
Villous adenoma
Ileostomy/uterosigmoidostomy
Fistulae
Ileus/intestinal obstruction

Magnesium (K&C, p. 709)

▌ Serum magnesium concentrations are determined by uptake in the small bowel and renal excretion
▌ Disordered magnesium concentrations occur in association with other electrolyte imbalance

Table 6.3 Causes of hyperkalaemia

Decreased excretion
Renal failure
Drugs
Spironolactone
Amiloride
Aldosterone deficiency
Renal tubular acidosis type 4
Addison's disease
ACE inhibitors
NSAIDs
Ciclosporin
Heparin
Acidosis
Increased release from cells
Acidosis
Diabetic ketoacidosis
Rhabdomyolysis
Tissue damage
Tumour lysis
Succinylcholine
Digoxin poisoning
Vigorous exercise

Increased extraneous load
Potassium chloride administration
Blood transfusion

Spurious
Increased *in vitro* release (either from abnormal cells e.g. leukaemia, or as a result of difficult phlebotomy)

Hypomagnesaemia
Aetiology

▌ See Table 6.4

Clinical features

▌ Irritability
▌ Tremor
▌ Ataxia
▌ Carpopedal spasm
▌ Hyperreflexia
▌ Confusion/hallucinations
▌ Convulsions
▌ ECG shows prolonged QT interval, flat T waves

Management

▌ Give supplements
▌ Treat underlying cause

Table 6.4 Causes of hypo/hypermagnesaemia

HYPOMAGNESAEMIA

Decreased magnesium absorption
Malabsorption
Malnutrition
Alcohol excess

Increased renal excretion
Drugs
Diuretics – loop and thiazide
Digoxin
Diabetic ketoacidosis
Bartter's syndrome
Hyperaldosteronism
SIADH
Alcohol excess
Hypercalciuria
1,25-(OH)-vitamin D deficiency
Drug toxicity
Amphotericin
Aminoglycosides
Cisplatin
Ciclosporin

GI losses
Prolonged nasogastric suction
Excessive purgatives
GI/biliary fistulae
Severe diarrhoea
Acute pancreatitis

HYPERMAGNESAEMIA

Impaired renal excretion
Chronic renal failure
Acute renal failure
Increased magnesium intake
Purgatives
Antacids
Haemodialysis with high magnesium concentration dialysate

Hypermagnesaemia
Aetiology

▌ See Table 6.4

Clinical features

▌ Lethargy
▌ Muscle weakness
▌ Hyporeflexia
▌ Narcosis
▌ Respiratory paralysis
▌ Cardiac conduction defects

Table 6.5 Causes of hypo/hyperphosphataemia

HYPOPHOSPHATAEMIA

Redistribution
Respiratory alkalosis
Treatment of diabetic ketoacidosis
Carbohydrate administration after starvation
(refeeding syndrome)
Post-parathyroidectomy

Renal losses
Hyperparathyroidism
Renal tubular defects
Diuretics

Decreased intake/absorption
Dietary
Malabsorption
Vomiting
Gut phosphate binders, e.g. aluminium hydroxide
Vitamin D deficiency
Alcohol withdrawal

HYPERPHOSPHATAEMIA

Chronic renal failure
Phosphate-containing enemas
Tumour lysis
Rhabdomyolysis
Myeloma

Management

▌ Calcium gluconate, dextrose and insulin
▌ Dialysis
▌ Remove cause

Phosphate (*K&C*, p. 711)

▌ The regulation of phosphate concentrations is closely linked to that of calcium

Hypophosphataemia
Aetiology

▌ See Table 6.5

Management

▌ If mild, rarely requires treatment
▌ If severe, give i.v. replacement slowly

Hyperphosphataemia
Aetiology

▌ See Table 6.5

Management

■ If acute, rarely requires treatment
■ If chronic, give gut phosphate binders or dialyse

ACID–BASE DISORDERS (*K&C*, P. 712)

■ Acid–base disturbance may be caused by:
  – Abnormal carbon dioxide removal in the lungs (respiratory alkalosis/acidosis)
  – Abnormalities of the regulation of bicarbonate and other buffers in the blood (metabolic alkalosis/acidosis)
■ Arterial blood gas analysis provides information on
  – pH
  – Bicarbonate concentrations
  – Partial pressures of oxygen and carbon dioxide

Respiratory acidosis

■ Caused by retention of carbon dioxide
■ Renal retention of bicarbonate may partly compensate (see Ch. 8)

Respiratory alkalosis

■ Caused by increased removal of carbon dioxide as a result of hyperventilation (see Ch. 8)

Metabolic acidosis

■ Caused by accumulation of acid
■ Demonstrated by a fall in plasma bicarbonate
■ Arises from:
  – Acid administration
  – Acid generation
  – Impaired acid excretion by kidneys
  – Bicarbonate losses from GI tract
■ Anion gap (unmeasured anions) helps differentiate the causes

$$\text{Anion gap} = ([Na^+] + [K^+]) - ([HCO_3^-] + [Cl^-])$$

■ Normal anion gap = $10–18\,mmol/L^{-1}$
■ Note that albumin is a major part of this anion gap; a fall in albumin will reduce the anion gap

Metabolic acidosis with a normal anion gap

▮ Suggests that either hydrochloric acid is being generated or bicarbonate is being lost
▮ In all cases plasma bicarbonate is low and plasma chloride high

Aetiology

▮ Increased GI bicarbonate losses
  – Diarrhoea
  – Ileostomy
  – Ureterosigmoidostomy
▮ Increased renal bicarbonate losses
  – Acetozolamide
  – Proximal (type 2) renal tubular acidosis
  – Hyperparathyroidism
  – Renal tubular damage – heavy metal poisoning, paraproteins, drugs
▮ Decreased renal hydrogen ion losses
  – Distal (type 1) renal tubular acidosis
  – Type 4 renal tubular acidosis
▮ Increased hydrochloric acid production
  – Ammonium chloride ingestion
  – Increased catabolism of lysine/arginine

Metabolic acidosis with a high anion gap

▮ Suggests presence of unmeasured endogenous or exogenous anions

Aetiology

▮ Renal failure
▮ Lactic acidosis
▮ Ketoacidosis
▮ Exogenous acid such as salicylate (aspirin)

Metabolic alkalosis

▮ Rarer than metabolic acidosis because renal excretion of bicarbonate is normally very efficient
▮ Can occur in
  – Extracellular fluid depletion
  – Potassium deficiency
  – Excess mineralocorticoids
  – Thiazide/loop diuretics
  – Vomiting
  – Exogenous alkalis, e.g. antacids plus one of the above

CARDIAC MARKERS (*K&C*, P. 809)

If you need more detailed explanation refer to Kumar & Clark, *Clinical Medicine*, Chapter 13.

These are markers whose elevated levels can be measured in the serum to help diagnose cardiac ischaemia. The cardiac enzymes are abnormal in cardiac ischaemia but are also elevated in other situations as listed below.

Cardiac troponin (troponin T and I)

- Regulatory proteins which have a high specificity for cardiac injury
- Not detectable in normal people
- Released early (2–4 hours) after injury and persist for up to 7 days
- If negative then repeat 9–12 hours after admission
- Very sensitive indicators of critical cardiac disease and when elevated in patients presenting with chest pain can be very useful for determining prognosis

Creatine kinase (CK)
Sources

- Heart, skeletal muscle and brain (MM/MB/BB isoforms)

Raised in

- Myocardial infarction
- Muscle dystrophies
- Polymyositis
- Pulmonary embolus
- Postoperative period
- Myocarditis
- Muscle trauma, e.g. fits, injections, exercise

Aspartate aminotransferase (AST)
Sources

- Heart, liver, muscle and kidney

Raised in

- Myocardial infarction
- Liver disease (hepatitis of any cause)
- Haemolytic anaemia
- Muscle trauma, e.g. fits, injections, exercise

Lowered in

❚ Renal failure

Lactate dehydrogenase (LDH)
Sources

❚ All cells release LDH when damaged

Raised in

❚ Myocardial infarction
❚ Tissue necrosis of any cause
❚ Liver disease
❚ Kidney disease
❚ Haematological diseases, e.g. lymphoma
❚ Muscle trauma, e.g. fits, injections, exercise

LIVER BIOCHEMISTRY (*K&C, P. 352*)

Liver function tests in the blood can be divided into 3 groups. Note that in severe disease the first two groups can both be elevated and that drugs can induce liver enzymes (see Ch. 4).

❚ Tests suggesting bile duct obstruction
  – Bilirubin
  – Alkaline phosphatase
  – γ-glutamyltranspeptidase
❚ Tests suggesting disease of hepatocytes
  – Aminotransferases ALT and AST
❚ Tests of liver synthetic function. Albumin and clotting factors are made in the hepatocyte and so reflect synthetic function
  – Albumin
  – Prothrombin time
Further information is given in Chapter 10.

Bilirubin
Sources

❚ Mainly haemoglobin destruction

Raised in

❚ Bile duct obstruction of any cause
❚ Hepatitis of any cause
❚ Haemolytic anaemia
❚ Gilbert's syndrome

Alkaline phosphatase
Sources

- Bile ducts, bone and placenta
- If source is the liver
  - γ-glutamyl transpeptidase is elevated
- If source is bone
  - γ-glutamyl transpeptidase is not elevated
  - Calcium/phosphate may be abnormal

Raised in

- Bile duct obstruction of any cause
- Liver malignancy/space-occupying lesion
- Bony metastases
- Osteomalacia
- Paget's disease of bone
- Haematological malignancy, e.g. lymphoma
- Heart failure (liver congestion)
- Also normally higher in children and pregnancy
- Hepatitis of any cause

Lowered in

- Hypothyroidism

Gamma glutamyl transpeptidase (γ-GT)
Sources

- Bile ducts and kidney

Raised in

- Alcohol excess
- Bile duct obstruction of any cause including malignancy/space-occupying lesion
- Hepatitis of any cause if severe
- Renal carcinoma
- Induction by drugs

Alanine aminotransferase (ALT)
Sources

- Liver and heart

Raised in

- Hepatitis of any cause
- Bile duct obstruction of any cause

TESTS OF RENAL FUNCTION (*K&C*, P.608)

This is covered in detail in Chapter 14. If you need more detailed explanation refer to Kumar & Clark, *Clinical Medicine*, Chapter 11.

Urea

▊ Plasma urea varies with protein intake and renal excretion

Raised in

▊ Renal disease of any cause
▊ Dehydration
▊ Upper GI bleeding
▊ Shock
▊ Cardiac failure
▊ Adrenal insufficiency
▊ Old age

Lowered in

▊ Liver failure
▊ Nephrotic syndrome
▊ Cachexia/kwashiorkor
▊ Pregnancy
▊ Overhydration

Creatinine

▊ Retention of creatinine indicates glomerular insufficiency

Raised in

▊ Renal disease of any cause
▊ Large meat intake
▊ Old age

Lowered in

▊ Muscle-wasting
▊ Pregnancy

Urate

▊ End-product of protein metabolism
▊ Excreted by kidneys

Raised in

- Gout
- Eclampsia
- Leukaemia/myeloma/lymphoma
- Renal insufficiency
- Thiazide diuretic therapy

Lowered in

- Allopurinol therapy
- Acute hepatitis of any cause
- Salicylate therapy

ACUTE PHASE REACTANTS

- Non-specific tests for inflammation/infection
- Include
  - Erythrocyte sedimentation rate (ESR)
  - C-reactive protein (CRP)

SELF-ASSESSMENT QUESTIONS

Best one of five questions

1. Persistent vomiting may result in:
   - **A.** Respiratory acidosis
   - **B.** Peripheral oedema
   - **C.** Metabolic acidosis
   - **D.** Hypokalaemia
   - **E.** Hypercalcaemia

2. Hyperkalaemia may be a result of the use of which of the following diuretics:
   - **A.** Furosemide
   - **B.** Bendroflumethiazide
   - **C.** Spironolactone
   - **D.** Metolozone
   - **E.** Bumetanide

3. Which of the following statements are correct for standard i.v. fluid solutions:
   - **A.** 0.9% saline distributes to all three fluid compartments
   - **B.** 5% dextrose remains in the vascular compartment
   - **C.** Colloid is used in hypovolaemia
   - **D.** 0.9% saline is indicated in most cases of hyponatraemia
   - **E.** 0.9% saline is useful i.v. fluid replacement therapy in patients with chronic liver disease

4. Which of these is a cause of a metabolic acidosis with a normal anion gap:
   - **A.** Sepsis
   - **B.** Diabetic ketoacidosis
   - **C.** Aspirin overdose
   - **D.** Acute renal failure
   - **E.** Type 4 renal tubular acidosis

5. Which of these is a cause of a metabolic acidosis with a high anion gap:
   - **A.** Diabetic ketoacidosis
   - **B.** Type 4 renal tubular acidosis
   - **C.** Diarrhoea
   - **D.** Lead poisoning
   - **E.** Hyperparathyroidism

6. In which of the following situations is the pH likely to be lower than normal:
   - **A.** Vomiting
   - **B.** Hypokalaemia
   - **C.** Conn's syndrome
   - **D.** Hyperventilating
   - **E.** Hyperparathyroidism

7. An elevated Troponin I occurs in the following circumstance:
   - **A.** 12 hours after the onset of pain in an acute coronary syndrome
   - **B.** Day 2 after hip replacement
   - **C.** Following a tonic-clonic seizure
   - **D.** Heart failure
   - **E.** Rhabdomyolysis

8. Serum bilirubin would be normal in patients with:
   - **A.** Gilbert's syndrome
   - **B.** A gallstone obstructing the common bile duct
   - **C.** Gallstones in the gallbladder
   - **D.** Autoimmune haemolytic anaemia
   - **E.** Acute fulminant hepatitis A

9. A low blood urea would be expected in:
   - **A.** Pregnancy
   - **B.** Upper GI bleeding

C. Cardiac failure
D. Acute renal failure
E. Dehydration

Extended matching questions

Question 1 *Theme: abnormal blood test results*

A. Shock
B. Cardiac failure
C. Cardiac failure treated with loop diuretics
D. Pneumonia
E. Renal failure
F. Nephrotic syndrome
G. Renal tubular acidosis
H. Diarrhoea
I. High ileostomy volumes

For each of the following questions, select the most likely answer from the list above:

I. An 84-year-old female presents with confusion and ankle oedema. Blood results show the following: Na^+ 132, K^+ 2.8, Urea 9.8, Creat 128. What is the most likely diagnosis?

II. A 37-year-old patient with Crohn's disease presents with malaise. Blood tests reveal the following: Na^+ 132, K^+ 2.8, Urea 10, Creat 60, Mg^{2+} 0.54 (low), Cl^- 105, pH 7.3, Bicarbonate 15. What is the most likely diagnosis?

III. A 56-year-old male presents with fever and malaise. Blood tests reveal the following: Na^+ 124, K^+ 4.5, Urea 7.6, Creat 98, pH 7.54, PO_2 8.2, PCO_2 3.2. What is the most likely diagnosis?

Question 2 *Theme: acid–base disturbance*

A. Acute renal failure
B. Acute liver failure
C. Aspirin overdose
D. Recurrent vomiting
E. Renal tubular acidosis
F. Diabetic ketoacidosis
G. Respiratory alkalosis
H. Type II respiratory failure

For each of the following questions, select the most likely answer from the list above:

I. A 64-year-old female presents with confusion and breathlessness. Blood gas analysis shows the following: pH 7.3, PCO_2 9.6, PO_2 4.5, Bicarbonate 28. What is the most likely diagnosis?

II. A 37-year-old patient with diabetes presents with a history of vomiting and confusion. Blood gas analysis shows the following: pH 7.15, PCO_2 2.5, PO_2 12.5, Bicarbonate 10. What is the most likely diagnosis?

III. An 18-year-old male is found collapsed at home. There is no history available. Blood tests reveal the following: pH 7.25, PCO_2 3.6, PO_2 13.5, Bicarbonate 8, Na^+ 135, K^+ 4, Cl^- 101. What is the most likely diagnosis?

Question 3 *Theme: abnormal blood test results*

A. Acute coronary syndrome
B. Cardiac failure
C. Polymyositis
D. Hodgkin's lymphoma

E. Haemolytic anaemia
F. Nephrotic syndrome
G. Renal tubular acidosis

For each of the following questions, select the most likely answer from the list above:

I.   A 74-year-old man presents with chest pains which he has had for 48 hours. Blood results which show elevation of CK, AST and Troponin I. What is the most likely diagnosis?

II. A 37-year-old patient presents with malaise. He has noticed a lump in his neck ever since he had an upper respiratory tract infection two weeks ago. Blood tests reveal the following: Haemoglobin 12.3 g/dl, CK 70 u/l, LDH 637 u/l, Troponin I not detected. What is the most likely diagnosis?

III. A 21-year-old male student presents with yellowness of the skin. He has recently been diagnosed with glandular fever. Blood tests reveal the following: Bilirubin 95 umol, ALT 24 u/l, AST 31 u/l, Haemoglobin 8.9 g/dl What is the most likely diagnosis?

Infectious diseases 7

Infectious disease remains the most common cause of morbidity and mortality worldwide. In order for an infectious agent to propagate within the population, there must be a reservoir of infection and a mode of transmission. Thus avoidance of infection starts with reduction of the reservoir and limiting or avoiding the transmission of an organism.

System-specific infections are discussed in the appropriate chapters.

DIAGNOSIS OF INFECTIOUS DISEASE (K&C, P. 26)

History

- Exposure to the causative agent
  - Travel to a high-risk area or environmental exposure
  - Contact with an infected individual
  - Occupation history
  - Animal exposure
  - Sexual history
  - Intravenous drug misuse
  - Blood transfusion
- Vaccination history

Examination

- Presence of a fever (Table 7.1)
- Rashes
- Lymphadenopathy
- Hepatosplenomegaly
- Evidence of septic shock (hypotension, tachycardia, peripheral vasodilatation)
- Delirium (confusion, hallucination)

Table 7.1 Causes of fever of unknown origin (FUO) (*K&C*, p. 30)

Infections (40%)	Immune (20%)
Abscess	Drugs
Tuberculosis	Connective tissue disease
Urinary infection	Sarcoidosis
Biliary infection	
Endocarditis	**Other**
Epstein–Barr virus	Thyrotoxicosis
	Ulcerative colitis
Malignancy (30%)	Crohn's disease
Lymphomas	Factitious
Leukaemia	*5–10% remain undiagnosed*
Solid tumours	

Investigations
Full blood count and blood film
- Neutrophilia suggests bacterial infection
- Lymphocytosis suggests viral infection
- Neutropenia may suggest viral infection
- Eosinophilia suggests parasitic infection

Thrombocytopenia
- Malaria or disseminated intravascular coagulation

Cell fragments – haemolysis
- Parasites on blood film, e.g. malaria

Blood culture
- Aerobic and anaerobic bottles
- Follow sterile procedure
- May require repeated samples

Liver function
- Elevated transferases in viral hepatitis

Microscopy, culture and sensitivity
- Can be performed on stool, urine, CSF, sputum, ascitic fluid, pleural fluid, joint aspirates
- Provides organism identification and antibiotic sensitivity

Immunological diagnosis
- Presence of antibodies against specific antigens
- Presence of specific antigens due to their reaction with a known antibody

Genetic diagnosis

- Detection of genome of organism, e.g. hepatitis C virus RNA
- Assessment of 'viral load' or replication e.g. HIV, Hepatitis B

Histological examination

- Pathology of specific infections on tissue biopsy

Imaging

- Localisation of an infection, e.g. by ultrasound or CT scanning
- Labelled white cell scanning localises the source of an infection

TREATMENT OF INFECTIOUS DISEASE
(*K&C*, P. 32)

Antibacterial drugs (Fig. 7.1) (*K&C*, pp. 33–40)

β-lactams
Penicillins

- Block cell wall growth
- Group 1: parenteral formulations
  - e.g. Benzylpenicillin
- Group 2: oral penicillin
  - e.g. Phenoxymethylpenicillin (penicillin V)
- Group 3: β-lactamase-stable penicillins
  - e.g. Flucloxacillin
  Group 4: extended spectrum
  - e.g. Amoxicillin, ampicillin
- Group 5: β-lactamase-resistant penicillin
  - e.g. Temocillin

Cephalosporins

- Inhibit cell wall synthesis
- Penicillinase-resistant
- Broader antibacterial range
- 10% of patients with penicillin allergy will have a reaction to cephalosporins

First generation
- Gram-positive cocci and Gram-negative
  - Cefalexin, Cefradrine

Second generation
- Gram-negative infections
  - Cefuroxime, cefaclor

Third generation
- Gram-negative infections
  - Ceftazidime, ceftriaxone

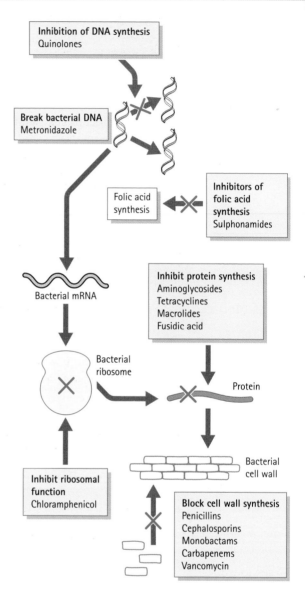

Fig. 7.1
Mechanism of
action of
antibacterial drugs.

Monobactams

❚ Aztreonam

Carbapenems

❚ Imipenem, meropenem

Aminoglycosides

❚ Inhibit bacterial protein synthesis

■ Gram negatives, e.g. *Pseudomonas*
  – Gentamicin, neomycin
■ N.B. Renal and ototoxicity, therefore serum levels
  need monitoring

Tetracyclines

■ Inhibit bacterial protein synthesis
■ Atypical pneumonias, acne
  – Tetracycline, doxycycline
■ N.B. Contraindicated in children and during
  pregnancy as they cause permanently stained teeth

Macrolides

■ Inhibit bacterial protein synthesis
■ Useful in atypical pneumonia
  – Erythromycin, clarithromycin
■ Gram-negative infection
  – Clarithromycin, azithromycin

Chloramphenicol

■ Inhibits bacterial ribosome function
■ Conjunctivitis (local therapy)

Fusidic acid

■ Inhibits bacterial protein synthesis
■ Staphylococcus aureus osteomyelitis

Sulphonamides

■ Inhibit bacterial folic acid synthesis
■ Used with trimethoprim in urinary tract and
  Pneumocystis carinii infection

Quinolones

■ Inhibit DNA synthesis
■ Gram-negative infections
  – Ciprofloxacin
  – Moxifloxacin

Nitroimidazoles

■ Break bacterial DNA
■ Anaerobic infections
  – Metronidazole

Glycopeptides

- Inhibit cell wall synthesis
- Gram-positive bacteria
  - Vancomycin

Side effects of anti-bacterials

- Sensitivity: rash/anaphylaxis
- Organism resistance, e.g. MRSA/VRE
- Disruption of normal gut flora → antibiotic related diarrhoea or pseudomembranous colitis

Antifungal drugs (*K&C*, p. 39)

Polyenes

- Disrupt fungal membranes
  - Amphotericin B – systemic disease
  - Nystatin – oral and enteric *Candida*

Azoles

- Broad-spectrum antifungals
  - Clotrimazole – ringworm
  - Ketoconazole – candidiasis

Triazoles

  - Fluconazole – penetrates CSF
  - Itraconazole

Others

  - Terbinafine
  - Griseofulvin

Side effects of anti-fungals

- Itraconazole – fulminant hepatic failure and hepatic dysfunction
- heart failure – avoid prescribing with calcium channel blockers

Antiviral drugs (*K&C*, p. 40)

Aciclovir

- Terminates viral DNA synthesis
- Herpes simplex and varicella zoster virus

Ganciclovir

- Cytomegalovirus infection

Amantadine

I Influenza virus

Interferons

I Hepatitis B and C
I Pegylated formulations are more effective and require less frequent dosing

Ribavirin

I Combination therapy (with interferon) for chronic hepatitis C

Antiretrovirals

I See page 149 See page 149

VACCINATION (TABLE 7.2) (K&C, P. 42)

Passive

I Antibody raised against the infecting organism, e.g. Tetanus immunoglobulin, diphtheria, rabies

Active

I Immunogenic antigen induces antibody production

Table 7.2 Vaccination schedule

2, 3 and 4 months
Diphtheria
Pertussis
Tetanus
Haemophilus influenzae b
Oral polio
Meningococcus gp C
Tuberculosis (BCG) for infants at high risk

13 months
Measles
Mumps   } MMR
Rubella

3 years, 4 months to 5 years
Diphtheria, tetanus
MMR and oral polio

13–18 years
Diphtheria, tetanus and oral polio

Live attenuated vaccines

▌ Measles, mumps, rubella
▌ BCG

Inactivated (killed) vaccines

▌ Hepatitis A
▌ Pertussis (whooping cough)
▌ *Haemophilus influenzae b*
▌ Meningococcus A and C
▌ Pneumococcus
▌ Influenza
▌ Polio

Toxoids

▌ Tetanus
▌ Diphtheria

Recombinant vaccines

▌ Hepatitis B

BACTERIAL INFECTION (*K&C*, P. 61)

Gram-positive cocci

Staphylococcus

▌ *Staph. aureus, epidermidis, saprophyticus* (Fig. 7.2)
▌ Skin:cellulitis, impetigo, necrotising fasciitis
▌ Lungs: pneumonia, abscesses
▌ Heart: endocarditis
▌ CNS: meningitis, abscesses
▌ Bones: osteomyelitis
▌ Gut: enterocolitis
▌ Staph. aureus produces a toxin, which may cause:
  – Food poisoning
  – Toxic shock syndrome
  – Scalded skin syndrome

Management

▌ Much community-acquired infection is penicillin-sensitive
▌ However, hospital spread of methicillin-resistant *Staph. aureus* (MRSA) is increasing

Streptococcus

▌ Majority of infections are due to β-haemolytic *Strep. pyogenes*
▌ Skin: impetigo, erysipelas

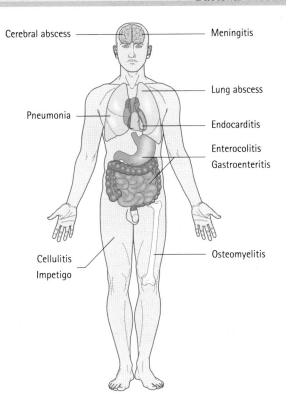

Fig. 7.2
Manifestations of
Staphylococcal
infection.

- Mouth: pharyngitis, tonsillitis
- Lungs: pneumonia – *Strep. pneumoniae*
- Other: endocarditis – *Strep. viridans*, scarlet fever, rheumatic fever

Management

- Majority are sensitive to penicillins

Gram-negative cocci

Neisseria

- *Neisseria meningitidis* → Meningitis and septicaemia (p. 494)
- *Neisseria gonorrhoeae* → gonorrhoea

Management

- Penicillin or cefotaxime

Gram-positive bacilli

Corynebacterium

- *C. diphtheriae*
- Toxin-producing forms → diphtheria

- Nasal discharge
- Pharyngeal inflammation
- Laryngeal inflammation → husky voice
- → Respiratory obstruction
- Myocarditis
- Neurological manifestations – cranial nerve palsies, polyneuropathy

Management

- Antitoxin + penicillin

Listeria

- *L. monocytogenes*
- → Abortions, meningitis or septicaemia

Management

- Ampicillin and gentamicin

Clostridium

- *C. botulinum, C. difficile* – see Ch. 10
- *C. tetani* → tetanus
  - Infects puncture wounds and bites
  - Neurotoxin production
  - → Neuromuscular blockade, lockjaw, muscle spasm, autonomic neuropathy

Management

- Antitoxin, penicillin, ITU care

Bacillus group

B. anthracis

- Anthrax
- → Erythematous skin lesion that ulcerates
- → Black central eschar
- Pulmonary and GI tract involvement

Management

- Penicillin

B. cereus

- → Toxin mediated food poisoning

Gram-negative bacilli

Brucella

- *B. abortus, melitensis, suis*
- Endotoxin → headache, fever, weakness
- Lymphadenopathy, hepatosplenomegaly

- Arthritis, encephalitis and endocarditis
- Contracted from non-pasteurised milk

Management

- Doxycycline

Bordetella

- *B. pertussis* – whooping cough
- Childhood disease
- Catarrhal phase – rhinorrhoea and conjunctivitis
- Paroxysmal phase – coughing attacks

Management

- Erythromycin in catarrhal phase

Haemophilus

- *H. influenzae, ducreyi, parainfluenzae*
- Increased risk of infection post-splenectomy
- Pneumonia, bronchitis
- Meningitis (*H. influenzae b*)
- Epiglottitis

Management

- Cefotaxime, cefuroxime

Prevention

- HiB vaccine

Cholera

- Vibrio cholerae (see Ch. 10)

Enterobacteria

- Escherichia coli
- Salmonella
- Campylobacter   see Chapter 10
- Shigella
- Helicobacter
- Yersinia

MYCOBACTERIAL DISEASE

Mycobacterium tuberculosis

- Acid-fast aerobic bacillus (Fig. 7.3)
- Droplet spread
- $\rightarrow$ Caseating granuloma
  - Lung

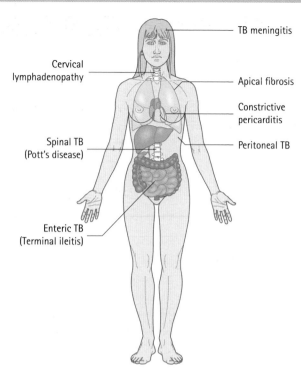

Fig. 7.3
Manifestations of
tuberculosis.

TB meningitis

Cervical
lymphadenopathy

Apical fibrosis

Constrictive
pericarditis

Spinal TB
(Pott's disease)

Peritoneal TB

Enteric TB
(Terminal ileitis)

– Adrenals
– Terminal ileum
– Lymph nodes
▌ → Cough, fever, weight loss, night sweats
▌ Immunosuppression → haematogenous spread
(miliary TB)

Complications

▌ TB meningitis
▌ TB peritonitis
▌ Arthritis and osteomyelitis
▌ Constrictive pericarditis

Investigations

▌ Imaging – X-ray/CT scan of the chest
▌ Microbiology – Ziehl–Nielsen staining of sputum
▌ Bronchoscopy and washings
▌ Biopsy of solid lesions
▌ CSF examination in meningitis
▌ Early morning urine

Management

▌ Combination therapy (Table 7.3)

Table 7.3 Drug regimens in tuberculosis

Pulmonary TB
Rifampicin and isoniazid for 6 months, pyrazinamide for first 2 months (add ethambutol if previously treated for TB)

TB osteomyelitis and ileal TB
Rifampicin and isoniazid for 9 months, pyrazinamide for 2 months

TB meningitis
Rifampicin, isoniazid for 12 months, pyrazinamide for 2 months

Drug resistance and HIV
Start standard therapy as above but alter based on sensitivities. Treat for a total of 2 years, or 1 year after the last positive culture result

Contact tracing

▮ X-ray and tuberculin testing in close contacts

Immunisation

▮ Bacille Calmette–Guérin (BCG)
▮ Bovine strain of TB with very low virulence after tuberculin testing

Mycobacterium leprae

▮ Leprosy (Hansen's disease)
▮ Immune response determines disease type (there are two ends of a clinical spectrum)

Tuberculoid

▮ High cell-mediated immunity
▮ Hypopigmented skin patches
▮ Loss of sensation over patch
▮ Tender thickened nerves

Lepromatous

▮ Macules, papules or nodules in the skin
▮ Laryngitis and hoarse voice
▮ Collapse of nasal cartilage
▮ Leonine face

Investigations

▮ Impossible to culture organism
▮ Diagnosis is basically clinical

Management

▮ Dapsone, rifampicin and clofazimine for 2 years

SPIROCHAETES

Syphilis

- *Treponema pallidum*

Primary syphilis (10–90 days post-infection)
- Painless ulcer (chancre) at infection site

Secondary syphilis (4–10 weeks)
- Lymphadenopathy
- Rash – papules or pustules
- Warty skin lesions (condylomata lata)
- Oral 'snail track' ulcers

Tertiary syphilis
- Granulomatous lesions
- Skin, bones, liver
- Aortic dilatation and valve regurgitation
- Neurosyphilis – meningitis, cerebral gumma
- Tabes dorsalis – dorsal root demyelination (Fig. 7.4)

Congenital syphilis
- Hutchinson's (notched) teeth
- Sabre tibia
- Long bone abnormalities
- Loss of nasal bridge

Management
- Procaine penicillin

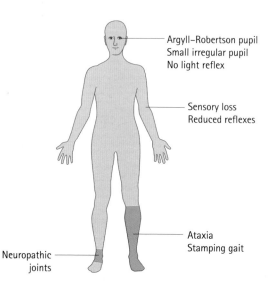

Argyll–Robertson pupil
Small irregular pupil
No light reflex

Sensory loss
Reduced reflexes

Ataxia
Stamping gait

Neuropathic joints

Fig. 7.4
Manifestations of tabes dorsalis.

Leptospirosis (Weil's disease)

- *Leptospira interrogans*
- Contact with animal reservoirs (rat's urine)
- Headache, fever, myalgia
- Conjunctival suffusion
- Hepatosplenomegaly and lymphadenopathy
- May progress to:
  - Jaundice
  - Haemolytic anaemia
  - Renal failure

Investigations

- IgM antibodies
- *Leptospira* cultured in blood

Management

- Penicillins
- Erythromycin

Lyme disease (Fig. 7.5)

- *Borrelia burgdorferi*
- Carried by ixodid ticks (from deer and sheep)

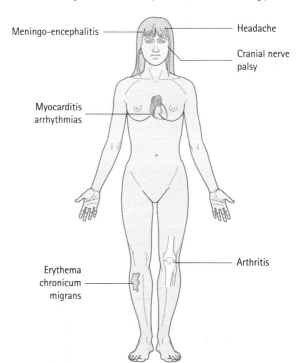

Meningo-encephalitis

Headache

Cranial nerve palsy

Myocarditis arrhythmias

Erythema chronicum migrans

Arthritis

Fig. 7.5 Manifestations of Lyme's Disease.

- Erythema chronicum migrans
- Headache, fever and malaise
- Meningoencephalitis
- Cranial nerve palsies
- Cardiac arrhythmias, myocarditis
- Arthritis

Investigations

- IgM antibodies against organism

Management

- Amoxicillin/penicillin

VIRAL INFECTIONS

- Viral hepatitis is discussed in Chapter 10

DNA viruses

Adenoviruses

- Croup
- Gastroenteritis
- Mesenteric adenitis in children

α-herpesvirus
Herpes simplex-1 (HSV-1)

- Stomatitis (primary infection)
- Cold sores
- Erythema multiforme

Herpes simplex-2 (HSV-2)

- Genital herpes

Varicella zoster virus (VZV)

- Chickenpox (primary infection)
- Shingles (see Ch. 12)

β-herpesvirus
Cytomegalovirus (CMV)

- Retinitis
- Pneumonitis   } in immunocompromised
- Gastrointestinal ulcers

Human herpes viruses 6 and 7

- Roseola infantum (children)

γ-herpesvirus
Epstein–Barr virus (EBV)

- Infectious mononucleosis
- Burkitt's lymphoma
- Nasopharyngeal carcinoma
- Gastric carcinoma

Human herpes virus 8

- Kaposi's sarcoma

Parvovirus B19

- Erythema infectiosum in children (fifth disease/slapped cheek syndrome)
- Aplastic crisis in sickle cell disease
- Anaemia, leucopenia and thrombocytopenia

Poxvirus

- Smallpox (now eradicated worldwide)
- Molluscum contagiosum

RNA viruses

PicoRNAviruses
Poliovirus

- Poliomyelitis
- 95% asymptomatic
- 0.1% suffer paralytic poliomyelitis
- Asymmetric paralysis
- No sensory involvement

Coxsackievirus

- Hand, foot and mouth disease (vesicular rash)
- Meningitis and encephalitis
- Myocarditis and pericarditis

Togaviruses
Rubella (German measles)

- Conjunctivitis
- Lymphadenopathy
- Macular pink/red rash
- Fetal infection → cardiac defect, cataracts, mental retardation and deafness

Yellow fever

- Mosquito spread
- Africa and Asia
- High fever

- Bradycardia
- Jaundice
- Clotting abnormalities → bleeding

Orthomyxovirus
Influenza

- Type A → epidemics and pandemics
- Type B → localised outbreaks
- Type C → rarely produces disease

Paramyxovirus
Measles (rubella)

- Incubation 8–14 days
- Malaise, fever, cough
- Koplik's spots in the mouth
- Erythematous rash
- Complications
  - Pneumonia
  - Myocarditis
  - Encephalomyelitis
  - Subacute sclerosing panencephalitis

Mumps

- Incubation 18 days
- Fever, headache, anorexia
- Parotid gland swelling ± submandibular involvement
- Epididymo-orchitis after puberty

Rhabdovirus
Rabies

- Contracted in animal bites
- Anxiety, agitation, hydrophobia and aerophobia
- Hyperreflexia and muscle spasm
- Death at 10–14 days
- No effective treatment

HUMAN IMMUNODEFICIENCY VIRUS (HIV) AND ACQUIRED IMMUNE DEFICIENCY SYNDROME (AIDS) (*K&C*, P. 129) (FIG. 7.6)

Epidemiology

- Young adults and children in developing world – heterosexual and vertical spread, breast-feeding

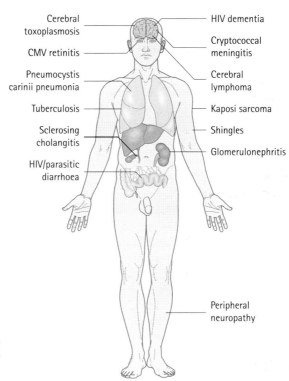

Cerebral toxoplasmosis

CMV retinitis

Pneumocystis carinii pneumonia

Tuberculosis

Sclerosing cholangitis

HIV/parasitic diarrhoea

HIV dementia

Cryptococcal meningitis

Cerebral lymphoma

Kaposi sarcoma

Shingles

Glomerulonephritis

Peripheral neuropathy

Fig. 7.6
Manifestations of HIV-AIDS.

❚ Sexual intercourse (vaginal and anal)
❚ Blood spread (shared needles, transfusions)

HIV

❚ Two subtypes:
  1. Europe/America and S.E. Asia
  2. Africa
❚ Retrovirus (reverse transcriptase allows DNA synthesis from RNA)
❚ Binds to CD4 lymphocyte surface marker
❚ Enters lymphocyte → viral synthesis

Clinical features

❚ Seroconversion illness 2 weeks after infection
❚ Fever, lymphadenopathy, headache

Investigations

❚ IgG against gp120
❚ IgG against p24 ⎤ after appropriate
❚ Viral p24 antigen ⎥ counselling
❚ Viral culture ⎦
❚ Viral load (RNA copies per ml)

Clinical latency

❚ Median time of 10 years until clinical presentation of AIDS

AIDS (*K&C*, p. 133)

❚ Infections due to low CD4 lymphocyte count
❚ Diagnosis based on low CD4 count and the presence of an AIDS-defining illness

Neurological disease

❚ HIV-related dementia
❚ Distal sensory polyneuropathy
❚ Autonomic neuropathy
❚ Progressive multifocal leucoencephalopathy
❚ Cryptococcal meningitis
❚ Cerebral lymphoma
❚ Cerebral toxoplasma

Eye disease

❚ CMV retinitis

Mucocutaneous disease

❚ Kaposi's sarcoma
❚ Molluscum contagiosum
❚ Shingles
❚ Oral hairy leucoplakia (tongue)
❚ Oral/oesophageal candidiasis
❚ Squamous cell carcinomas

Haematological disease

❚ Low CD4 (< 200)
❚ Anaemia
❚ Neutropenia
❚ Isolated thrombocytopenia

Gastrointestinal disease

❚ Weight loss
❚ *Cryptosporidium*
❚ *Microsporidium*
❚ HIV enteropathy
❚ CMV colitis
❚ Bacterial infection
❚ *Mycobacterium*
❚ Sclerosing cholangitis
❚ Oesophageal candidiasis

HIV-related diarrhoea

Renal disease

❚ HIV nephropathy
❚ Focal glomerulonephritis

Table 7.4 Post-exposure prophylaxis

Post-needlestick injury
Blood from patient and injured person

Then 4–6 weeks of
Zidovudine
Lamivudine
± Indinavir

Respiratory disease
- Pneumonia
- Pneumocystis carinii pneumonia (PCP)

Disease monitoring
- CD4 lymphocyte count
- HIV viral load (HIV RNA)

Management (Table 7.4)
Antiretroviral drugs
- Nucleoside analogues, e.g. zidovudine/abacavir/lamivudine
- Protease inhibitors, e.g. ritonavir/saquinovir
- Non-nucleoside reverse transcriptase inhibitors (only active against HIV 1) e.g. nevirapine/efavirenz
- HIV cell fusion inhibitors e.g. enfuvirtide
- HAART: highly active antiretroviral therapy – combination therapy that significantly reduces viral load and improves survival
- Complications of anti-retroviral therapy: Lipodystrophy syndrome (insulin resistance/dyslipidaemia/fat redistribution)

Early management of opportunistic infections
- Screening for infection, e.g. ophthalmoscopy for CMV retinitis

Monitoring
- Immune status (CD4 count)
- Viral replication (HIV DNA measurement)

Prevention of infection
- Safe sex practices
- Needle exchanges
- Screening of blood transfusions

FUNGAL DISEASE (*K&C*, P. 91)

Candidiasis
- *Candida albicans*
- Vaginal and oral thrush
- Oesophagitis
- Increased in the immunocompromised, by antibiotics and steroids and in the elderly

Diagnosis
- Microscopy
- Clinical appearance

Management
- Nystatin for oral lesions
- Ketoconazole

Histoplasmosis
- *Histoplasma capsulatum*
- Pulmonary focus
- Erythema nodosum and multiforme
- TB-like disease

Aspergillosis
Bronchopulmonary allergic aspergillosis
- Mimics asthma
- Bronchiectasis and eosinophilia

Aspergilloma
- Fungus ball in cavity in lung
- Often in old TB focus

Invasive aspergillosis
- Immunocompromised patients
- Pneumonia
- Meningitis and intracerebral abscess

PROTOZOAL DISEASE (*K&C*, P. 95)

Leishmaniasis
Visceral leishmaniasis (kala-azar)
- Fever, cough, diarrhoea
- Pigmented rough skin
- Splenomegaly (often massive)

- Hypersplenism → pancytopenia
- Hepatomegaly

Cutaneous leishmaniasis
- Transmitted by sandfly
- Multiple painless nodules → ulceration

Trypanosomiasis
Sleeping sickness (African disease)
- Tsetse fly transmission
- Meningoencephalitis
- Apathy and somnolence

Chagas disease (American disease)
- Lymphadenopathy
- Hepatosplenomegaly
- Conjunctivitis
- GI motility disturbance
- Neurological complications

Toxoplasmosis
- *Toxoplasma gondii*
- Transmission by cats
- Lymphadenopathy
- Neck stiffness and headache
- Acute febrile illness

Malaria
Epidemiology
- 250 million people worldwide
- Hot humid countries

Aetiology
- *Plasmodium – vivax, ovale, falciparum, malariae*
- Transmitted by ♀ *Anopheles* mosquito

Clinical features
- High fever
- Splenomegaly
- *Vivax, ovale* and *malariae* → milder chronic disease
- *Falciparum* → more serious acute disease:
- Blackwater fever: haemolysis → black urine
- Cerebral malaria: convulsions, coma
- Severe malaria: 1% erythrocytes infected (*falciparum* malaria)
- → Cerebral, renal and GI involvement
  - Risk of splenic rupture

Table 7.5 Prevention of malaria

Avoid insect bites
Repellents
Impregnated mosquito nets

Chemoprophylaxis
Seek advice prior to travel due to changes in resistance patterns

Proguanil daily + chloroquine weekly
or
Mefloquine weekly
or
Maloprim daily + chloroquine weekly

- Renal failure
- Haemolysis and thrombocytopenia
- Hypoglycaemia and acidosis

Investigations

- Thick and thin blood film shows parasites and allows identification
- Quantification of percentage of infected red cells
- Blood count, liver function tests, urea and electrolytes for complications

Management

- Falciparum: quinine sulphate orally (consider i.v. quinine if severe malaria) plus single dose of pyrimethamine and sulfadoxine (Fansidar®) (N.B. contra-indicated in G-6 PD deficiency)
- Other species: chloroquine

Prevention

- See Table 7.5

NEMATODE, TREMATODE AND CESTODE INFECTIONS (*K&C*, P. 106)

Nematodes

Filariasis

- Lymphangitis and elephantiasis

Toxocara

- Transmitted by dogs and cats
- Abdominal pain and hepatomegaly

Intestinal infections
▌ See Chapter 10

Trematodes
Schistosomiasis (bilharzia)
Schistosoma japonicum/mansoni
▌ Intestinal ulceration and fibrosis
▌ Granulomatous hepatitis
▌ Hepatosplenomegaly
▌ Portal hypertension

S. haematobium
▌ Dysuria and haematuria
▌ Bladder carcinoma

Cestodes
▌ Tapeworms

SEXUALLY TRANSMITTED DISEASE (*K&C*, P. 117)

Gonorrhoea
▌ *Neisseria gonorrhoeae*
▌ ♂ Urethritis and urethral discharge
▌ ♀ 40% asymptomatic
▌ Dysuria and vaginal discharge
▌ Conjunctival infection in the newborn
▌ Arthritis and rash in systemic disease

Investigations
▌ Microscopy and culture of urethral or vaginal swabs

Management
▌ Amoxicillin or cefixime
▌ Ciprofloxacin

Chlamydia
▌ *Chlamydia trachomatis*
▌ ♂ Urethritis with discharge
▌ ♀ Acute salpingitis → subfertility
▌ Ophthalmic trachoma → blindness
▌ Reiter's syndrome – oral ulcers, arthritis, conjunctivitis, urethritis (see p. 313)

Table 7.6 Diseases notifiable under the Public Health (Infectious Diseases) Regulations 1988

Acute encephalitis	Ophthalmia neonatorum
Acute poliomyelitis	Paratyphoid fever
Anthrax	Plague
Cholera	Rabies
Diphtheria	Relapsing fever
Dysentery	Rubella
Food poisoning	Scarlet fever
Leptospirosis	Smallpox
Malaria	Tetanus
Measles	Tuberculosis
Meningitis	Typhoid fever
Meningococcal	Typhus fever
Pneumococcal	Viral haemorrhagic fever
Haemophilus influenzae	Viral hepatitis A, B, C
Viral	Whooping cough
Unspecified	Yellow fever
Mumps	

Investigations ∎ Serology (IgM) or antigen detection

Management ∎ Tetracycline or erythromycin

Syphilis

∎ See p. 142

HIV

∎ See p. 146

Human papilloma virus (HPV)

∎ Sexual transmission
∎ Results in cervical dysplasia
∎ Cervical carcinoma
∎ Vaccine available

NOTIFIABLE DISEASES

∎ See Table 7.6

SELF-ASSESSMENT QUESTIONS

Multiple choice questions

1. The following diseases are paired with their correct mode of transmission:
   A. Leishmaniasis – sandfly bites
   B. Hepatitis A – intravenous drug use
   C. Giardiasis – faecal–oral spread
   D. *Taenia solium* – infected meat products
   E. *Neisseria gonorrhoeae* – sexual intercourse

2. The following antibiotics act by disrupting bacterial cell wall synthesis:
   A. Amoxicillin
   B. Metronidazole
   C. Cefuroxime
   D. Ciprofloxacin
   E. Gentamicin

3. The following are live attenuated vaccines:
   A. Oral polio vaccine
   B. Tetanus
   C. Bacille Calmette–Guérin (BCG)
   D. *Haemophilus influenzae b*
   E. Hepatitis B vaccine

4. The following are recognised side-effects of the named antibiotic:
   A. Ampicillin – rash in infectious mononucleosis
   B. Gentamicin – renal toxicity
   C. Flucloxacillin – ototoxicity
   D. Sulphonamides – erythema multiforme
   E. Fusidic acid – seronegative arthropathy

5. The following may result in atypical lymphocytes on a blood film:
   A. Epstein–Barr virus
   B. Cytomegalovirus
   C. Influenza A
   D. Toxoplasmosis
   E. Salmonellosis

6. The following are manifestations of staphylococcal disease:
   A. Osteomyelitis
   B. Scarlet fever
   C. Impetigo
   D. Infective endocarditis
   E. Cerebral abscesses

7. The following are true of *Mycobacterium tuberculosis*:
   A. It may cause a terminal ileitis
   B. Tuberculous meningitis results in a low protein and glucose in CSF
   C. Pyrazinamide is useful in eradicating organisms in macrophages
   D. Infection may cause lupus vulgaris
   E. Miliary infection results from haematogenous spread

8. The following organisms release a neurotoxin:
   A. *Clostridium botulinum*
   B. *Clostridium difficile*
   C. *Clostridium tetani*
   D. *Corynebacterium diphtheriae*
   E. *Yersinia*

9. The following belong to the herpesvirus family:
   A. Cytomegalovirus
   B. Epstein–Barr virus

C. Coxsackievirus
D. Varicella zoster virus
E. Rhabdovirus

10. The following are of use in chronic viral hepatitis:
    A. Lamivudine
    B. Azathioprine
    C. Ribavirin
    D. Interferon-a
    E. Zidovudine

11. In the following diseases animal vectors constitute an important mode of transmission:
    A. Yellow fever (togavirus)
    B. Fifth disease (parvovirus B19)
    C. Rabies (rhabdovirus)
    D. Hand, foot and mouth disease (paramyxovirus)
    E. Molluscum contagiosum (pox virus)

12. The following are recognised complications of the named infection:
    A. Measles virus – subacute sclerosing panencephalitis
    B. Rabies – aerophobia
    C. Varicella – pneumonia
    D. Cytomegalovirus – retinitis
    E. Parvovirus B19 – aplastic anaemia

13. The following are causes of abnormal liver function tests in HIV infection:
    A. Zidovudine
    B. Lamivudine
    C. Sclerosing cholangitis
    D. Cytomegalovirus infection
    E. *Mycobacterium avium intracellulare*

14. The following drugs are paired with the appropriate mechanism of action:
    A. Ritonavir – protease inhibitor

B. Zidovudine – nucleoside analogue
C. Nevirapine – viral RNA inhibitor
D. Lamivudine – inhibition of cell wall synthesis
E. Saquinavir – protease inhibitor

15. The following increase the risk of systemic candidiasis:
    A. Diabetes mellitus
    B. Oral prednisolone
    C. Chronic renal failure
    D. Acute viral hepatitis
    E. Intravenous cephalosporin therapy

16. The following are not features of falciparum malaria:
    A. Thrombocytopenia
    B. Intravascular haemolysis
    C. Bronchospasm
    D. Hyposplenism
    E. Hypoglycaemia

17. The following are indicators of severe malaria:
    A. Fever >38°C
    B. Parasitaemia >2%
    C. Dark urine
    D. Glucose-6-phosphate deficiency
    E. Convulsions

18. The following may cause conjunctivitis in the newborn babies of infected mothers:
    A. Syphilis
    B. Chlamydia
    C. Gonorrhoea
    D. HIV
    E. Rubella

19. The following are true of syphilis infection:
    A. Acute infection usually presents as a painless ulcer

B. A rash involving the palms of the hands suggests a secondary streptococcal infection

C. Neurological signs may be due to intracerebral abscesses

D. Syphilis meningitis may complicate tertiary syphilis

E. Congenital infection results in an internuclear ophthalmoplegia

20. The following may result in oral ulceration:
   A. Syphilis
   B. Ulcerative colitis
   C. Behçet's syndrome
   D. Mumps infection
   E. *Toxoplasma gondii*

Best one of five questions

21. The following are true of sexually transmitted disease:
   A. The incidence of non-specific urethritis is falling
   B. Gonorrhoea infection is asymptomatic in 90% of infections in males
   C. Chlamydia is an important cause of male infertility
   D. Gonorrhoea may result in a pustular rash
   E. Reactive arthritis is not associated with chlamydia infection

22. Which one of the following is true of HIV infection:
   A. *Pneumocystis carinii* pneumonia is an AIDS-defining illness
   B. The CD4-positive lymphocyte count is a poor marker of immune status

C. The median duration of infection prior to the development of AIDS is 2 years

D. HIV dementia is due to a parvovirus infection

E. Kaposi's sarcoma is an indication of adenovirus infection

23. Which one of the following causes an acute hepatitic illness:
   A. Rhabdovirus
   B. Parvovirus B19
   C. Togaviruses
   D. Dane particle
   E. Epstein–Barr virus

24. Which one of the following is a Gram-positive organism?
   A. *Staphylococcus aureus*
   B. *Escherichia coli*
   C. *Helicobacter pylori*
   D. *Salmonella typhi*
   E. Giardia lamblia

25. A 23-year-old man presents with a cough, with rust coloured sputum, peri-oral Herpes Simplex and findings of left lower lobe consolidation on chest X-ray. What is the most likely cause of his pneumonia?
   A. *Staph. aureus*
   B. *Strep. pneumoniae*
   C. *H. influenzae*
   D. *Pneumocystis carinii pneumonia*
   E. *M. tuberculosis*

26. A 76-year-old man presents with a fever, shortness of breath and a cough. On examination he has a pan-systolic murmur that radiates to the axilla.

On testing he has microscopic haematuria. What is the most likely diagnosis?

A. Interstitial glomerulonephritis
B. Pyleonephritis
C. Bacterial endocarditis
D. Cordae tendonae rupture
E. Mycoplasma pneumonia

27. A 43-year-old woman was referred with weight loss, sweats and a fever. Investigations revealed lypmphopenia. A CD4 lymphocyte count was recorded as < 100. What is the most likely underling cause?

A. Parvovirus B19
B. Epstein–Barr Virus
C. Human Immunodeficiency Virus
D. Human papilloma virus
E. Cytomegalovirus

28. A 67-year-old man is being treated with steroids and antibiotics for an infective exacerbation of chronic obstructive pulmonary disease. He reports pain and difficulty in swallowing. What is the most likely diagnosis?

A. Peptic oesophageal stricture
B. *Helicobacter pylori* induced ulceration
C. Oesophageal cytomegalovirus
D. Oesophageal candidiasis
E. Eosinophilic oesophagitis

29. A 14-year-old boy presents with a 3-day history of a non-productive cough followed by the appearance of multiple erythematous spots on the torso, arms and legs. On examination he has white spots on the buccal mucosa. What is the most likely cause?

A. Chicken pox
B. Rubella
C. Erythema infectiosum
D. Scarlet fever
E. Measles

Extended matching questions

Question 1 Theme: fever of unknown origin

A. Acute bronchopulmonary aspergillosis
B. *Pneumocystis carinii*
C. Staphylococcal pulmonary abscess
D. Aspergilloma
E. *Mycobacterium tuberculosis*
F. Falciparum malaria
G. Leishmaniasis
H. Liver abscess
I. Acute hepatitis A
J. *Streptococcus pneumoniae* pneumonia
K. *Mycoplasma* pneumonia
L. Schistosomiasis

For each of the following questions, select the best answer from the list above:

I. A 42-year-old Ugandan woman with known HIV infection and a CD4 lymphocyte count of 86 is admitted with a cough, haemoptysis, weight loss and cervical lymphadenopathy. A chest X-ray reveals diffuse apical shadowing of the left lung. What is the most likely diagnosis?

II. An 18-year-old man is admitted with a cough with rust-coloured sputum, anorexia, a temperature of 38.6°C and marked shortness of breath. On examination he is noted to have perioral herpes and coarse crackles at the right upper zone with some bronchial breathing. What is the most likely diagnosis?

III. A 28-year-old woman is admitted with a fever and jaundice. She has recently returned from India after visiting her family. She has a moderately enlarged liver and spleen. On full blood count she is noted to have a platelet count of 76. What is the most likely diagnosis?

Question 2 Theme: Investigation of pyrexia

A. Full blood count
B. Thick and thin blood film
C. Urea and electrolytes
D. Liver function tests
E. Serum calcium
F. Blood glucose
G. Blood cultures
H. Urine microscopy and culture
I. Sputum culture
J. Chest X-ray
K. Abdominal X-ray
L. Ultrasound of the liver
M. CT scan of the head
N. CT scan of the liver and pancreas
O. Endoscopic retrograde cholangiopancreatogram

For each of the following questions, select the best answer from the list above:

I. A 57-year-old woman is admitted with right upper quadrant pain, jaundice and a fever. On examination, she is tender in the right hypochondrium. What single investigation would be most useful in reaching a diagnosis?

II. A 28-year-old man returns from a trip to Kenya. He has a fever and is jaundiced. He has moderate splenomegaly. What single investigation would you choose to make the diagnosis?

III. A 76-year-old man develops a fever and cough with white frothy sputum a week after a mitral valve replacement. On examination he has fine crackles in both lung bases and a pansystolic murmur. Which investigation will be of most use in guiding treatment?

Respiratory medicine 8

If you need more detailed explanation refer to Kumar & Clark, *Clinical Medicine*, Chapter 14.

STRUCTURE AND FUNCTION

The structure of the respiratory system facilitates its role in extracting oxygen from the environment and disposing of waste gases (primarily carbon dioxide):

▌ The lungs provide a large surface area for gas exchange

▌ The alveoli walls present minimal resistance to gas exchange

▌ Efficient gas transfer is facilitated by matching ventilation to perfusion in the pulmonary capillary bed

▌ Host defences protect against inhaled gases, dusts and infectious agents

SMOKING (*K&C*, P. 893)

Cigarette smoke contains polycyclic aromatic hydrocarbons and nitrosamines which are potent carcinogens and mutagens. Smoking also causes release of enzymes from neutrophils and macrophages which destroy elastin leading to lung damage. Smoking is addictive. The dangers of smoking and the effects on the lungs are listed in Tables 8.1 & 8.2.

Table 8.1 The dangers of cigarette smoking

General
Lung cancer
COPD
Carcinoma of the oesophagus
Ischaemic heart disease
Peripheral vascular disease
Bladder cancer
An increase in abnormal spermatozoa
Memory problems

Maternal Smoking
Decreased infant birthweight
Increased fetal and neonatal mortality
Increase in asthma

Passive Smoking
Risk of asthma, pneumonia and bronchitis in infants of smoking parents
An increase in cough and breathlessness in smokers and non-smokers with CPOD & asthma
Increased cancer risk

Table 8.2 The effects of cigarette smoking on the lungs

Large Airways
Increase in submucosal gland volume
Increase in number of goblet cells
Chronic inflammation
Metaplasia & dysplasia of the surface epithelium

Small Airways
Increase in number and distribution of goblet cells
Airway inflammation and fibrosis
Epithelial metaplasia/dysplasia
Carcinoma

Parenchyma
Proximal acinar scarring
Increase in alveolar macrophage numbers
Emphysema (pan- and centri-acinar)

EXAMINING THE RESPIRATORY SYSTEM
(*K&C*, P. 883)

Examination should contain all of the following and be done in roughly this order:

Look for

▌ Clues around the bed
  – Oxygen
  – Inhalers

Table 8.3 Some common causes of finger clubbing

Respiratory
Lung cancer
Fibrosis, e.g. cryptogenic fibrosing alveolitis (CFA)
Chronic lung sepsis
Bronchiectasis
Lung abscess
Empyema
Mesothelioma

Cardiovascular
Cyanotic heart disease
Infective endocarditis
Atrial myxoma

Gastrointestinal
Cirrhosis
Inflammatory bowel disease (IBD)

Others
Congenital

      – Nebulisers
      – Peak flow meter

Expose the chest

- Maintain the dignity of the patient
- Act professionally (e.g. avoid showing embarrassment about exposing the breasts in female patients)
- Look for:
  - Cyanosis
  - Breathlessness/use of accessory muscles
  - Weight loss
  - Chest wall scars or deformity
  - Prominent veins on the chest wall (suggesting superior vena cava (SVC) obstruction)

Hands

- Flapping tremor of CO_2 retention – hold arms outstretched with wrists fully extended and fingers splayed and watch for movements of fingertips
- Clubbing (Table 8.3)
- Peripheral cyanosis
- Nicotine staining

Face

- Anaemia
- Central cyanosis

Neck

- Examine JVP (remember a fixed distended JVP suggests SVC obstruction)
- Check for lymphadenopathy

Thorax (Table 8.4)

- Locate tracheal position and apex beat
- Check for lymphadenopathy (axilla)

Assess chest expansion
Anterior

- Place hands on upper aspect of chest either side of sternum
- Ask patient to breathe in and out and watch your thumbs move laterally
- Do they move symmetrically?
- Repeat with your hands over lateral lower aspect of chest

Posterior

- Place hands over lateral lower aspect of chest and repeat the above

Percussion

- Hand firmly on chest wall
- Compare left with right anteriorly and posteriorly
- Don't forget apices and under arms
- Tap distal i.p. joint with middle finger

Listen to breath sounds

- Use diaphragm of stethoscope and again compare left with right
- Listen for added sounds (wheeze, crackles) (Table 8.5)

Check for vocal resonance and fremitus

- Ask patient to say 99 and listen with stethoscope (resonance) or palpate (vocal fremitus)

Measure peak flow

- See Chapter 3, p. 33
- Normal values
  - 40-year-old 175 cm tall ♂ = 620 L/min
  - 40-year-old 155 cm tall ♀ = 460 L/min

Table 8.4 Physical signs of respiratory disease

Pathology	Chest wall movement	Tracheal deviation	Percussion note	Breath sounds	Vocal resonance	Added sounds
Consolidation (pneumonia)	Reduced on affected side	None	Dull	Bronchial	Increased	Crackles
Collapse (major bronchus)	Reduced on affected side	Towards lesion	Dull	Diminished/absent	Reduced/absent	None
Fibrosis (generalised)	Reduced	None	Normal	Vesicular	Increased	Crackles
Pleural effusion (>500 mL)	Reduced	Away if massive	Stony dull	Diminished/absent	Reduced/absent	None
Pneumothorax (large)	Reduced	Away from lesion	Normal or hyper-resonant	Diminished/absent	Reduced/absent	None
Chronic obstructive pulmonary disease (COPD)	Reduced	None	Normal	Prolonged expiration	Normal	Expiratory wheeze
Asthma	Reduced	None	Normal	Prolonged expiration	Normal	Expiratory wheeze Crackles

Table 8.5 Abnormal breath sounds

Pathogenic process	Description of breath sounds	Auscultatory features
Airways obstruction	Wheezes	High-pitched end-expiratory 'squeaking' noises Monophonic = single airway obstruction Polyphonic = many small airways obstruction
Consolidation	Bronchial breathing	Breath sounds with prolonged expiratory phase (similar to breath sounds heard over trachea)
Fibrosis	Fine crackles	Short-lived end-inspiratory high-pitched added sounds 'like bubbles popping'
Fluid in alveoli (pulmonary oedema)	Fine crackles	Short-lived end-inspiratory high-pitched added sounds 'like bubbles popping'
Pleural inflammation	Pleural rub	Localised creaking/groaning added sounds

INVESTIGATIONS IN LUNG DISEASE

Radiology

▌ Chest X-ray (see Chapter 5)
▌ CT scan of the chest
  – Mass lesions
  – Interstitial lung disease
  – Bronchiectasis
▌ Ventilation perfusion ($\dot{V}/\dot{Q}$) scan
  – Diagnosis of pulmonary embolus
▌ PET (Positron Emission Topography) scanning
  – Assessment of lymph node involvement and metastases in lung cancer

Endoscopy

▌ Bronchoscopy
  – Allows direct visualisation of bronchi
  – Biopsies and cytology

Table 8.6 Abnormalities of blood gases in respiratory failure

	Pao_2	$Paco_2$	pH	HCO_3
Type I e.g. Severe asthma, pneumonia, acute respiratory distress syndrome (ARDS)	↓	↓ or →	↑ or →	→ or ↓
Type II e.g. COPD, CNS depression (opiates), respiratory muscle weakness	↓	↑	↓	↑

MEASURING RESPIRATORY FUNCTION
(*K&C*, P. 888)

Peak flow rate

- See above
- ↓ in airflow limitation (used to monitor the condition and its treatment)

Blood gas analysis (*K&C*, p. 890) (Table 8.6)

- Arterial blood sample (usually radial artery) measures partial pressure of O_2 and CO_2
- Essential to manage acute severe asthma and respiratory failure

Pulse oximetry

- Measures the difference in absorption of light by oxyhaemoglobin and deoxyhaemoglobin
- Used to assess and monitor arterial oxygen saturation

Spirometry (*K&C*, p. 889)

- Involves a maximum inspiration then forced expiration into a spirometer. Measures FEV_1 and FVC
- Forced expiratory volume in 1 second (FEV_1) = volume of air expired in first second
- Forced vital capacity (FVC) = maximum volume of air expired
- The FEV_1:FVC ratio ↓ in airflow limitation, e.g. asthma

■ Both FEV_1 and FVC ↓ in restrictive diseases, e.g. fibrosis

Transfer factor

■ Measures transfer of gas across the alveolar–capillary membrane
■ Decreased in alveolar disease/loss
  – Fibrosing alveolitis
  – Sarcoidosis
  – Asbestosis
  – Emphysema
■ Increased in pulmonary haemorrhage

SAMPLING PLEURAL TISSUE

Pleural biopsy

■ Pleural lesions
  – Malignancy
  – Tuberculosis

Pleural aspirate

■ Removing pleural effusion fluid
■ Microscopy and culture in infection
■ Protein content (transudate vs exudates)
■ Cytology (malignancy)
■ LDH

PULMONARY INFECTION

Pneumonia

■ Lung infections are classified by site (e.g. lobar pneumonia or bronchopneumonia) or by aetiology

Aetiology (Table 8.7)

■ Bacterial
■ Viral
■ Opportunistic organisms
■ Chemical (e.g. aspiration of vomit)
■ Radiotherapy
■ Allergic mechanisms

Clinical features (Table 8.8)

■ Cough
■ +/−Purulent sputum
■ Fever

Table 8.7 Aetiology of pneumonia in the UK

Infecting agent	%	Clinical circumstance
Streptococcus pneumoniae	50	Community pneumonia patients usually previously fit
Mycoplasma pneumoniae	6	As above
Influenza A	5	As above
Haemophilus influenzae	5	Pre-existing lung disease, e.g. COPD
Chlamydia pneumoniae	5	Community-acquired in institutions/families
Chlamydia psittaci	3	Contact with birds (not inevitable)
Staphylococcus aureus	2	Children/i.v. drug users/flu outbreaks
Legionella pneumophila	2	Institutional outbreaks (hospitals/hotels)
Coxiella burnetii	1	Abattoir and hide workers
Pseudomonas aeruginosa	<1	Cystic fibrosis
Pneumocystis carinii	<1	AIDS/lymphomas/leukaemias/use of immunosuppressant drugs
Actinomyces israelii		
Nocardia asteroides		
Cytomegalovirus		
Aspergillus fumigatus		
Anaerobic organisms	<1	Inhalation pneumonia/alcohol excess/postoperative
None isolated	20	

Table 8.8 CURB 65 score for community acquired pneumonia

Each of the following scores 1:

Confusion (MTS <9, new disorientation in time/person/place

Urea > 7 mmol/l

Respiratory rate =30/minute

Blood pressure (SBP < 90 mmHg or DBP = 60 mmHg)

Age > 65 years

Score 0 or 1: Mortality low (1.5%) – could go home
Score 2: Mortality intermediate (9.2%)
Score 3–5: Mortality high (22%) – consider ITU care

❚ Pleuritic chest pain
❚ Breathlessness

Specific features

Strep. pneumoniae ❚ Rust-coloured sputum
❚ Peri-oral HSV

Mycoplasma ❚ White cell count normal, cold agglutinins occur in 50%
❚ Extra-pulmonary complications e.g. rash, myocarditis, pericarditis, haemolytic anaemia, myalgia, neurological abnormalities, abnormal liver function, diarrhea

Staphylococcus aureus	∎ Abscesses – in lung and elsewhere
Coxiella burnetii	∎ Multiple lesions on chest X-ray

Investigations

∎ Chest X-ray
∎ Arterial blood gases or oxygen saturation
∎ Blood/sputum culture
∎ Microbiological: urine for pneumococcal or legionella antigen, serology

Management

∎ Antibiotics choice depends on severity (Table 8.8)
  – Mild: amoxicillin 500 mg three times a day (or clarithromycin if allergic)
  – Moderate: IV amoxicillin 500 mg three times a day and clarithromycin 500 mg twice a day
  – Severe: IV cefuroxime 1.5 g four times a day and clarithromycin 500 mg twice a day
  – Adjust as appropriate if particular organism suspected or known
∎ Oxygen
∎ Correct/prevent dehydration

Complications

∎ Respiratory failure
  – Type 1 – low PaO_2, low/normal $PaCO_2$
∎ Lung abscess
  – Particularly aspiration pneumonia, staphylococcal or *Klebsiella* infection, bronchial obstruction (cancer or foreign body)
∎ Empyema
  – Pus in the pleural space

Prognosis

∎ Overall 5% mortality for hospital inpatients
∎ >25% mortality for *staph. aureus* pneumonia
∎ 50% mortality for severe community acquired pneumonia (see Table 8.8)

Tuberculosis (*K&C*, p. 930)

∎ Caseating granulomatous infection due to *Mycobacterium* tuberculosis in the lung
∎ TB is a notifiable disease and contact tracing is important

Patients at risk

- Those from developing countries (including contacts)
- Immunosuppressed patients
- HIV, steroids, malignancy
- Alcoholics/homeless people/people living in overcrowded conditions

Clinical features

- See Fig. 8.1
- May be none
- Malaise and lethargy
- Anorexia/weight loss
- Fever
- Cough
- Haemoptysis

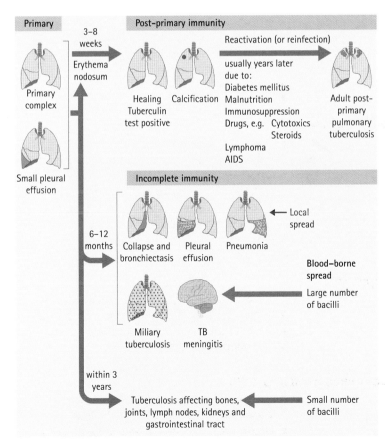

Fig. 8.1 Manifestations of primary and post-primary tuberculosis. (K&C, p. 931)

■ Signs of
  – Pleural effusion
  – Pneumonia
  – Fibrosis

Investigations

■ Chest X-ray
  – Affects upper zones particularly
  – +/– Calcification
  – +/– (*K&C*, p. 932) Cavitation
■ Sputum microscopy (Ziehl–Nielsen stain) and culture
■ Lung tissue microscopy and culture: bronchoscopy and washings or lung/pleural biopsies

Management

■ 6 months of combination of antibiotics, usually
  – Rifampicin and isoniazid
  – + Pyrazinamide for first 2 months +
  – Add ethambutol if risk of drug resistance is increased
■ Compliance is vital
■ Multi-resistant TB does occur, particularly in HIV, and may require more antibiotics (according to sensitivities) over a longer period

Side-effects of anti-TB drugs

Rifampicin ■ Liver dysfunction
           ■ Discoloration of body fluids
           ■ Reduced effectiveness of oral contraceptives and other drugs
Isoniazid ■ High doses cause polyneuropathy
           ■ Pyridoxine is added to prevent this
Pyrazinamide ■ Liver dysfunction
Ethambutol ■ Retrobulbar neuritis (patients need ophthalmology monitoring)
Streptomycin ■ Vestibular nerve damage

Other mycobacteria

M. kansasii ■ Usually less severe disease than *M. tuberculosis*
            ■ Particularly middle-aged men
            ■ COPD and working in dusty conditions (e.g. miners)
M. avium intracellulare (MAI) ■ Immunosuppressed patients, e.g. HIV

PULMONARY MALIGNANCY (K&C, P. 947)

Bronchial carcinoma

▌ Malignant tumour of bronchial tree

Epidemiology

▌ Most common malignancy (32 000 deaths/year in UK)
▌ Third most common cause of death in UK

Cell types

▌ Small cell (20–30%)
▌ Non-small cell
  – Squamous (40%)
  – Large cell (25%)
  – Adenocarcinoma (10%)
  – Bronchoalveolar cell (1–2%)

Aetiology

▌ Smoking (including passive)
  – Squamous
▌ Urban > rural
▌ Occupational
  – Adenocarcinoma
  – Asbestos, coal, chromium, arsenic, petroleum products and oils, radiation

Clinical features

▌ See Table 8.9
▌ Often no clinical signs
▌ Clubbing
▌ Supraclavicular nodes (small cell)
▌ Signs of:
  – Pleural effusion or collapse
  – Unresolved chest infection
  – Chronic lung disease (e.g. asbestosis)

Table 8.9 Frequency of common presenting symptoms of bronchial carcinoma

Symptom	Frequency (%)
Cough	41
Chest pain	22
Cough and pain	15
Haemoptysis	7
Chest infection	<5
Others (malaise, breathlessness etc)	<5

Spread of bronchial carcinoma

Direct
- Pleura and ribs
- Erosion of ribs and involvement of lower brachial plexus nerves in apical tumours (Pancoast's tumour)
- Sympathetic ganglion (Horner's syndrome – small pupil and ptosis)
- Recurrent laryngeal nerve palsy with unilateral vocal cord paralysis (hoarseness, bovine cough)
- Spinal cord compression
- Oesophagus (dysphagia)
- SVC obstruction (headache, facial congestion, fixed distended veins)

Metastatic
- Bones (spinal cord compression can complicate)
- Liver
- Brain
- Adrenal glands (usually asymptomatic)

Non–metastatic extrapulmonary manifestations

- Ectopic hormone production, adrenocorticotrophic hormone (ACTH), e.g. (small cell)
- Neurological, e.g. myasthenic syndrome
- Hypertrophic pulmonary osteoarthropathy (HPOA)
- Vascular/thrombotic/haematological
- Cutaneous, e.g. dermatomyositis

Investigations

- Chest X-ray
- Blood tests
  - Hyponatraemia
  - Polycythaemia
  - Anaemia
- CT scan and PET scanning for staging
- Bronchoscopy biopsy (proximal lesions) or percutaneous biopsy (peripheral lesions)

Management

- Multidisciplinary team approach

Surgery
- Only 5–10% of cases suitable
- For non-small cell

Radiotherapy
- Particularly for squamous cell
- Can be useful for symptom control
- Used for SVC obstruction

Chemotherapy
- Combination chemotherapy
  - Particularly useful for small cell
  - Also used for non-small cell

Prognosis

- 55–67% 5-year survival for those with local disease only
- 23–40% 5-year survival for those with locally advanced disease
- 1–3% 5-year survival for those with advanced disease

OBSTRUCTIVE LUNG DISEASE

Asthma (*K&C*, p. 912)

- Chronic inflammatory disease of the airways
- Three components
  - Reversible airflow limitation
  - Airway hyper-responsiveness to stimuli
  - Inflammation of the bronchi

Epidemiology

- Prevalence increasing

Aetiology and precipitating factors

- Atopy and allergy
- Increased airway responsiveness
- Cold air, exercise, pollution
- Occupational, e.g. isocyanates (paint-sprayers)
- Drugs, e.g. NSAIDs, Beta-blockers

Clinical features

- Cough
- Wheeze
- Breathlessness
- Chest tightness

Investigations

- Chest X-ray
- Lung function tests
- Peak flow charts
- Skin testing of allergies

Management (Table 8.10)

- Self-management plan
- Avoid precipitants
- Stepwise drug treatments
- β_2-agonists (short & long acting)
- Antimuscarinics
- Anti-inflammatories, e.g. sodium chromoglicate

Table 8.10 Acute severe asthma

Clinical features
Inability to complete a sentence in one breath
Respiratory rate = 25/min
Tachycardia = 110 beats/min
Peak flow <50% of predicted normal or best

Life-threatening features
Silent chest, cyanosis or feeble respiratory effort
Exhaustion, confusion or coma
Bradycardia or hypotension
Peak flow <30% of predicted normal or best

Very severe life-threatening features
A high $P_aCO_2 > 6\,kPa$
A very low $P_aO_2 < 8\,kPa$ despite oxygen
A low and falling arterial pH

Management
Reassure the patient and monitor pulse oximetry and arterial blood gases
Give oxygen 40–60%
Nebulised β_2 agonist e.g. salbutamol 5 mg and repeat if no improvement otherwise use 4 hourly
Add nebulised anti-muscarinics e.g ipratropium bromide 0.5 mg
Give IV steroids e.g. hydrocortisone 200 mg IV every 4 hours
Exclude pneumothorax on chest X-ray
If no improvement consider IV infusion of magnesium sulphate or salbutamol and ventilation

I Corticosteroids
I Leukotriene antagonists (selected cases)

Chronic obstructive pulmonary disease (COPD) (*K&C*, p. 900)

I Progressive airflow limitation that is not fully reversible

Aetiology

I Smoking accounts for 90% of cases
I Rarely, α_1-antitrypsin deficiency

Clinical features

I Cough and sputum
I Wheeze
I Breathlessness
I Exacerbating factors
  – Upper respiratory tract infection
  – Cold/foggy weather
  – Pollution
I Tachypnoea with prolonged expiration
I Use of accessory muscles

- Intercostal muscle recession on inspiration
- Pursed lips on expiration
- Reduced chest expansion
- Hyperinflation
- Cyanosis
- Signs of:
  - Right ventricular failure (oedema, hepatomegaly, ↑ JVP)
  - CO_2 retention (bounding pulse, peripheral vasodilatation, tremor, confusion, coma)

Investigations

- Spirometry
- Chest X-ray
- Blood gases
- ECG (P pulmonale, right branch bundle block, right ventricular hypertrophy)
- Haemoglobin and packed cell volume
- White cell count
- α_1-antitrypsin level

Management

- **Stop smoking**
- Flu and pneumococcal vaccines
- β_2-agonists
- Antimuscarinics e.g. tiotropium
- Corticosteroids
- Prompt antibiotics if infection present
- Diuretics for right ventricular failure
- Assisted ventilation with bilevel positive airway pressure ventilatory support – (BiPAP)
- Home oxygen (if meets recognised criteria for benefit)

Surgery

- Lung volume reduction in carefully selected patients

Prognosis

- 50% of patients with severe breathlessness die within 5 years
- Stopping smoking improves prognosis

Obstructive sleep apnoea (*K&C*, p. 907)

- Occurs in patients who are overweight
- 30% have other correctable factors, e.g. ENT problems, drugs (sedatives), alcohol, acromegaly

Clinical features

- Snoring/nocturnal choking
- Daytime sleepiness
- Unrefreshed or restless sleep
- Morning headaches or 'drunkeness'
- Reduced libido
- Ankle swelling

Investigations

- Sleep study (measure oximetry, abdominal/thoracic movement and EEG during sleep)

Management

- Weight loss, ENT surgery, or correction of other factors listed above
- CPAP ventilation at night

Bronchiectasis (*K&C*, p. 908)

- Abnormal and permanently dilated airways

Aetiology

- See Table 8.11

Clinical features

- Cough and excessive sputum
- Recurrent chest infections
- Halitosis
- Haemoptysis
- Clubbing
- Coarse crackles in affected areas
- Hyperinflation (resonant percussion note, impalpable apex)

Investigations

- Chest X-ray
- High-resolution CT of the lung
- Sputum examination
- Sinus X-rays
- Immunoglobulins
- Sweat electrolytes for cystic fibrosis
- Mucociliary clearance

Management

- Postural drainage
- Antibiotics
- Bronchodilators if airflow limitation
- Steroids
- Heart/lung transplant

Table 8.11 Causes of bronchiectasis

Congenital
Deficiency of bronchial wall elements
Pulmonary sequestration

Mechanical bronchial obstruction
Intrinsic
Foreign body
Inspissated mucus
Post-tuberculous stenosis
Tumour

Extrinsic
Lymph node
Tumour

Postinfective bronchial damage
Bacterial and viral pneumonia, including pertussis, measles and aspiration pneumonia

Granuloma and fibrosis
Tuberculosis, sarcoidosis and fibrosing alveolitis

Immunological over-response
Allergic bronchopulmonary aspergillosis
Post-lung transplant

Immune deficiency
Primary
Panhypogammaglobulinaemia
Selective immunoglobulin deficiencies (IgA and IgG$_2$)

Secondary
HIV and malignancy

Mucociliary clearance defects
Genetic
Primary ciliary dyskinesia (Kartagener's syndrome with dextrocardia and situs inversus)
Cystic fibrosis

Acquired
Young's syndrome – azospermia, sinusitis

Cystic fibrosis (*K&C*, p. 909)

❙ Autosomal recessive disorder of the cystic fibrosis transmembrane conductance regulator (CFTR) which induces low salt and chloride excretion into airways leading to increased viscosity of airway secretions

Clinical features

Respiratory
- Recurrent chest infections
- Clubbing
- Sinusitis
- Haemoptysis
- Nasal polyps
- Spontaneous pneumothorax
- Respiratory failure
- Right ventricular failure

Gastrointestinal
- Steatorrhoea (pancreatic insufficiency)
- Meconium ileus
- Gallstones
- Cirrhosis

Investigations

- Sweat electrolyte test
- DNA analysis for genotype

Management

- Antibiotics
- Pancreatic/nutritional supplements
- Amiloride or adenosine to improve hydration of secretions
- Inhaled antibiotics, corticosteroids and recombinant human DNase
- CFTR gene therapy
- Lung transplant

Prognosis

- Median survival 40 years

OCCUPATIONAL LUNG DISEASE (K&C, P. 944)

Exposure to dusts, gases, vapours and fumes at work can lead to:

- Acute bronchitis and pulmonary oedema from irritants, e.g. SO_2, chlorine
- Pulmonary fibrosis due to mineral dust, e.g. coal
- Occupational asthma
- Extrinsic allergic bronchiolar alveolitis
- Bronchial carcinoma due to industrial agents, e.g. asbestos, radon

Coal-worker's pneumoconiosis (K&C, p. 945)

- Patients may qualify for industrial injuries benefit

Aetiology

▌ Deposition of dust particles in small airways

Clinical features

▌ Breathlessness
▌ Cough +/− black sputum

Investigations

▌ Chest X-ray – fine micronodular shadowing
▌ Spirometry – mixed restrictive and obstructive pattern with reduced gas transfer

Complications

▌ Progressive massive fibrosis
  – Large round masses in upper lobes +/− necrotic centres
  – May be associated with rheumatoid factor and antinuclear factor
  – Respiratory failure

Asbestosis (*K&C*, p. 945)

▌ Ubiquitous use of asbestos put many at risk
▌ Particular problems with roofers, shipyard workers, those making gas masks in World War II

Aetiology

▌ Deposition of inhaled blue fibres in airways
▌ Synergistic effect of smoking

Clinical features

▌ Breathlessness
▌ Cough
▌ Chest pain

Investigations

▌ Chest X-ray
  – Fine reticulonodular shadowing
  – Honeycomb lung
  – Pleural plaques/effusion
▌ Spirometry – restrictive +/− ↓ gas transfer

Diseases caused by asbestos

▌ Pleural plaques
▌ Pleural effusion
▌ Bilateral diffuse pleural thickening*
▌ Mesothelioma* occurs 20–40 years after exposure to asbestos dust
▌ Asbestosis (restrictive fibrotic lung disease)*

■ Carcinoma of the bronchus*

* Patients eligible for industrial injuries benefit.

PULMONARY INFLAMMATION AND FIBROSIS

Sarcoid (*K&C*, p. 935)

■ A multisystem granulomatous disorder presenting usually as
  - Bilateral hilar lymphadenopathy
  - Pulmonary infiltration
  - Skin/eye lesions

Epidemiology

■ 19 in 100 000
■ Female > male
■ More severe in blacks than whites

Aetiology

■ Unknown

Clinical features (Table 8.12)

■ Commonly presents in third or fourth decade

Extrapulmonary features

■ Skin
  - Erythema nodosum
  - Lupus pernio
■ Eye
  - Uveitis
  - Conjunctivitis
  - Keratoconjunctivitis sicca
■ Face
  - Parotitis
  - Facial nerve palsy
■ Metabolic
  - Hypercalcaemia (10%)

Table 8.12 Presenting symptoms of sarcoid	
Presentation	%
Respiratory symptoms/abnormal chest X-ray	50
Fatigue or weight loss	5
Peripheral lymphadenopathy	5
Fever	4
Normal chest X-ray	20

- CNS
  - Meningoencephalitis
  - Spinal cord disease
  - Myopathy
  - Polyneuropathy
- Gastrointestinal
  - Hepatosplenomegaly
- Cardiovascular
  - Cardiomyopathy

Investigations

- Chest X-ray
- CT chest
- Blood tests
  - FBC (normocytic anaemia)
  - ↑ ESR
  - ↑ Ca^{++}
  - ↑ Serum angiotensin-converting enzyme (ACE)
- Transbronchial biopsy
- Spirometry
  - Restrictive defect
  - ↓ Gas transfer

Management

- Steroids

Pulmonary involvement in systemic diseases
Rheumatoid arthritis (Fig. 8.2)

- Rheumatoid factor always present
- Lung features may precede arthropathy

Systemic lupus erythematosus

- Pleurisy/pleural effusion

Systemic sclerosis

- Pulmonary fibrosis/honeycomb lung

Wegener's granulomatosis

- Granulomatous vasculitis of small arteries
- Rhinorrhoea
- Nasal ulceration
- Nodular masses (+/−cavitation)
- Migratory pulmonary infiltrates
- Associated with antineutrophil cytoplasmic antibodies (ANCA)
- Treated with cyclophosphamide

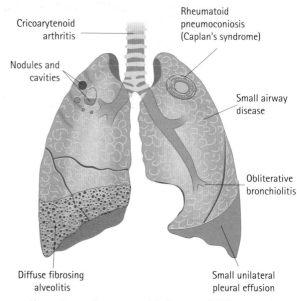

Fig. 8.2 Respiratory manifestations of rheumatoid disease. (K&C, p. 937)

Churg–Strauss syndrome

▌ Systemic vasculitis
▌ Asthma
▌ Rhinitis
▌ Eosinophilia
▌ Associated with ANCA
▌ Treated with steroids

Goodpasture's syndrome

▌ Disease associated with anti-glomerular basement membrane (GBM) antibodies which cross-react with the glomerulus and the lung
▌ Cough
▌ Haemoptysis (can be massive)
▌ Intrapulmonary haemorrhage
▌ Glomerulonephritis
▌ Treated with steroids

Pulmonary fibrosis and honeycomb lung

▌ See Table 8.13

Cryptogenic fibrosing alveolitis (*K&C*, p. 941)
Clinical features

▌ Breathlessness
▌ Cyanosis

Table 8.13 **The main causes of honeycomb lung**

Localised	Diffuse
Systemic sclerosis	Cryptogenic fibrosing alveolitis
Sarcoidosis	Rheumatoid lung
Tuberculosis	Langerhans' cell histiocytosis
Asbestosis	Tuberous sclerosis
Berylliosis	Neurofibromatosis

▊ Clubbing
▊ Bilateral fine inspiratory crackles
▊ Signs of:
  – Respiratory failure
  – Pulmonary hypertension
  – Right heart failure

Disease associations

▊ Autoimmune e.g. autoimmune hepatitis
▊ Coeliac disease
▊ Ulcerative colitis
▊ Renal tubular acidosis

Investigations

▊ Chest X-ray – reticulonodular shadowing
▊ High-resolution CT
▊ Spirometry
  – Restrictive pattern with ↓ gas transfer
▊ Bronchoalveolar lavage – hypercellular
▊ Transbronchial biopsy

Management

▊ Oxygen
▊ Steroids
▊ Immunosuppressants, e.g. azathioprine
▊ Single lung transplant

Complications

▊ Respiratory failure

Prognosis

▊ Median survival 5 years

Extrinsic allergic alveolitis (*K&C*, p. 942)
Aetiology

▊ See Table 8.14

Table 8.14 Extrinsic allergic (bronchiolar) alveolitis – some causes

Disease	Situation	Antigens
Farmer's lung	Forking mouldy hay/ mouldy vegetable material	Actinomycetes e.g. *Micropolyspora faeni* and fungi e.g. *Aspergillus*
Bird fancier's lung	Handling pigeons, cleaning lofts or budgerigar cages	Proteins present in the 'bloom' on the feathers and in excreta
Maltworker's lung	Turning germinating barley	*Asperigillus clavatus*
Humidifier fever	Contaminated humidifying systems in air conditioners or humidifiers in factories (especially in printing works)	Possibly a variety of bacteria or amoeba (e.g. *Naegleria gruberi*), Actinomycetes
Mushroom workers	Turning mushroom compost	Actinomycetes
Cheese maker's lung	Mouldy cheese	Penicillin casei, aspergillus clavatus
Wine maker's lung	Mould on grapes	Botrytis

Clinical features

- Fever
- Malaise
- Breathlessness
- Cough
- Tachypnoea
- Coarse inspiratory crackles
- Wheeze

Investigations

- Chest X-ray – fluffy nodular shadowing
- Precipitating antibodies (e.g. pigeon protein)
- Spirometry
  - restrictive pattern with ↓ gas transfer
- Bronchoalveolar lavage – hypercellular

Management

- Avoid precipitant
- Steroids

PNEUMOTHORAX (*K&C*, P. 953)

- Air in the pleural space leading to lung deflation

Aetiology

- Spontaneous
- Chest trauma
- Intubation and ventilation

Clinical features

- See Table 8.4
- Pleuritic chest pain
- Breathlessness

Specific features

- Young patients: $\male > \female$ 6:1, often tall and thin
- >40 years usually associated with COPD
- Rarely caused by asthma, carcinoma, lung abscess, severe pulmonary fibrosis
- If severe can present as tension pneumothorax (mediastinal shift and respiratory compromise)

Investigations

- Chest X-ray

Management

- Simple aspiration (second intercostal space mid-clavicular line)
- Intercostal drain if recurs after aspiration
- See algorithm (Fig. 8.3)
- Surgery for recurrent pneumothorax

Complications

- Bronchopleural fistula

CARBON MONOXIDE POISONING (K&C, P. 1010)

- Carbon monoxide combines readily with haemoglobin and prevents the formation of oxyhaemoglobin

Aetiology

- Gas appliances with poor ventilation

Clinical features

- Mental impairment
- Nausea and vomiting
- Headache
- Hallucinations
- Fits
- Drowsiness and coma

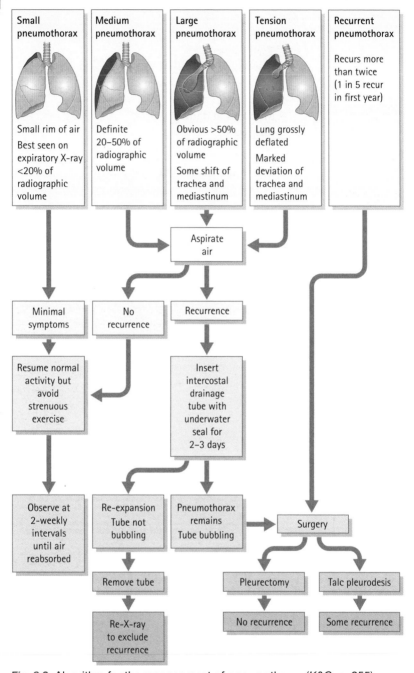

Fig. 8.3 Algorithm for the management of pneumothorax (*K&C*, p. 955).

▌ Mild–moderate toxicity
  – Tachycardia
  – Tachypnoea
▌ Severe toxicity
  – Hypotension
  – Bradycardia
  – Myocardial damage
  – Respiratory distress

Investigations

▌ Blood carboxyhaemoglobin level

Management

▌ Remove the source
▌ High-flow oxygen
▌ Hyperbaric oxygen if
  – Coma
  – Carboxyhaemoglobin level >10%

SELF-ASSESSMENT QUESTIONS

Best one of five questions

1. Clubbing is commonly seen in:
   A. Empyema
   B. Asthma
   C. COPD
   D. Diverticular disease
   E. Mesothelioma

2. The clinical findings of a pleural effusion are:
   A. Hyper-resonant percussion note
   B. Stony dull percussion note
   C. Increased tactile vocal fremitus
   D. Increased vocal resonance
   E. Tracheal deviation even with small effusions

3. In asthma:
   A. Peak flow rate is low during exacerbations
   B. Patients always have reduced air entry on chest auscultation
   C. FEV_1:FVC ratio is normal
   D. FVC is low
   E. JVP is elevated

4. In pneumonia:
   A. *Strep. pneumoniae* is an unusual cause
   B. *Haemophilus influenzae* pneumonia usually occurs in patients with normal lungs
   C. Pneumonia is only caused by bacteria
   D. *Pneumocystis carinii* pneumonia occurs in patients who are immunosuppressed
   E. Extrapulmonary abscesses do not occur in *Staph. aureus* pneumonia

5. In pneumonia:
   A. *Coxiella Burneti* is associated with contact with birds
   B. Cold agglutinins are rare in *Mycoplasma* pneumonia
   C. Patients with *Staph. aureus* pneumonia have a good prognosis
   D. *Mycobacterium kansasii* usually presents in young adults
   E. *Staph. aureus* is associated with recent influenza infection

6. Tuberculosis:
   A. Treatment is with combination antibiotics
   B. Prevalence is reducing
   C. Mycobacteria are identified by haematoxylin and eosin stain
   D. Pneumonia usually affects the lower zones of the lungs
   E. Treatment with isoniazid causes eye problems

7. Lung cancer:
   A. Is the most common cause of malignancy-related death in the UK
   B. Most commonly is an adenocarcinoma
   C. Never occurs in non-smokers
   D. Patients usually present with haemoptysis
   E. Patients always have clinical signs

8. In lung cancer:
   A. A Pancoast's tumour presents with pain in the chest
   B. Recurrent laryngeal nerve palsy is not a result of direct tumour spread

C. Horner's syndrome is associated with ptosis and a dilated pupil

D. Spread to bone is uncommon

E. Dermatomyositis may occur

9. In the treatment of lung cancer:

A. Surgery is appropriate for most patients

B. Radiotherapy is used for SVC obstruction

C. Chemotherapy is most successful in adenocarcinoma

D. A 20% 5-year survival is the norm for those with local disease only

E. Radiotherapy is not used for palliation

10. In asthma:

A. Airway hyper-responsiveness is a major feature

B. Exacerbations are not precipitated by particular weather conditions

C. Attacks can be precipitated by use of paracetamol

D. Peak flow is elevated during exacerbations

E. Intravenous magnesium sulphate is used for mild cases

11. In COPD:

A. A common cause is α_1-antitrypsin deficiency

B. Disease occurs in smokers

C. A small volume pulse suggests CO_2 retention

D. Stopping smoking will not improve prognosis in severe cases

E. Home oxygen is used in patients with PaO_2 <12 kPa

12. Obstructive sleep apnoea:

A. Is treated with inhaled steroids

B. Can present with morning headaches

C. Commonly affects people with a low body mass index

D. ENT assessment is rarely necessary

E. Is treated with single lung transplant

13. Pneumothorax:

A. Can be a complication of mechanical ventilation

B. Leads to a dull percussion note on the affected side

C. Is usually treated with chest drain insertion

D. Always requires chest drain insertion

E. Usually presents with haemoptysis

14. In cryptogenic fibrosing alveolitis:

A. Coarse crackles are heard on auscultation

B. Spirometry shows a reduced FVC

C. There is a good prognosis

D. Clubbing is not a clinical feature

E. There is an association with Crohn's disease

15. Regarding occupational lung disease:

A. In coal-worker's pneumoconiosis large round opacities are usually seen on the chest X-ray

B. Patients may qualify for industrial injury benefits

C. Mesothelioma usually occurs 5–10 years after exposure to asbestos fibres

D. The risk of lung cancer is not increased

E. Cigarette smoking in patients exposed to asbestosis only slightly increases the risk of bronchial adenocarcinoma

Extended matching questions

Question 1 *Theme: breathlessness*

A. Adenocarcinoma of the lung
B. Asthma
C. Chronic obstructive pulmonary disease
D. Extrinsic allergic alveolitis
E. Cryptogenic fibrosing alveolitis
F. Mesothelioma
G. Heart failure
H. Iron deficiency anaemia
I. Pneumothorax

For each of the following questions, select the best answer from the list above:

I. A 23-year-old female has intermittent episodes of breathlessness and cough. She has a past history of eczema and her FEV_1:FVC ratio is reduced. What is the most likely diagnosis?

II. A 50-year-old male smoker who works on a farm presents with progressive increasing breathlessness and weight loss over 6 months. He has finger clubbing. What is the most likely diagnosis?

III. An 80-year-old female presents with episodes of breathlessness

on exertion. She takes ibuprofen for joint pains and nifedipine for hypertension. She has normal pulmonary function tests and the PA chest X-ray is also normal. What is the most likely cause of her symptoms?

Question 2 *Theme: pneumonia*

A. *Streptococcus pneumoniae*
B. *Mycobacterium tuberculosis*
C. *Haemophilus influenzae*
D. *Mycoplasma pneumoniae*
E. *Pneumocystis carinii*
F. *Staphylococcus aureus*
G. *Chlamydia psittaci*
H. *Legionella pneumophila*
I. *Coxiella burnetii*
J. Influenza A

For each of the following questions, select the best answer from the list above:

I. A 28-year old female who has previously been well and takes the oral contraceptive pill presents with a fever and a cough productive of rust-coloured sputum. A chest X-ray reveals a right middle lobe pneumonia. What is the most likely microbiological causal agent?

II. A 50-year-old male who is known to have HIV with a low CD4 count presents with a history of fever and breathlessness. The chest X-ray looks normal and there are few clinical findings apart from marked hypoxia. What is the most likely microbiological causal agent?

III. An 80-year-old female presents with fever and cough. She lives in an old people's home where there has recently been a flu outbreak. A chest X-ray shows right lower zone shadowing with an area suggesting a cavity. What is the most likely microbiological causal agent?

Question 3 *Theme: abnormal chest X-rays*

A. Sarcoid
B. Goodpasture's syndrome
C. Cryptogenic fibrosing alveolitis
D. Pneumothorax
E. Pneumocystis pneumonia
F. Extrinsic allergic alveolitis
G. Cystic fibrosis
H. Mesothelioma
I. Asbestosis
J. Tuberculosis

For each of the following questions, select the best answer from the list above:

I. A 20-year old student who has previously been well, takes a summer job on a local farm when she is travelling. Since she started working on the farm she has had a fever and malaise each afternoon but feels well again each morning. A chest X-ray shows fluffy nodular shadowing. What is the most likely diagnosis?

II. A 34-year-old female from South Africa who has been in the UK for 20 years saw her GP with a troublesome cough. Her GP arranged a chest X-ray which has shown bilateral hilar lymphadenopathy. What is the most likely diagnosis?

III. An 82-year-old man presents with chest pain and cough. He lives in the East End of London and was exposed to asbestos during the war years. He has previously been told his chest X-ray is abnormal but not to be concerned. He completed a 4 week course of steroids for some arthralgia symptoms one week previously. A chest X-ray shows pleural plaques and a pleural effusion. What is the most likely diagnosis?

Cardiology 9

EXAMINING THE CARDIOVASCULAR SYSTEM
(*K&C*, P. 735)

Examination should contain all of the following and be done in roughly this order:

▌ Position the patient at 30–45° to the horizontal with the chest and upper body exposed

General inspection

▌ Look for central cyanosis
▌ Note breathlessness
▌ Count the respiratory rate

Hands

▌ Peripheral cyanosis
▌ Nicotine stains
▌ Clubbing (congenital cyanotic heart disease, infective endocarditis)
▌ Splinter haemorrhages and nail fold infarcts (infective endocarditis)

Face

▌ Central cyanosis (blue lips and tongue)
▌ Malar flush (mitral valve disease)
▌ Pallor

Chest

▌ Scars (sternotomy, pacemaker, mitral valvotomy)
▌ Visible pulsations

Radial pulse (Table 9.1)

▌ Time it with the minute hand on a watch or clock

Table 9.1 The radial pulse

Character of radial pulse	Cause
Low volume	Low BP
	Aortic stenosis
Collapsing pulse	Aortic regurgitation
Pulsus alternans	Variable volume due to cardiac failure
Pulsus paradoxus	Volume reduces on inspiration in acute asthma

BOX 9.1 COLLAPSING PULSE

With the flats of your fingers over the radial pulse, raise the patient's arm above the level of the heart (without causing discomfort)
Normally there is no change or there is a reduction in the impulse
If the pulse is collapsing you will feel a strong, fast impulse which falls away immediately

BOX 9.2 BLOOD PRESSURE

Use an appropriately sized cuff
Apply the cuff 25 mm above the antecubital fossa and palpate brachial artery. Inflate cuff until pulsation not palpable, place the diaphragm of the stethoscope over the artery, then deflate at a rate of 2–5 mmHg/second
When a sound is heard with each pulse (Korotkoff 1) this is the systolic pressure
The point at which the sound disappears (Korotkoff 5) represents the diastolic pressure
Record each to the nearest 2 mmHg

Rate

▌ Record the rate as beats per minute (be exact)
▌ Feel both radial pulses

Rhythm

▌ Regular or irregular
 – Atrial fibrillation
 – Multiple ventricular ectopics

Radiofemoral delay

▌ Coarctation of the aorta

Blood pressure

▌ See information box

Carotid pulse

▌ Feel each carotid artery separately
▌ Character (slow rising in aortic stenosis, collapsing in aortic regurgitation)

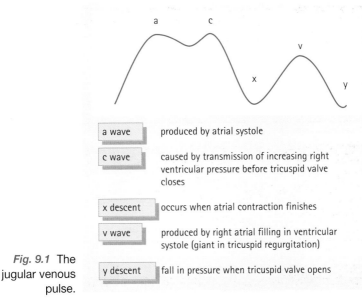

a wave	produced by atrial systole
c wave	caused by transmission of increasing right ventricular pressure before tricuspid valve closes
x descent	occurs when atrial contraction finishes
v wave	produced by right atrial filling in ventricular systole (giant in tricuspid regurgitation)
y descent	fall in pressure when tricuspid valve opens

Fig. 9.1 The jugular venous pulse.

Table 9.2 Features which differentiate the jugular venous pulse from the carotid pulse

JVP has double impulse
JVP not seen on sitting up and inspiration, when normal
JVP is impalpable
JVP fills from above if the internal jugular vein is occluded by light pressure at the base of the neck
Hepatojugular reflux – if pressure is put on the abdomen it increases venous return from the liver and the JVP becomes more prominent

Table 9.3 Causes of an abnormal jugular venous pressure

Right ventricular failure
Fluid overload
Tricuspid regurgitation (large v wave)
Pericardial effusion or restrictive pericarditis (pulsus paradoxus)
Complete heart block (giant a waves due to atrial contraction against a closed tricuspid valve)
Superior vena caval obstruction (non-pulsatile)

Jugular venous pulse (JVP) (*K&C*, p. 737)

I See Fig. 9.1 and Tables 9.2 and 9.3

Apex beat (Table 9.4)

I Position in terms of intercostal space and mid-clavicular line
I Most lateral and inferior position of palpable beat

BOX 9.3 JUGULAR VENOUS PULSE

With the patient at 45° turn the face to the left to relax the neck strap muscles
Assess the internal jugular venous pulsation
The height of the JVP is measured vertically from the sternal angle. Use a ruler or finger breadths to measure the height accurately
The upper limit of normal is 4 cm

Table 9.4 The apex beat

Quality	Haemodynamics	Causes
Hyperdynamic (thrusting)	Volume overload	Aortic regurgitation
		Mitral regurgitation
Sustained (heaving)	Pressure overload	Aortic stenosis
		Hypertension
Tapping	Palpable first heart sound	Mitral stenosis
Dyskinetic segment		Left ventricular aneurysm

Reasons for failure to locate the apex beat

▌ Fat or muscular chest wall
▌ Left pneumothorax or pleural effusion
▌ Emphysema
▌ Pericardial effusion
▌ Dextrocardia

Precordium

▌ Palpate over each valvular area with the palm of the hand for thrills (palpable murmurs)
▌ Right ventricular hypertrophy may cause a sustained impulse (heave) at the left sternal edge

Auscultation (Table 9.5 and Fig. 9.2)

▌ Listen with both the bell and the diaphragm to each valvular area
▌ Time any abnormal sounds with the carotid pulse

Mitral valve

▌ After the apex, listen in the left axilla for radiation of mitral murmurs

Table 9.5 Cardiac auscultation
High-pitched sounds (diaphragm)
S_1 and S_2
Opening snap
Ejection murmurs
Early diastolic murmur of aortic regurgitation
Low-pitched sounds (bell)
S_3 and S_4
Mid-diastolic murmur of mitral stenosis

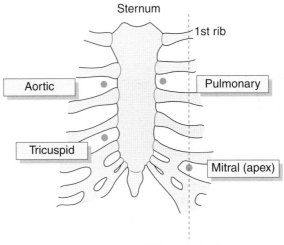

Fig. 9.2 Valvular areas.

■ Turn the patient on to the left side and listen to the apex and axilla again in held expiration to accentuate difficult-to-detect murmurs, especially the 'rumbling' mid-diastolic murmur of mitral stenosis

Aortic valve

■ When listening at the left sternal edge sit the patient forward in held expiration to accentuate the early diastolic murmur of aortic regurgitation
■ Listen for radiation of aortic murmurs to the carotids with the diaphragm followed by the bell for carotid bruits

Lung bases

■ While the patient is sitting forward examine the lung bases for crackles indicating pulmonary oedema

Heart sounds

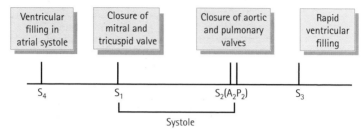

Fig. 9.3 Heart sounds.

Abdomen

❙ Liver enlargement in right ventricular failure
❙ Pulsation of liver in tricuspid regurgitation
❙ Abdominal aortic aneurysm
❙ Aortic and renal bruits

Peripheral pulses

❙ Examine all of them and listen for femoral and carotid bruits

Peripheral oedema

❙ Check for dependent pitting oedema at ankles and sacrum

Normal and abnormal signs in cardiovascular examination

Heart sounds

❙ See Fig. 9.3

S_1

❙ Closure of mitral and tricuspid valves at the onset of systole

S_2 (A_2 P_2)

❙ Closure of the aortic and pulmonary valves at the end of systole

S_3

❙ Occurs in early diastole and is due to rapid ventricular filling
❙ Normal in young people, or if the left ventricle is stiff
❙ Volume overload in mitral regurgitation

S_4

❙ Occurs in late diastole due to ventricular filling in atrial systole

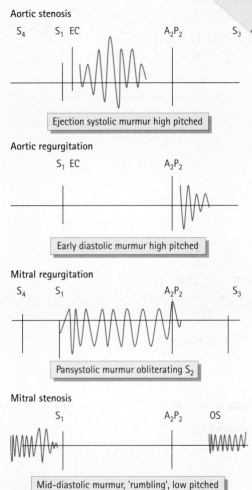

Fig. 9.4 Common murmurs.
EC: Ejection click.
OS: opening snap.

⬛ Always abnormal due to reduced ventricular distensibility, e.g. aortic stenosis, acute myocardial infarction (MI)

Prosthetic valve sounds

⬛ Mechanical valves make loud heart sounds often audible without a stethoscope

Common murmurs

⬛ See Fig. 9.4

INVESTIGATIONS IN CARDIOLOGY (*K&C*, P. 741)

Chest x-ray (see Ch. 5)

▮ Heart size and shape
▮ Lung fields
   – Rib-notching in coarctation of aorta

Electrocardiography (*K&C*, p. 744)

▮ The electrocardiogram (ECG) is a recording of the electrical activity of the heart
▮ It is the vector sum of all the depolarisation and repolarisation potentials of all the myocardial cells

Limb leads

▮ Six of the leads are obtained by recording from the limbs (Fig. 9.5)

Chest leads

▮ The other six leads record potentials between points on the chest wall (Fig. 9.5) and an average of the three limbs

Aspects of the heart (Fig. 9.5)

▮ V_1 and V_2 – right ventricle
▮ V_3 and V_4 – interventricular septum
▮ V_5 and V_6 – left ventricle
▮ Leads II, III and AVF – inferior aspect
▮ Leads I and AVL – lateral left ventricle

BOX 9.4 PERFORMING AN ECG

Connect the ECG machine to a power point and switch on
Connect the leads
Limb leads
Red to right arm
Yellow to left arm
Green to left leg
Black (neutral) to right leg
Chest leads
V_1 Fourth intercostal space just to right of sternum
V_2 Fourth intercostal space just to left of sternum
V_3 Halfway between V_2 and V_4
V_4 Fifth intercostal space left of mid-clavicular line
V_5 On same horizontal as V_4 in anterior axillary line
V_6 On same horizontal as V_4 in mid-axillary line
Check that there is paper and that the paper speed is correct (25 mm/s)
Ask the patient to keep still
Press record/acquire ECG
Label the ECG with the patient's name, and the date and time

ECG paper

▌ The standard paper speed is 25 mm/s
▌ This means each small square = 0.04 s
▌ Each large square = 0.2 s

Normal ECG waveform (Fig. 9.6)

▌ P wave is atrial depolarisation
▌ QRS is ventricular depolarisation
▌ T wave is ventricular repolarisation

(A) The bipolar leads

(B) The augmented bipolar leads

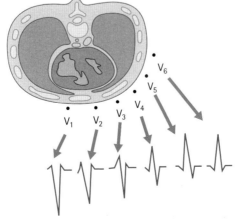

(C) The chest (unipolar) leads

Fig. 9.5 The connections or directions that comprise the 12-lead ECG.

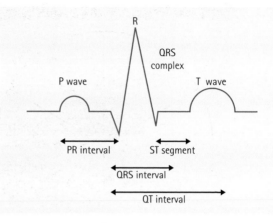

Fig. 9.6 Waves and intervals of the normal ECG.

Normal ECG intervals

- P wave duration = 0.12 s
- PR interval 0.12–0.22 s
- QRS complex duration = 0.1 s

Axis

- The normal axis of the heart is −30° and +90°
- Axis deviation can be identified by looking at the positive and negative deflections in leads I, II and III (Fig. 9.7)

The normal 12-lead ECG

- See Fig. 9.8

The exercise ECG

- Assesses cardiac response to exercise
- Detects myocardial ischaemia (ST depression and T wave changes) during exertion

Indications

- Investigation of chest pain
- Risk assessment after MI

Contraindications

- Recent MI or troponin positive ACS (within 1 week)
- Unstable angina
- Aortic stenosis
- Hypertrophic obstructive cardiomyopathy

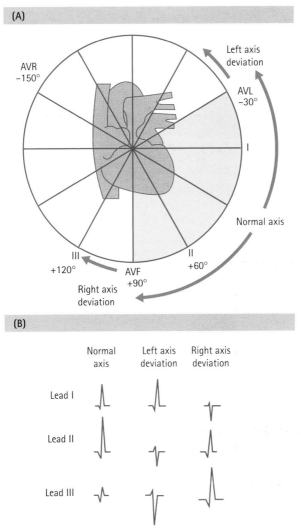

(A)

AVR
−150°

Left axis
deviation

AVL
−30°

I

Normal axis

III
+120°

AVF
+90°

II
+60°

Right axis
deviation

(B)

	Normal axis	Left axis deviation	Right axis deviation
Lead I			
Lead II			
Lead III			

Fig. 9.7 The cardiac axis. A. The hexaxial reference system, illustrating the six leads in the frontal plane, e.g. lead I is 0°, lead II is +60°, lead III is +120°. B. Calculating the direction of the cardiac vector. In the first column the QRS complex with zero net amplitude (i.e. when the positive and negative deflections are equal) is seen in lead III. The mean QRS vector is therefore perpendicular to lead III and is either −150° or +30°. Lead I is positive, so the axis must be +30°, which is normal. In left axis deviation (second column) the main deflection is positive (R wave) in lead I and negative (S wave) in lead III. In right axis deviation (third column) the main deflection is negative (S wave) in lead I and positive (R wave) in lead III. The frontal plane QRS axis is normal only if the QRS complexes in leads I and II are predominantly positive.

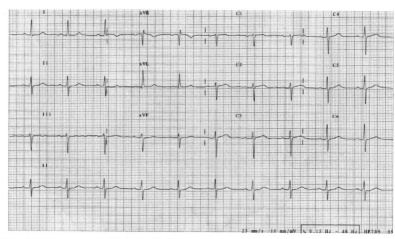

Fig. 9.8 The normal 12-lead ECG.

BOX 9.5 PROCEDURE FOR EXERCISE ECG

Continuous recording of pulse rate and 12-lead ECG and intermittent BP recordings (every 60 seconds)

The patient walks on a treadmill or cycles an exercise bike, slowly on the flat at first then graduating to high-speed walking (or running or cycling) on a gradient until a predesignated target heart rate (according to age) is reached or until symptoms or ECG abnormalities prevent further exertion

The ECG is analysed for ischaemic changes

24-hour ambulatory taped ECG (*K&C*, p. 747)

▮ 24-hour recording of ECG via a portable recorder
▮ Records transient changes, e.g. paroxysmal tachycardias or rhythm pauses
▮ Event recording can link symptoms to changes in the ECG

Echocardiography (*K&C*, p. 749)

▮ Non-invasive ultrasound examination of the heart
▮ Records dynamic anatomy of the four chambers and the valves
▮ Doppler echo gives information about
    – Blood flow
    – Ejection fraction
    – Pressure gradients

Abnormalities detected on echocardiography

▮ Valve stenosis
▮ Valve regurgitation

Table 9.6 Cardiac catheterisation

Functions of cardiac catheter	Chambers and vessels examined
Direct pressure measurements	Right atrium Aorta Right ventricle Left ventricle Pulmonary artery
Indirect pressure measurements	Left atrium using pulmonary capillary wedge pressure
Blood sampling for P_aO_2	From all chambers to detect right to left shunts

▌ Aortic root dissection
▌ Valve vegetations
▌ Cardiac failure (reduced ejection fraction)
▌ Cardiomyopathies
▌ Pericardial effusion
▌ Masses in heart chambers, e.g. thrombus, myxoma
▌ Left ventricular aneurysm
▌ Congenital heart disease

Nuclear imaging (e.g. thallium scan) (K&C, p. 755)

▌ Used to measure myocardial function and perfusion defects and position
▌ Detects reversible ischaemia, e.g. resting or stress-induced, and irreversible ischaemia, e.g. MI

Cardiac catheterisation (Table 9.6) (K&C, P. 757)

▌ Uses intraluminal catheter inserted via peripheral blood vessel to perform pressure measurements and contrast imaging from within the heart chambers, great vessels and coronary arteries

Coronary angiography

▌ X-ray contrast medium is injected directly into the main coronary arteries via an intracardiac catheter

Indications

▌ Angina refractory to medical therapy
▌ Strongly positive exercise test
▌ Troponin positive acute coronary syndrome (ACS)
▌ Angina after MI
▌ Young patients with angina or MI
▌ Uncertain diagnosis
▌ For primary percutaneous intervention for ACS, e.g. stenting/angioplasty

VALVULAR HEART DISEASE (K&C, P. 817)

Investigations

- Chest X-ray
- ECG
- Echocardiogram
- Cardiac catheterisation

Management

- Antibiotic prophylaxis
  - Required for patients with congenital abnormalities of heart or great vessels or valve disease for procedures which may cause a significant bacteraemia. Example regime: gentamicin 160 mg plus amoxicillin 1 g
- Medical
- Surgical

Mitral stenosis
Aetiology

- Rheumatic fever

Clinical features

- Progressive breathlessness ⎫
- Paroxysmal nocturnal dyspnoea ⎪ Secondary to
- Orthopnoea ⎬ pulmonary venous
- Haemoptysis ⎪ hypertension
- Recurrent bronchitis ⎭
- Mitral facies (malar flush – a cyanotic purple discoloration over the upper cheeks)
- Small-volume pulse
- Atrial fibrillation
- Tapping apex beat
- Loud first heart sound
- Opening snap (OS)
- 'Rumbling' mid-diastolic murmur at apex with presystolic accentuation (if in sinus rhythm)
- Signs of right ventricular failure

Investigations

- Chest X-ray
  - Large left atrium (widened carina)
  - Convex left heart border
- ECG
  - Bifid P wave or atrial fibrillation
  - Right ventricular hypertrophy

– Right axis deviation
▌ Echocardiogram

Management

Medical ▌ Diuretics
▌ Digoxin
▌ Anticoagulation for atrial fibrillation
Surgery ▌ For non-responsive or severe disease
▌ Balloon valvotomy
▌ Closed valvotomy
▌ Open valvotomy
▌ Mitral valve replacement

Complications

▌ Atrial fibrillation
▌ Systemic embolisation
▌ Pulmonary hypertension
▌ Pulmonary infarction
▌ Chest infections
▌ Tricuspid regurgitation
▌ Right ventricular failure

Mitral regurgitation (*K&C*, p. 820)
Aetiology

▌ Mitral valve prolapse
▌ Rheumatic fever
▌ Ischaemic heart disease
▌ Dilated cardiomyopathy
▌ Infective endocarditis

Clinical features

▌ Palpitations
▌ Exertional breathlessness
▌ Fatigue
▌ Cardiac failure
▌ Apex (laterally displaced, hyperdynamic, systolic thrill)

Heart sounds

▌ Soft first heart sound
▌ Loud pansystolic murmur at apex radiating to axilla
▌ Third heart sound
▌ Signs of cardiac failure

Investigations

▌ Chest X-ray
▌ Echocardiography
▌ Cardiac catheterisation

Management

- Surgery (valve replacement)
- Symptomatic
  - ACE inhibitors, diuretics

Aortic stenosis (*K&C*, p. 822)
Aetiology

- Congenital
- Rheumatic fever
- Calcific

Clinical features

- Often no symptoms
- Exercise-induced angina, syncope, breathlessness
- Sudden death
- Small-volume slow-rising pulse
- Sustained apex beat
- Systolic thrill in aortic area

Heart sounds

- Ejection murmur in aortic area radiating to carotids
- Ejection click
- Soft second heart sound
- Fourth heart sound

Investigations

- ECG – left ventricular hypertrophy/strain

Management

- Avoid exercise
- Avoid vasodilators
- β-blockers for angina
- Surgery – aortic valve replacement

Aortic regurgitation (*K&C*, p. 824)
Aetiology

- Rheumatic fever
- Marfan's syndrome
- Syphilitic aortitis
- Connective tissue disorders
- Aortic dissection
- Hypertension

Clinical features

- No symptoms
- Palpitations

- Angina
- Left ventricular failure
- Collapsing pulse
- Pistol shot femorals
- Wide pulse pressure

Heart sounds

- Apex (displaced, diffuse, hyperdynamic)
- Soft high-pitched early diastolic murmur at left sternal edge
- Maybe systolic aortic flow murmur
- Visible carotid or head nodding

Management

- Medical – treat heart failure
- Surgery – valve replacement

Tricuspid regurgitation (*K&C*, p. 826)
Aetiology

- Infective endocarditis in intravenous drug users
- Chronic lung disease
- Pulmonary hypertension
- Dilatation of right ventricle
- Carcinoid syndrome

Clinical features

- Exertional breathlessness
- Gastrointestinal upset secondary to congestion
- Elevated JVP with giant v wave
- Enlarged pulsatile liver
- Peripheral oedema
- Ascites
- Pleural effusions
- Right ventricular impulse at left sternal edge

Heart sounds

- Pansystolic murmur at lower left sternal edge, louder in inspiration

Management

- Medical – treat right ventricular failure
- Surgical valve resection – for infective endocarditis
- Valve surgery
- Valve repair
  - Maintains anatomy of heart muscle
  - Avoids anticoagulation

ISCHAEMIC HEART DISEASE (K&C, P. 798)

Aetiology

- Occlusive coronary artery disease
- Atheroma
- Thrombosis
- Spasm

Risk factors for coronary artery disease

- Age
- Male sex
- Family history
- Hyperlipidaemia
- Smoking
- Hypertension
- Diabetes mellitus
- COX 2 inhibitors

Angina (K&C, p. 803)
Clinical features

- Chest pain – heavy, tight, gripping
- Central, radiates to arms and jaw ⎫
- Breathlessness ⎬ Exertional — relieved by rest
- Usually no signs ⎭

Investigations

- Resting ECG (normal or signs of previous MI)
- Exercise ECG (ST depression > 1 mm during exercise which reverts to normal – Fig. 9.9)
- Thallium scan
- Coronary angiography and intervention

Management

- Eliminate risk factors
  - Patient should stop smoking
  - Treat hypertension
  - Optimise diabetes treatment
  - Treat hyperlipidaemia
- Aspirin
- Nitrates, e.g. glyceryl trinitrate (GTN), isosorbide mononitrate
- β-blockers, e.g. atenolol
- Calcium channel blockers, e.g. amlodipine
- Potassium channel blockers, e.g. nicorandil

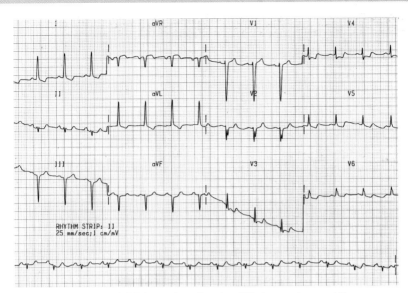

Fig. 9.9 Twelve-lead ECG in angina showing ST depression and T wave inversion.

■ Revascularisation
- Percutaneous transluminal coronary angioplasty (PTCA)
- Intracoronary stents
- Coronary artery bypass grafting (CABG)

Acute coronary syndrome (see box) (*K&C*, p. 808)

■ NSTEMI – non ST elevation myocardial infarction
■ STEMI – ST elevation myocardial infarction
■ unstable angina

Aetiology

■ Coronary atheroma

Clinical features

■ Chest pain
- Severe
- Sudden onset at rest
- Persists several hours
■ 'Silent' in 20%
■ Sweating
■ Breathlessness
■ Nausea and vomiting

BOX 9.6 ACS – NSTEMI AND UNSTABLE ANGINA

Clinical features
Pain at rest
'Crescendo' angina

Management
Admission for bed rest with cardiac monitoring
High-flow oxygen
Aspirin 300 mg chewed stat then 75–150 mg daily

Pain relief
Diamorphine 2.5–5 mg i.v. (plus antiemetic)
Heparin
Low molecular weight heparin subcutaneously to full
anticoagulant dose, e.g. enoxaparin 1 mg/kg/day

Standard medical anti-anginal therapy
β-blockers unless contraindicated
Atenolol 50 mg orally
Nitrates
GTN i.v. infusion titrated to pain
Isosorbide mononitrate 60 mg orally daily
Consider – glycoprotein IIb/IIIa receptor inhibitors
Prompt angiography and revascularisation

▮ Patient is pale, sweaty and grey
▮ Tachycardia
▮ Heart failure
▮ hypotension

Investigations

ECG ▮ See Figs 9.10–9.12 and Table 9.7
Cardiac enzymes ▮ Creatine kinase (CK) peaks 24 hours after ACS
▮ Cardiac-specific troponins (very high specificity for myocardial ischaemia) rise early (max at 12 hours, also raised in unstable angina)
▮ Aspartate aminotransferase (AST) and lactate dehydrogenase (LDH) rise 2–5 days after MI

Assessment of infarct site
▮ See Table 9.8

Acute management
▮ See information box

Aftercare
Ongoing pain ▮ I.v. β-blocker or nitrate
after thrombolysis ▮ Emergency angiography and revascularisation

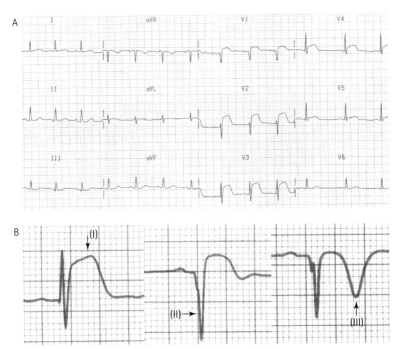

Fig. 9.10 Myocardial infarction. A. Twelve-lead ECG showing full-thickness anterior MI with S–T elevation (STEMI). B. Progressive ECG changes with time during an acute STEMI. ST elevation (i); Q waves (ii); T inversion (iii).

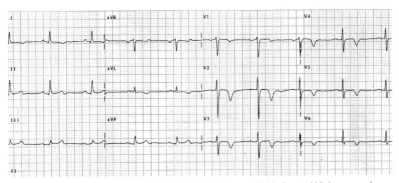

Fig. 9.11 Twelve-lead ECG showing subendocardial infarct. Widespread T wave inversion, no Q waves (NSTEMI).

Pain-free with signs of heart failure	▮ Nitrate +/− diuretic ▮ ACE inhibitor long-term
Pain-free with no complications	▮ β-blocker long-term ▮ Return to work in 2–3 months

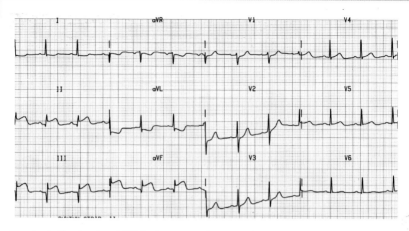

Fig. 9.12 Twelve-lead ECG showing inferior MI (S–T elevation) (STEMI).

Table 9.7 Typical ECG changes in acute MI

STEMI	NSTEMI
Q waves	No Q waves
>1 mm broad and 2 mm deep	Deep ST depression
Negative deflection at start of QRS complex	T wave inversion
Normal in AVR and V_1	
ST elevation	
T wave inversion	

Table 9.8 Assessment of infarct site

Infarct site	Leads showing main changes
Anterior	V_2–V_5
Antero-septal	V_1–V_3
Antero-lateral	V_4–V_6, I and AVL
Lateral	I, II and AVL
Inferior	II, III and AVF
Posterior	V_1 and V_2 (reciprocal)
Subendocardial	Any

All patients
- Aspirin 75–150 mg/day
- β-blocker if no contraindications
- Statin
- Risk factor stratification
- Exercise ECG +/− angiography
- Structured rehabilitation
- No driving for 1 month

Complications

Early
- Arrhythmias
- Sudden death

BOX 9.7 ACUTE MANAGEMENT OF SUSPECTED MI

Clinical features
Chest pain
Sweating
Breathlessness
Vomiting
Pale, sweaty, grey

ECG
See Fig. 9.10

Immediate treatment
Fast Track through A&E
Continuous cardiac monitoring
Oxygen 60%
Diamorphine 2.5–5 mg i.v.
Metoclopramide 10 mg i.v.
Aspirin 300 mg chewed
Emergency primary PTCA or thrombolysis according to availability

No contraindications to thrombolysis
Aim for rapid 'door to needle time'
Streptokinase 1.5 million units i.v. over 1 hour
Or
Recombinant tissue plasminogen activator (rtPA) accelerated protocol

With contraindications to thrombolysis
Emergency primary PTCA

Follow up with
Coronary care and monitoring for 48 hours

I Pericarditis
I Cardiac failure
I Cardiogenic shock
I Ruptured papillary muscle or chordae tendinae
I Ventricular septal defect (VSD)
I Cardiac rupture

Late I Deep venous thrombosis (DVT), pulmonary embolism (PE)
I Mural thrombus
I Cardiac aneurysm
I Dressler's syndrome (fever, chest pain, pericarditis secondary to autoimmune carditis)

Sudden cardiac death
I See Figs 9.13 and 9.14

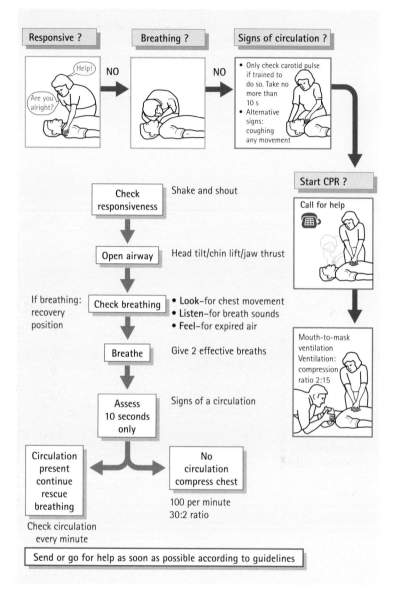

Fig. 9.13 Basic life support.

Prognosis

- 50% die acutely
- 6–7% die in hospital
- 20% die within 2 years
- 30 day mortality depending on other risk factors 1–35%

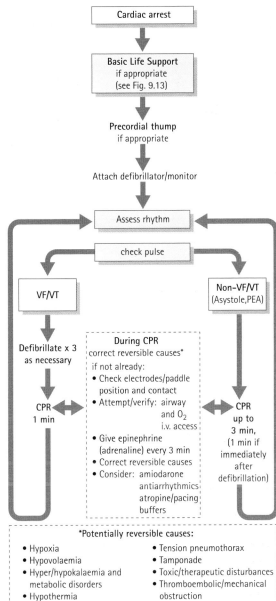

Fig. 9.14 Universal advanced life support algorithm. Reproduced by permission of the European Resuscitation Council and Laerdal Medical Ltd. CPR: Cardiopulmonary resuscitation. PEA: Pulseless electrical activity. VF/VT: Ventricular fibrillation/ Ventricular tachycardia.

The figure contains the following text:

Cardiac arrest

Basic Life Support
if appropriate
(see Fig. 9.13)

Precordial thump
if appropriate

Attach defibrillator/monitor

Assess rhythm

check pulse

VF/VT

Non–VF/VT
(Asystole, PEA)

Defibrillate x 3
as necessary

CPR
1 min

During CPR
correct reversible causes*
if not already:
- Check electrodes/paddle position and contact
- Attempt/verify: airway and O_2 i.v. access
- Give epinephrine (adrenaline) every 3 min
- Correct reversible causes
- Consider: amiodarone antiarrhythmics atropine/pacing buffers

CPR
up to
3 min,
(1 min if
immediately
after
defibrillation)

*Potentially reversible causes:
- Hypoxia
- Hypovolaemia
- Hyper/hypokalaemia and metabolic disorders
- Hypothermia
- Tension pneumothorax
- Tamponade
- Toxic/therapeutic disturbances
- Thromboembolic/mechanical obstruction

CARDIAC FAILURE (K&C, P. 784)

❚ Occurs when the heart is unable to maintain sufficient cardiac output to meet the demands of the body despite adequate venous filling pressures

BOX 9.8 ACUTE PULMONARY OEDEMA

Clinical features
Extreme breathlessness (often in middle of night)
Wheeze
Anxiety
Cold sweat
Cough with frothy pink sputum
Grey and/or cyanosed
Tachypnoea
Peripherally shut down and cold
Raised JVP
Gallop rhythm
Crackles and wheeze throughout chest
Hypotension

Immediate investigations
Chest X-ray – exclude pneumothorax
Arterial blood gases – low PO_2, $\pm$ high PCO_2
ECG – arrhythmia

Immediate management
Sit up
High-flow oxygen
I.v. furosemide (frusemide) 40–80 mg
I.v. diamorphine 2.5–5 mg (not if BP < 80 systolic)
I.v. metoclopramide 10 mg
I.v. GTN (if not hypotensive)
Nebulised salbutamol 2.5 mg if bronchospasm

Aetiology

▌ See Table 9.9

Left heart failure (*K&C*, p. 787)
Aetiology

▌ Ischaemic heart disease
▌ Hypertension
▌ Mitral valve and aortic valve disease
▌ Cardiomyopathy

Clinical features

▌ Fatigue
▌ Exertional breathlessness
▌ Orthopnoea
▌ Paroxysmal nocturnal dyspnoea (PND)
▌ Pulmonary oedema pink frothy sputum
▌ Distress

Table 9.9 Causes of cardiac failure

Myocardial dysfunction	High cardiac output
Ischaemic heart disease	Thyrotoxicosis
Cardiomyopathy	Anaemia
Hypertension	Paget's disease
	Left to right shunts
Volume overload	
Valve disease	**Compromised ventricular filling**
Fluid overload	Constrictive pericarditis
	Pericardial tamponade
Obstruction to flow	
Aortic stenosis	**Altered rhythm**
Chronic lung disease	Atrial fibrillation

- Tachycardia
- Enlarged heart
- Gallop rhythm (triple fast rhythm due to third or fourth heart sound)
- Fine crackles at lung bases

Right heart failure (*K&C*, p. 788)
Aetiology

- Chronic lung disease = cor pulmonale
- Pulmonary emboli
- Pulmonary hypertension
- Left to right shunts
- Tricuspid regurgitation

Clinical features

- Tiredness
- Anorexia, nausea
- Gastrointestinal upset
- Raised JVP
- Dependent pitting oedema
- Pleural effusions
- Hepatic enlargement
- Ascites
- Functional tricuspid regurgitation

Investigation and treatment of cardiac failure
(*K&C*, p. 789)
Investigations

- Chest X-ray
- ECG

221

■ Echocardiogram
  – Left ventricular ejection fraction < 45%
■ cardiac catheter and coronary angiography

Management

■ Identify and treat causes or aggravating factors
■ Drugs
  – Diuretics (spironolactone, furosemide)
  – ACE inhibitors (reduce mortality)
  – β-blockers (reduce mortality)
  – Digoxin
  – Nitrates
  – Anticoagulation
■ Surgery
  – CABG
  – Valve replacement
  – Pacemaker
  – Heart transplant

HYPERTENSION (*K&C*, P. 857)

■ See Fig. 9.15

Primary 'essential' hypertension
Aetiology

■ Genetic
■ Obesity
■ Alcohol
■ Sodium intake
■ Stress

Secondary hypertension
Aetiology

Renal   ■ Diabetic nephropathy
          ■ Renovascular disease
          ■ Adult polycystic disease
          ■ Chronic glomerulonephritis
Endocrine   ■ Conn's syndrome
              ■ Adrenal hyperplasia
              ■ Phaeochromocytoma
              ■ Cushing's syndrome
              ■ Acromegaly

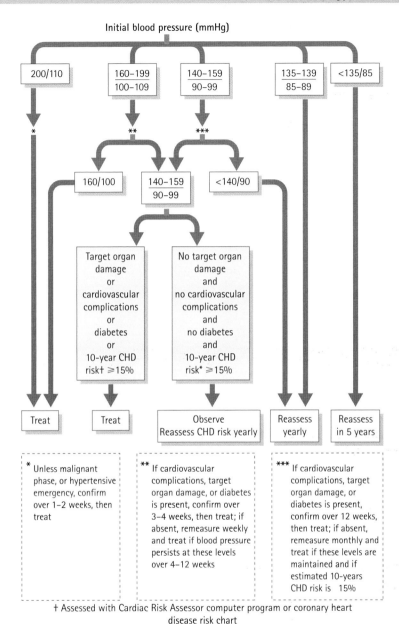

Fig. 9.15 Blood pressure thresholds and drug treatment in hypertension. From Ramsay LE *et al.* (1999) *British Medical Journal* 309: 630.

Cardiovascular Drugs	▌ Coarctation of the aorta
	▌ Oral contraceptive pill
	▌ Steroids
	▌ NSAIDS

Pregnancy
- Second half of pregnancy
- Pre-eclampsia
- Hypertension and proteinuria

Clinical features

- Usually no symptoms
- Features of underlying cause
- Headaches
- Nose bleeds
- Nocturia
- Complications (see below)
- Elevated blood pressure
- Renal artery bruit
- Radiofemoral delay (coarctation of the aorta)
- Left ventricular hypertrophy

Retinal changes

- Grade 1 – tortuosity of retinal arteries and 'silver wiring'
- Grade 2 – grade 1 plus arteriovenous nipping
- Grade 3 – grade 2 plus flame haemorrhages and soft 'cotton wool' exudates
- Grade 4 – grade 3 plus papilloedema

Investigations

- Chest X-ray
- ECG (left ventricular hypertrophy and strain)
- Echocardiogram (left ventricular hypertrophy)
- Urinalysis for casts, protein and red cells
- Fasting blood glucose and lipids
- Serum urea, creatinine and electrolytes

Complications

- Cerebrovascular disease
- Coronary artery disease
- Retinopathy
- Renal disease

Management
General measures
- Weight loss
- Alcohol reduction
- Salt restriction
- Exercise
- low fat diet
- reassess after 6 months

Drug therapy
- See Table 9.10

Table 9.10 Drug treatment of secondary hypertension

Class	Example	Side-effects
Thiazide diuretics	Bendroflumethiazide (bendrofluazide)	Hypokalaemia
β-blockers	Atenolol	Bronchospasm Nightmares Cold peripheries Erectile dysfunction
ACE inhibitors	Enalapril	Dry cough Profound first-dose hypotension Renal function deterioration
ACE II receptor antagonists	Losartan	
Calcium channel blockers	Amlodipine	Erectile dysfunction Hypotension
α-blockers	Doxazosin	Hypotension

Malignant hypertension (*K&C*, p. 859)
Clinical features

▌ Diastolic BP > 140 mmHg
▌ Progressive renal failure, proteinuria and haematuria
▌ Cerebral oedema or haemorrhage
▌ Grade 4 retinopathy
▌ Hypertensive encephalopathy

Management

▌ Aim to reduce diastolic BP to 100–110 mmHg over 24–48 hours
▌ Oral treatment is usual
▌ In urgent situations, e.g. aortic dissection
▌ i.v. sodium nitroprusside or β-blockers

CONGENITAL HEART DISEASE (*K&C*, P. 832)

▌ Affects 1% of live births

Disease associations

▌ Maternal rubella infection
▌ Maternal alcohol abuse

- Chromosomal abnormalities, e.g.
  - Down's syndrome
  - Turner's syndrome

Acyanotic – Left to right shunt (*K&C*, p. 834)

Ventricular septal defect (VSD)

- 1:500 live births

Clinical features

- Often no symptoms
- Fatigue
- Dyspnoea
- Loud pansystolic murmur at lower left sternal edge
- Thrill at lower left sternal edge
- Pulmonary hypertension

Management

- Antibiotic prophylaxis for procedures
- Surgical closure

Complications

- Pulmonary hypertension
- Reversal of shunt
- Eisenmenger's syndrome
  - Blood bypasses the lungs

Atrial septal defect (ASD)

Clinical features

- Usually none until adulthood
- Breathlessness
- Fatigue
- Right ventricular heave
- Loud pulmonary second sound
- Fixed splitting of second heart sound (A_2–P_2)
- Mid-diastolic murmur at left sternal edge

Management

- angiographic transcatheter closure
- Surgical closure

Complications

- Pulmonary hypertension

Persistent ductus arteriosus

- Continuous aorta to pulmonary artery shunt

Aetiology

- Idiopathic
- Prematurity

Clinical features

- Left heart failure
- Congestive heart failure
- Infective endocarditis
- Continuous 'machinery' murmur

Management

- Surgical closure
- Angiographic ligation
- Aspirin
- indomethacin in premature infants

Cyanotic – right to left shunt

Fallot's tetralogy (*K&C*, p. 838)

- VSD
- Overriding aorta
- Right ventricular outflow obstruction
- Right ventricular hypertrophy

Clinical features

- Breathlessness
- Fatigue
- Hypoxia on exertion – cyanosis +/− syncope
- Squatting – to improve venous return and reduce shunt
- Right parasternal heave
- Systolic ejection murmur
- Central cyanosis
- Finger clubbing
- Polycythaemia

Management

- Surgical correction
- Antibiotic prophylaxis

Eisenmenger's syndrome

- Reversal of shunt in large VSD due to secondary pulmonary hypertension giving right to left shunt and cyanosis

No shunt

Coarctation of the aorta (*K&C*, p. 837)

- ♂ > ♀
- Turner's syndrome
- Associated with bicuspid aortic valve and aortic stenosis

Clinical features

- Hypertension in upper limbs
- Radiofemoral delay
- Mid to late systolic murmur over the back

Investigations

- CXR
  - Dilated aorta
  - Rib notching (due to large collateral arteries eroding ribs)

Management

- Surgical excision

INFLAMMATORY AND INFECTIVE DISEASES OF THE HEART

Acute pericarditis (*K&C*, p. 854)
Aetiology

- Viral (Coxsackie virus)
- Post-MI (acute in 20% of full-thickness anterior MI)
- Dressler's syndrome (type 3 hypersensitivity about 3 weeks after MI)
- Uraemic
- Tuberculous
- Malignant

Clinical features

- Chest pain
  - Substernal
  - Sharp
  - Worse on breathing
  - Relieved by sitting forward
  - Worse on lying flat
- Fever
- Malaise
- Pericardial friction rub (sounds like 'walking on snow')

Investigations

▌ ECG (widespread 'saddle-shaped' ST elevation)

Management

▌ Anti-inflammatory drugs
▌ Rest
▌ Treat underlying cause
▌ 20% recur

Pericardial effusion (*K&C*, p. 855)
Aetiology

Acute ▌ MI with ventricular rupture
▌ Aortic dissection
▌ Post cardiac surgery
▌ Post transeptal puncture at cardiac catheterisation

Sub acute and ▌ Metastatic malignant disease
chronic ▌ Tuberculous pericarditis
▌ Dressler's syndrome

Clinical features

▌ Raised JVP
▌ Kussmaul's sign (JVP elevates during inspiration)
▌ Pulsus paradoxus
▌ Failure to locate apex beat
▌ Quiet heart sounds

Investigations

▌ ECG (low-voltage complexes)
▌ Chest X-ray (large globular heart)
▌ Echocardiogram
▌ Pericardiocentesis for diagnosis and to treat incipient tamponade

Myocarditis (*K&C*, p. 847)
Aetiology

▌ Viral
  – Coxsackie
  – Influenza
  – Rubella
  – Polio
▌ Protozoal
  – *Trypanosoma cruzi* (Chagas disease)
  – *Toxoplasma gondii*
▌ Toxins
  – Lead poisoning
  – Radiation injury

- Bacterial infection
  - Diphtheria
  - Q fever
  - *Coxiella burneti*
- Autoimmune disease

Clinical features

- Acute cardiac failure
- Fever

Investigations

- Chest X-ray
- ECG
  - ST and T wave abnormalities
  - Arrhythmias
- Cardiac enzymes elevated
- Echocardiography
- Endomyocardial biopsy
- Viral antibody titres

Management

- Treat heart failure
- Treat underlying cause

Rheumatic fever (*K&C*, p. 76)
Aetiology

- Group A streptococcal infection

Clinical features (Table 9.11)

- General
  - Fever
  - Malaise
- Carditis
  - New or changing murmurs
  - Cardiac failure
  - Pericardial effusion
- Arthritis
  - Fleeting polyarthritis of large joints
- Sydenham's chorea (St Vitus' dance)
  - Choreoathetoid movements
- Skin
  - Erythema marginatum
  - Subcutaneous nodules (painless)

Investigations

- Throat swab
- Antistreptolysin-O titre

Table 9.11 Duckett Jones diagnostic criteria in rheumatic fever

Two or more major *or* one major *plus* two or more minor *plus* evidence of recent streptococcal infection

Major	Minor
Carditis	Fever
Polyarthritis	Arthralgia
Chorea	Previous rheumatic fever
Erythema marginatum	Raised erythrocyte sedimentation rate (ESR)/
Subcutaneous nodules	C-reactive protein (CRP)
	Raised white cell count
	Prolonged PR interval

∎ ESR
∎ CRP

Management

∎ Penicillin to eradicate streptococci
∎ Bed rest
∎ High-dose aspirin
∎ Corticosteroids (prednisolone 60–120 mg/day)

Infective endocarditis (*K&C*, p.828)

∎ Most commonly affects rheumatic or congenitally abnormal valves, VSD or patent ductus
∎ Prosthetic valves may also be affected

Aetiology

∎ Streptococcus viridans (50% of cases)
∎ *Enterococcus faecalis*
∎ *Staphylococcus aureus*
 – Often acute
 – Associated with central venous catheters, temporary pacing wires and in i.v. drug users
 – Poor prognosis
∎ *Staphylococcus epidermidis*
 – I.v. drug users
 – Alcoholics
∎ *Coxiella burneti* (Q fever)

Clinical features

∎ (*Seen in > 50% of cases)
∎ General
 – Malaise*
 – Clubbing

- Cardiac
  - Murmurs*
  - Cardiac failure*
- Arthralgia
- Pyrexia*
- Skin lesions
  - Osler's nodes
  - Splinter haemorrhages
  - Janeway lesions
  - Petechiae*
- Eyes
  - Roth spots
- Splenomegaly
- Neurological (cerebral emboli)
  - Mycotic aneurysm
  - Renal (haematuria*)

Investigations

Blood	- Anaemia
	- Raised serum CRP and ESR
	- Mildly abnormal liver biochemistry
	- Raised total serum immunoglobulins
	- Raised total complement and C3
Urinalysis	- Proteinuria with casts
	- Microscopic haematuria
Blood cultures	- At least six sets from different veins at different times (positive in 75% of cases)
Echocardiography	- Trans-oesophageal echocardiography (TOE) is best for visualizing vegetations and is mandatory in non-native valves

Management

Antibiotics	- Bactericidal antibiotics chosen on the basis of blood culture results and sensitivities
	- I.v. antibiotics for 2–6 weeks with back-titrations to confirm bactericidal serum levels
Indications for surgery	- Significant extensive valve damage
	- Early infection of prosthetic valve
	- Persistent infection with negative blood cultures
	- Embolisation
	- Progressive cardiac failure
	- Tricuspid valve infection in i.v. drug users
Prophylaxis	- See page 208

See page 208

CARDIAC ARRHYTHMIAS (K&C, P. 764)

- Bradycardia – heart rate <60 bpm
- Tachycardia – heart rate >100 bpm

Sinus arrhythmia

- Due to normal changes in autonomic tone
- Heart rate increases in inspiration and falls in expiration

Sinus bradycardia
Aetiology

- Hypothermia
- Hypothyroidism
- Raised intracranial pressure
- Drugs (β-blockers, digoxin)
- Ischaemia

Sinus tachycardia
Aetiology

- Fever
- Exertion
- Emotion
- Pregnancy
- Anaemia
- Cardiac failure
- Thyrotoxicosis
- Drugs (sympathomimetics)

Sinus node disease (sick sinus syndrome)
Aetiology

- Ischaemia
- Infarction
- Degenerative disease

Clinical features

- Combinations of fast and slow supraventricular rhythms

Investigations

- ECG – long interval between P waves > 2 seconds

Management

- Permanent pacemaker
- Antiarrhythmic drugs to combat tachycardia
- Anticoagulation

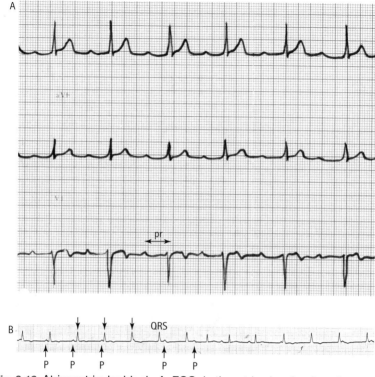

Fig. 9.16 Atrioventricular block. A. ECG rhythm strip showing first-degree heart block with prolongation of the PR interval. B. Complete heart block with dissociation of the P waves and QRS complexes.

Atrioventricular block (*K&C*, p. 767)
First-degree

■ Prolonged PR interval (Fig. 9.16)

Second-degree

■ Some P waves conduct to ventricles
■ Mobitz type 1 ('Wenckebach' – Fig. 9.17)
  – Progressive elongation of PR interval until failure to conduct
■ Mobitz type 2
  – Dropped QRS conduction without progressive PR elongation
■ 2:1 or 3:1 block
  – every second or third P wave conducts to ventricles (Fig. 9.18)

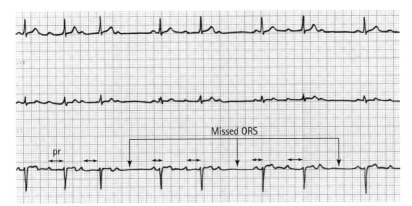

Fig. 9.17 ECG rhythm strip showing second-degree 'Wenckebach' heart block, with prolongation of the PR interval and missed QRS.

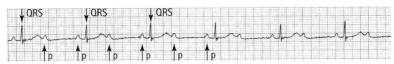

Fig. 9.18 ECG rhythm strip showing second-degree '2:1' heart block.

Third-degree (complete heart block)

■ No P waves conduct
■ Ventricular rhythm is maintained by spontaneous escape rhythm from ventricular myocardium with broad complexes

Aetiology

■ Ischaemic heart disease
■ Cardiac surgery
■ Dilated cardiomyopathy
■ Drugs

Clinical features

■ Maybe no symptoms (first- and second-degree)
■ Dizziness
■ Syncope
■ Blackouts (Stokes–Adams attacks) (third-degree)
■ Cannon 'a' waves in JVP in third-degree

Management

■ Permanent pacemaker for symptomatic bradycardias

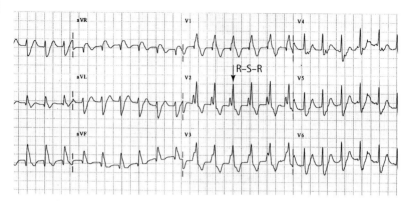

Fig. 9.19 Twelve-lead ECG showing right bundle branch block and right axis deviation.

Bundle branch block (*K&C*, p. 768)
Aetiology

Right bundle branch block (RBBB – Fig. 9.19)	∎ Congenital heart disease ∎ Cor pulmonale ∎ Pulmonary embolus ∎ Myocardial infarction ∎ Cardiomyopathy ∎ Hyperkalaemia ∎ Can be normal
Left bundle branch block (LBBB – Fig. 9.20)	∎ Aortic stenosis ∎ Hypertension ∎ Acute MI ∎ Severe coronary artery disease ∎ Cardiomyopathy

Management

∎ Permanent pacemaker for symptomatic cases

Atrial tachyarrhythmias (*K&C*, p. 773)
Aetiology

∎ Ischaemic heart disease
∎ Rheumatic heart disease
∎ Thyrotoxicosis
∎ Cardiomyopathy
∎ Wolff–Parkinson–White syndrome
∎ Pneumonia
∎ Atrial septal defect
∎ Pericarditis
∎ Pulmonary embolus

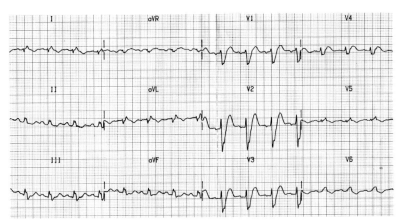

Fig. 9.20 Twelve-lead ECG showing left bundle branch block.

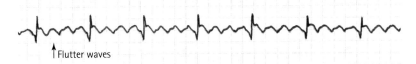

Fig. 9.21 ECG rhythm strip showing atrial flutter.

Atrial flutter

▌ Atrial rate about 300/min with 2:1 or 3:1 AV conduction

Investigations

▌ ECG (Fig. 9.21) – sawtooth atrial flutter waves between QRS complexes

Management

▌ Electrical cardioversion
▌ Class III antiarrhythmic drugs
▌ Radiofrequency catheter ablation

Atrial fibrillation

▌ Uncoordinated rapid continuous activation of atria from multiple foci

Aetiology

▌ See above

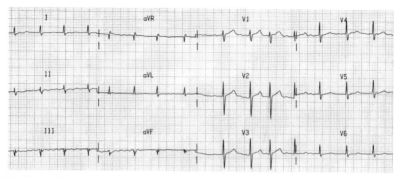

Fig. 9.22 Twelve-lead ECG showing atrial fibrillation with controlled ventricular rate (no P waves).

Clinical features

▌ No symptoms
▌ Reduced exercise tolerance
▌ Palpitations
▌ Heart failure
▌ Embolic events
▌ Completely irregular pulse

Investigations

▌ ECG (Fig. 9.22)
  – No p waves
  – Irregular rapid QRS rhythm

Management

▌ Treat the cause
▌ Control ventricular rate
  – β-blockers
  – Digoxin
  – Verapamil
▌ Cardioversion
  – Electrical DC cardioversion
  – Drugs (amiodarone, flecainide)
▌ Prophylaxis against thrombotic events
  – Warfarin
▌ AV node ablation and permanent pacemaker insertion

Supraventricular tachycardia (*K&C*, p. 770)

▌ AV junctional tachycardias

Aetiology

▌ Provoked by
  – Exertion

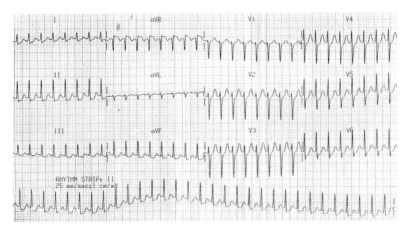

Fig. 9.23 Supraventricular tachycardia.

- Caffeine
- Alcohol
- β_2-agonists

▍ Congenital
- Wolff–Parkinson–White syndrome
- Lown–Ganong–Levine syndrome

Clinical features

▍ Palpitations
▍ Chest pain
▍ Breathlessness
▍ Syncope
▍ Polyuria
▍ Rapid regular pulse 140–280/min

Investigations (Fig. 9.23)

▍ ECG
- Narrow complex QRS tachycardia
- Occasionally broad complex when associated with interventricular conductance disturbances

Management (Fig. 9.24)

▍ Vagotonic manoeuvres
▍ Carotid sinus massage
▍ Ocular pressure
▍ Valsalva manoeuvre
▍ Drugs

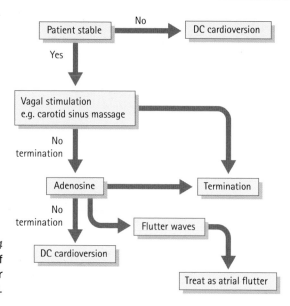

Fig. 9.24
Management of
supraventricular
tachycardia.

      – Adenosine in increasing i.v. doses with
        continuous rhythm monitoring (avoid in
        asthma)
▌ Prophylaxis
▌ Accessory pathway ablation

Ventricular tachyarrhythmias (*K&C*, p. 776)

Sustained ventricular tachycardia
▌ Rapid ventricular rhythm at 120/min for more
than 30 sec

Clinical features
▌ Palpitations
▌ Dizziness
▌ Syncope
▌ Angina

Investigations (Fig. 9.25)
▌ ECG – broad complex tachycardia

Acute management
▌ See Fig. 9.26

Long term management
▌ Drugs – class III antiarrhythmics
▌ Accessory pathway ablation
▌ Implantable cardioverter defribrillator = ICD

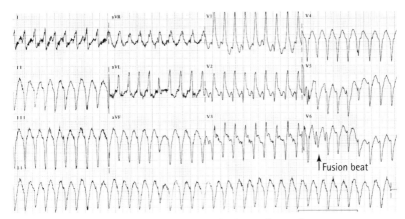

Fig. 9.25 Twelve-lead ECG showing ventricular tachycardia.

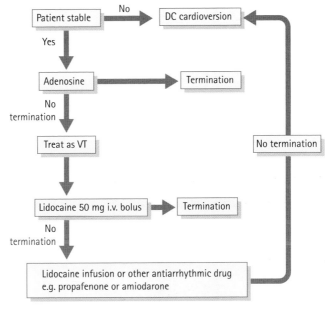

Fig. 9.26 Management of broad complex tachycardia.

Torsades de pointes
Causes

- Congenital long QT
- Electrolyte disturbances
- Drugs

Investigations

- ECG VT with alternating polarity
- Prolonged QT

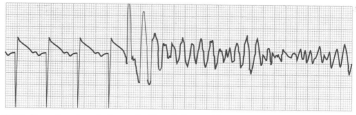

Fig. 9.27 Four beats of sinus rhythm followed by a ventricular ectopic beat that initiates ventricular fibrillation. The ST segment during sinus rhythm is elevated owing to acute MI in this case.

Management

▮ ICD

Ventricular fibrillation

▮ See Fig. 9.27
▮ Pulseless rapid irregular ventricular activity with no mechanical effect

BEST ONE OF FIVE QUESTIONS

Multiple choice questions

1. The following are features of aortic stenosis:
   A. Collapsing pulse
   B. Pan-systolic murmur
   C. Syncope on exertion
   D. Austin flint murmur
   E. Opening snap

2. The following are features of mitral stenosis:
   A. Atrial fibrillation
   B. Tapping apex beat
   C. Pulmonary hypertension
   D. Right axis deviation on ECG
   E. All of the above

3. In mitral regurgitation:
   A. The pulse is characteristically collapsing
   B. There is an apical pansystolic murmur radiating to the axilla
   C. The ECG shows left ventricular hypertrophy
   D. The commonest cause is hypertension
   E. Atrial fibrillation is uncommon

4. In tricuspid regurgitation:
   A. There is a pansystolic murmur radiating to the axilla
   B. Pulmonary hypertension is a cause
   C. There may be pulsatile splenomegaly
   D. Cannon waves are seen in the jugular venous pulse
   E. Complete heart block is common

5. In acute myocardial infarction:
   A. The ECG always shows raised ST segments
   B. The pain is characteristically left-sided and worse on inspiration
   C. Diamorphine is contraindicated
   D. Creatine kinase levels are maximally elevated 2–4 hours after the onset of pain
   E. Treatment with streptokinase reduces mortality

6. The following are signs of congestive cardiac failure:
   A. Raised jugular venous pressure
   B. Splinter haemorrhages
   C. Splenomegaly
   D. Papilloedema
   E. All of the above

7. In unstable angina:
   A. The most common heart rhythm is atrial fibrillation
   B. The ECG shows ST depression and T wave inversion
   C. Creatine kinase is elevated
   D. Treatment of choice is anticoagulation with warfarin
   E. Thirty-day mortality is 50%

8. In systemic hypertension:
   A. The commonest cause is renal artery stenosis
   B. Complications include diabetes mellitus
   C. Effective treatment reduces the incidence of stroke
   D. Presents most commonly with headache
   E. The first-line treatment is methyldopa

9. The following are usual features of tetralogy of Fallot:
   A. Episodes of cyanosis
   B. Atrial septal defect
   C. Ebstein's anomaly
   D. Normal life expectancy
   E. Right ventricular dilatation

10. The following are features of acute rheumatic fever:
    A. Recent staphlococcal throat infection
    B. Clubbing
    C. Roth spots
    D. Sydenham's chorea
    E. Osler's nodes

11. In acute pericarditis:
    A. The chest pain is characteristically crushing and radiates down the right arm
    B. The ECG shows widespread concave ST elevation
    C. There is usually pulsus paradoxus
    D. Viral infections are an uncommon cause
    E. High-dose prednisolone is the treatment of choice

12. The following are features of infective endocarditis:
    A. Spider naevi
    B. Osler's nodes
    C. Huntingdon's chorea
    D. Jaundice
    E. Past history of pulmonary TB

13. In patients with atrial fibrillation:
    A. The cardiac rhythm becomes more regular with exertion
    B. Common causes include rheumatoid arthritis and obstructive jaundice
    C. A fourth heart sound is always absent

D. Digoxin should always be given
E. Complications include stroke and mesenteric infarction

14. In supraventricular tachycardia:
    A. The onset is characteristically sudden
    B. The QT interval is prolonged
    C. Carotid sinus massage causes the heart rate to accelerate
    D. First-line treatment is atropine
    E. There is often underlying heart disease

15. The following are features of complete heart block:
    A. Syncopal attacks
    B. Giant V waves in the jugular venous pulse
    C. A delta wave on ECG
    D. It responds to an atrial pacemaker
    E. All of the above

Extended matching questions

Question 1 Theme: central chest pain
A. Reflux oesophagitis
B. Angina
C. Acute coronary syndrome
D. Dissecting thoracic aortic aneurysm
E. Mitral valve prolapse
F. Costochondritis
G. Gallstones
H. Duodenal ulcer
I. Pneumothorax
J. Mesothelioma
K. Pulmonary embolus

For each of the following questions, select the best answer from the list above:

I. A 20-year-old male with Marfan's syndrome presents with severe chest pain at rest associated with nausea and shortness of breath. Blood pressure is decreased in the right arm compared with the left arm. What is the most likely diagnosis?

II. A 55-year-old male smoker with diabetes presents with a history of self-limiting central chest pain lasting 2 minutes, associated with nausea and shortness of breath which starts every time he plays football with his grandson. What is the most likely diagnosis?

III. A 45-year-old obese female smoker presents with episodic burning chest pain, worse at night and after spicy foods. What is the most likely diagnosis?

Question 2 Theme: ankle swelling

A. Left ventricular failure
B. Cardiomyopathy
C. Deep venous thrombosis
D. Nephrotic syndrome
E. Cellulitis
F. Ruptured Baker's cyst
G. Liver failure
H. Gout
I. Charcot's joints

For each of the following questions, select the best answer from the list above:

I. A 60-year-old male alcoholic present with a 3-month history of swelling of the abdomen and ankles, and shortness of breath on exertion. On examination there are no signs of chronic liver disease. His pulse is 120/minute with atrial fibrillation and the apex beat is displaced laterally and inferiorly; he has ascites and ankle oedema. What is the most likely diagnosis?

II. A 70-year-old female with a history of myocardial infarction 10 years ago, and who returned from Australia 1 week ago, presents with swollen ankles, worse on the right, and shortness of breath on exertion. What is the most likely diagnosis?

III. A 50-year-old diabetic female on enalapril presents with a painful swollen right ankle which started 10 days ago. Examination reveals erythema and oedema, with a small painless ulcer on the right heel. What is the most likely diagnosis?

Question 3 Theme: palpitations

A. Supraventricular tachycardia
B. Atrial fibrillation
C. Wolff–Parkinson–White syndrome
D. Anxiety
E. Thyrotoxicosis
F. Hypertension
G. Stokes–Adams attacks
H. Digoxin toxicity
I. β_2-agonists
J. Cocaine abuse

For each of the following questions, select the best answer from the list above:

I. A 69-year-old female smoker being investigated for chest pains presents with sudden onset of rapid palpitations associated with dizziness and shortness of breath. Her pulse is irregular, rate 160/minute, and BP is 90/60. The ECG shows no P waves. What is the most likely diagnosis?

II. A 68-year-old female recently saw her GP for wheeze and shortness of breath, and was prescribed some treatment. She now presents with episodes of dizziness, palpitations and tremor. On examination her pulse is regular, 130/min. The ECG shows a sinus tachycardia. What is the most likely diagnosis?

III. A 22-year-old law student presents with intermittent episodes of palpitations, shortness of breath and tingling in his fingers and round his lips. Examination is normal. Thyroid function tests a year ago (for similar symptoms) were normal. What is the most likely diagnosis?

Gastroenterology and hepatology 10

I For a more detailed description, see Kumar and Clark, *Clinical Medicine*, 6th edn. Chapters 6 & 7

The gastrointestinal tract, liver and pancreas have multiple functions:

Nutrition

- Processing of dietary components
- Nutrient absorption
- Water homeostasis

Endocrinology

- Control of blood glucose
- Steroid hormone metabolism

Detoxification

- Waste products of metabolism
- Chemical processing (e.g. drugs)
- Non-digestible dietary components

Storage

- Glycogen
- Vitamin B_{12}

Immunological

- Lymphoreticular (liver)
- Innate (barrier) immunity
- Cellular immunity (Peyer's patches)

Synthetic

- Proteins, lipids
- E.g. coagulation factors, albumin

EXAMINING THE ABDOMEN (K&C, P. 267)

Examination should include all of the following and be done in this order:

Expose the abdomen

▌ Xiphisternum to the suprapubic area
▌ Maintaining the dignity of the patient is vital

Look for

▌ Jaundice (Table 10.1)
▌ Weight loss/malnutrition
▌ Stigmata of chronic liver disease (Table 10.2)
▌ Shape of the abdomen and signs of distension

Table 10.1 Causes of jaundice

Pre-hepatic	Haemolysis	Autoimmune haemolytic anaemia
		Malaria
Hepatic	Abnormal bilirubin metabolism	Gilbert's syndrome and others
	Hepatocellular dysfunction	Viral hepatitis
		Drugs/alcohol
Post-hepatic	Cholestasis	Primary biliary cirrhosis
	Biliary obstruction	Sclerosing cholangitis
		Gallstones
		Pancreatic carcinoma

Table 10.2 Stigmata of chronic liver disease

Skin	Abdomen
Jaundice	Ascites
Spider naevi	Hepatomegaly
Caput medusae	Splenomegaly
Distended abdominal veins	
Bruising	**Eyes**
Striae	Anaemia
	Jaundice
Hands	
Liver flap	**Mouth**
Leuconychia	Fetor hepaticus
Dupuytrens contractures	Bleeding gums
Palmar erythema	
Clubbing	
Muscle wasting	

■ Stomas
  – Bowel: ileostomy or colostomy
  – Urinary: ileal conduit
■ Operation scars

Hands

■ Anaemia
■ Clubbing
■ Palmar erythema
■ Dupuytren's contractures
■ Liver flap
  Koilonychia – iron deficiency anaemia – concave nails
■ Leuconychia – hypoalbuminaemia – white nails

Face

■ Anaemia
■ Jaundice
■ Fetor hepaticus
■ Spider naevi

Thorax

■ Spider naevi – demonstrate filling from the central arteriole by pressing in the centre
  – >5 in men or 7 in women pathological
■ Lymphadenopathy – supraclavicular fossae (a node in the left fossa may indicate oesophageal or gastric cancer)

Abdomen

■ Obvious masses
■ Visible peristalsis
■ Scratch marks due to obstructive jaundice
■ Stretch marks
■ Caput medusae – distended abdominal veins radiating from umbilicus
■ Scars
■ Hernias (periumbilical, inguinal and femoral)

Palpation

■ Ask if the abdomen is tender and, if so, where
■ Start palpating away from this point
■ Start gently, with the flat of the fingers, eliciting tenderness and obvious masses

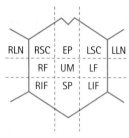

Fig. 10.1 Anatomical regions of the abdomen. EP: Epigastrium. SC: Subcostal. LN: Loin. UM: Umbilical. F: Flank. SP: Suprapubic. IF: Iliac fossa.

Table 10.3 Causes of hepatomegaly	
Infective	**Metabolic**
Acute viral hepatitis	Haemochromatosis
Epstein–Barr virus	
Malaria	
Kala-azar	**Malignant**
	Hepatocellular cancer
	Chronic leukaemia
Inflammatory	Secondary malignancy
Alcoholic liver disease	
Primary biliary cirrhosis	
Infiltration	**Cardiovascular**
Amyloid fat	Right ventricular failure
	Tricuspid regurgitation

▌ Then palpate more deeply in an ordered way around the abdomen looking for deep masses
▌ Describe the location of findings as per the regions shown in Fig. 10.1

Liver (Tables 10.3 and 10.4)

▌ The normal liver is only just palpable in slim people on inspiration
▌ Start from the right inguinal ligament
▌ Use the pulps of the finger or the side of the index finger (with the hand flat)
▌ Ask the patient to take deep breaths in and out
▌ As the patient breathes in, the diaphragm flattens, pushing the liver down on to your fingers. Note the position of the lowest palpable point
▌ The upper limit is defined by percussing in the mid-clavicular line from the nipple and noting the boundary between resonance and dullness (normally the sixth intercostal space)
▌ Note any tenderness or palpable texture

Table 10.4 Causes of hepatosplenomegaly

Hepatic Chronic liver disease with portal hypertension	**Infection** Viral hepatitis Epstein–Barr infection Schistosomiasis
Malignancy Leukaemia Lymphoma	**Infiltration** Amyloid Sarcoid

Table 10.5 Causes of splenomegaly

Malignancy Myelofibrosis Lymphoma Chronic myeloid leukaemia	**Infective** Malaria Kala-azar EBV
Infiltration Gaucher's disease Amyloid	**Chronic liver disease** Portal hypertension

Table 10.6 Causes of enlarged kidneys

Bilateral	**Unilateral**
Polycystic kidney disease	Renal carcinoma
Hydronephrosis	Hydronephrosis
Amyloid	Large renal cyst

Spleen (Tables 10.4 and 10.5)

▌ Start from the right inguinal region
▌ Palpate towards the left hypochondrium
▌ The normal spleen is not palpable
▌ Ask the patient to roll on to his or her right side to bring the spleen forward, making it easier to feel
▌ You will not be able to feel the upper margin
▌ You may just feel the splenic notch in the anterior aspect and the spleen is dull to percussion

Kidneys (Table 10.6)

▌ Place your hand under the loin just below the level of the costal margin
▌ Use this hand to push the kidney up towards your other hand (balloting)

Table 10.7 Causes of ascites

Hepatic	Hypoalbuminaemia
Chronic liver disease	Nephrotic syndrome
(Portal hypertension)	Protein-losing enteropathy
	Protein malnutrition
Peritoneal	
Peritoneal malignancy	**Vascular**
	Hepatic vein thrombosis
Infection	Budd-Chiari syndrome
Tuberculosis	

▌ If you are able to feel the kidney, just below the hypochondrium, it is enlarged

▌ You should be able to feel the upper pole of an enlarged kidney

▌ Always check for a transplanted kidney, usually in the right iliac fossa

▌ Check for an arteriovenous fistula (for haemodialysis) on the forearm

Ascites (Table 10.7)

▌ Eliciting shifting dullness is the easiest and most appropriate test

Shifting dullness

▌ Percuss the abdomen from the umbilicus laterally until the boundary between resonance and dullness is apparent

▌ Position your hand so that this boundary is between the middle and ring fingers of your splayed hand

▌ Ask the patient to roll towards you keeping your hand on the abdomen

▌ Allow the fluid to settle (at least 15–20 seconds), then percuss again to demonstrate that the boundary has moved

Fluid thrill

▌ (Do not do this in an exam unless asked to by the examiner)

▌ Ask the examiner or the patient to place the lateral aspect of his or her hand firmly on the abdomen in the midline, then flick or tap the lateral aspect of the abdomen with one hand

I The other hand is placed on the opposite side to detect the vibration

Hernial orifices

I Palpate the hernial orifices
I Ask the patient to cough and feel for an impulse
I Repeat with the patient standing

Tell the examiner

I That you would like to examine the genitalia and carry out a rectal exam

GASTROINTESTINAL INVESTIGATIONS
(*K&C*, P. 268)

Radiology

I See Chapter 5

Endoscopy

Gastroscopy

I Examines the oesophagus, stomach and parts one and two of the duodenum
I Allows macroscopic diagnosis
I Biopsies for histology
I Therapeutic procedures
  – Dilatation of strictures
  – Injection of bleeding ulcers

Endoscopic retrograde cholangiopancreatography (ERCP)

I Outlines the pancreatic duct and biliary tree

Stones

I Gallbladder or bile duct

Strictures

I Carcinoma of the pancreas
I Cholangiocarcinoma
I Sclerosing cholangitis

Stents

I Tubes inside the bile duct, used to bypass obstructions

Colonoscopy

I Examines the colon and terminal ileum

- Allows biopsies and therapeutic procedures, e.g. polypectomy
- Screening for colorectal cancer

Sigmoidoscopy

- Examines the rectum and sigmoid colon
- Investigation of rectal bleeding/symptoms

Proctoscopy

- Examines the anus
- Haemorrhoids
- Anal fissure

Enteroscopy

- Examines the stomach and proximal small bowel
- Allows biopsies and therapeutic procedures, e.g. polypectomy

Wireless capsule

- Swallowed capsule incorporating camera, light source and transmitter
- Allows for examination of entire small bowel mucosa
- Cannot be used to biopsy mucosa

Breath tests

^{13}C urea breath test

- Diagnosis of *Helicobacter pylori* infection
- Urea split by *H. pylori* $\rightarrow$ ammonia + $^{13}CO_2$
- $^{13}CO_2$ exhaled and detected in breath
- Sensitivity 98%; specificity 99%

H_2 breath test

- Diagnosis of bacterial overgrowth
- Lactulose meal
- Bacteria ferment carbohydrate, releasing hydrogen
- Breath hydrogen peaking at <2 hours indicates overgrowth

Stool tests

Microscopy and culture

- Infections

Faecal occult blood

▮ Screening for malignancy

Faecal elastase

▮ Pancreatic insufficiency

OESOPHAGEAL DISEASE

Hiatus hernia (Fig. 10.2) (*K&C*, p. 274)

▮ Herniation of the stomach into the thorax
▮ Sliding: gastro-oesophageal junction above diaphragm
▮ Rolling: fundus herniates beside oesophagus
▮ Disrupts lower oesophageal sphincter → gastro-oesophageal reflux

Clinical features

▮ Usually none
▮ Heartburn due to reflux

Management

▮ Treat reflux (see below)
▮ Surgery for large hernias/severe reflux

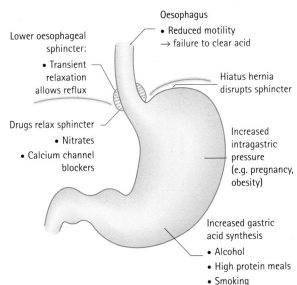

Oesophagus
• Reduced motility
→ failure to clear acid

Lower oesophageal sphincter:
• Transient relaxation allows reflux

Hiatus hernia disrupts sphincter

Drugs relax sphincter
• Nitrates
• Calcium channel blockers

Increased intragastric pressure (e.g. pregnancy, obesity)

Increased gastric acid synthesis
• Alcohol
• High protein meals
• Smoking

Fig. 10.2 Aetiology of gastro-oesophageal reflux disease.

Gastro-oesophageal reflux disease (GORD) (*K&C*, p. 275)

- Passage of gastric contents into the oesophagus due to relaxation of the lower oesophageal sphincter
- Acid or bile causes mucosal irritation

Aetiology (Fig. 10.2)

- Ineffective lower oesophageal sphincter
- Hiatus hernia
- Obesity
- Alcohol (increased acid secretion)
- Oesophageal dysmotility
- Pregnancy
- Drugs: nifedipine/isosorbide mononitrate

Clinical features

- Retrosternal burning pain (heartburn)
- Often during the night or when bending over
- Associated bitter taste in the mouth
- Sore throat/dysphonia
- Excessive salivation (water-brash)
- Nocturnal cough or bronchospasm (aspiration)
- Dysphagia (difficulty in swallowing)
- Peptic strictures

Investigations

- Trial of antacid/proton pump inhibitor
- Upper GI endoscopy
- Oesophageal pH studies & manometry

Management

- Lifestyle changes: reduce smoking/alcohol
- Lose weight
- Antacids
- Histamine$_2$-receptor blockers, e.g. ranitidine
- Proton Pump inhibitors, e.g. omeprazole
- (Laparoscopic) Nissen fundoplication

Complications

- Peptic oesophageal strictures
- Barrett's oesophagus
- Oesophageal adenocarcinoma

Barrett's oesophagus (*K&C*, p. 277)

- Columnar epithelium with intestinal metaplasia replaces normal squamous mucosa
- Increased risk of adenocarcinoma ($\male \gg \female$)

- Associated with gastro-oesophageal reflux
- Endoscopic screening of patients with Barrett's may reduce cancer mortality

Oesophageal carcinoma (*K&C*, p. 279)

- 40% squamous cell carcinomas
- 60% adenocarcinomas
- Prevalence: 10–15/100 000 and increasing

Clinical features

- Dysphagia
- Progressive: solids then liquids
- Weight loss
- Anorexia
- Virchow's node in supraclavicular fossa

Investigations

- Upper GI endoscopy and biopsy
- Endoscopic ultrasound
- CT to stage tumour ($\pm$PET)

Management

- 10% 5-year survival
- Squamous cell cancer
  - Radiotherapy $\pm$ chemotherapy
  - Surgery
- Adenocarcinoma
  - Surgery
  - Palliative or neo-adjuvant chemotherapy
- Palliation: oesophageal stents reduce dysphagia
- Thermal ablation (endoscopically)
- Radiotherapy

Achalasia (*K&C*, p. 277)

- Rare: 1/100 000/year
- Failure of relaxation of lower oesophageal sphincter
- $\rightarrow$ Dysphagia (intermittent to solids and liquids)

Investigations

- Barium swallow – rat's tail appearance
- Endoscopy – to exclude malignancy
- Oesophageal manometry
  - Measurement of sphincter pressure (raised, non-relaxing)
  - Aperistalsis or non-propulsive contractions

Management

- Endoscopic balloon dilatation of sphincter
- Injection of Botulinum toxin into sphincter
- Surgery (Heller's procedure: division of muscle)

THE STOMACH

Dyspepsia

- Symptoms referable to the upper gastrointestinal tract

Epidemiology

- 75–90% of population get symptoms
- 4% of all GP consultations

Aetiology

- Non-ulcer (functional) dyspepsia
- GORD
- Gastritis (NSAIDs, *H. pylori*, bile)
- Peptic ulcer disease
- Gastric malignancy

Clinical features

- Heartburn
- Epigastric pain
- Pain, discomfort or 'fullness' after eating
- Nausea
- Bloating

Alarm signals

- Weight loss
- Vomiting
- Haematemesis, melaena or anaemia
- Dysphagia
- Previous gastric ulcer or gastric surgery
- Non-steroidal anti-inflammatory drugs (NSAIDs)

Investigations

- ^{13}C urea breath test for *H. pylori*
- *H. pylori* serology
- Upper GI endoscopy if over 45 years old

Management

- Depends on cause
- Consider a trial of proton pump inhibitors if no alarm signals and age <50

Peptic ulceration (*K&C*, p. 284)

▌ Breaches in the mucosa in the stomach or duodenum

Aetiology

▌ Gastric ulcers
  – *H. pylori* (60%)
  – NSAIDs
  – Adenocarcinoma
  – Lymphoma
  – Steroids
  – Bisphosphonates
  – Selective COX II inhibitors
  – Chronic renal failure
  – Hypercalcaemia
▌ Duodenal ulcers
  – *H. pylori* (80%)
  – NSAIDs
  – Zollinger–Ellison syndrome

Clinical features

▌ Upper abdominal pain
▌ Pain at night often related to food
▌ Nausea
▌ GI haemorrhage (haematemesis or melaena)
▌ Anaemia
▌ Tender abdomen

Investigations

▌ Upper GI endoscopy
▌ Barium meal
▌ Urease test at endoscopy
▌ Biopsy for histology

Management

▌ *H. pylori* eradication therapy (proton pump inhibitor and two antibiotics for 7 days)
▌ Stop NSAIDs
▌ Proton pump inhibitors for 8 weeks

Complications

▌ Haemorrhage → haematemesis/melaena
▌ Perforation → peritonism and air under diaphragm on chest X-ray
▌ Gastric outlet obstruction

Gastritis (*K&C*, p. 287)

- Inflammation of the gastric mucosa
- Often asymptomatic

Aetiology

- *H. pylori*
- NSAIDs
- Autoimmune (pernicious anaemia)
- Chemical (bile)

Management

- *H. pylori* eradication
- Avoid NSAIDs

Upper GI bleeding (*K&C*, p. 291)

Aetiology

- Oesophageal causes
  - Varices
  - Ulceration
  - Reflux disease → erosions
  - Mallory–Weiss tear (associated with vomiting)
  - Malignancy
- Gastric causes
  - Ulcers
  - Erosions
  - Malignancy
- Duodenal causes
  - Ulceration

Clinical features

- Nausea
- Haematemesis
- Melaena
- Dizziness due to hypovolaemia
- Hypotension
- Tachycardia
- Stigmata of chronic liver disease
  - Splenomegaly ⎫
  - Ascites ⎬ Portal hypertension
  - Spider naevi ⎪
  - Caput medusae ⎭

Investigations

- Full blood count – low haemoglobin, high platelets
- Urea and electrolytes – high urea
- Liver biochemistry – abnormal in liver disease

BOX 10.1 UPPER GASTROINTESTINAL HAEMORRHAGE

Haematemesis and/or melaena is indicative of gastrointestinal bleeding:
I.v. access: two large bore lines in big veins
Measure blood pressure and pulse
Immediate fluid resuscitation with colloid
Blood for full blood count/urea and electrolytes/coagulation
Immediate blood group and cross-match
Request senior review
Assess for evidence of perforation
Assess medical risk – age/heart disease/diabetes
Assess causal factors – NSAIDs/liver disease
Fluid-resuscitate with blood once available
Consider endoscopy or surgical intervention

- Coagulation – elevated prothrombin time
- Upper GI endoscopy to identify and treat cause

Management

- See box
- 80% will stop spontaneously
- Upper GI endoscopy
- Therapy depends on cause (see below)

Varices
- Endoscopic therapy
  - Inject sclerosant
  - Elasticated band around varix
- Non-endoscopic therapy
  - Vasopressin analogues
  - Sengstaken tube
  - Transjugular intrahepatic portosystemic shunt (TIPS)

Ulcers
- Adrenaline (epinephrine) injection
- clipping of bleeding vessel
- Thermal coagulation
- Angiography and embolisation of feeding vessel

Surgery
- Required for uncontrollable bleeding

Medical therapy
- Intravenous PPI infusions reduce rebleeding following endoscopy

Gastric tumours (*K&C*, p. 288)

Stromal tumours

- GI stromal tumours (GIST)
- May ulcerate → bleeding

Adenocarcinoma

Epidemiology

- Fourth most common cause of cancer-related death
- 15/100 000 men/year
- Wide geographical variation, e.g. common in Japan

Aetiology

- *H. pylori*
- Low dietary vitamin C and β-carotene
- Smoking
- Family history
- Pernicious anaemia
- Previous gastric surgery

Clinical features

- Abdominal pain
- Early satiety
- Weight loss
- Nausea and vomiting
- Upper GI bleeding
- Palpable epigastric mass
- Left supraclavicular lymph node (Virchow's)
- Enlarged liver due to metastases

Investigations

- Upper GI endoscopy or
- Barium swallow and meal
- CT ⎫ To stage
- Laparoscopy ⎬ tumour

Management

- Surgery for low-stage tumours
- Palliation for high-stage tumours
- Poor response to chemotherapy/radiotherapy
- 10% 5-year survival

MALT lymphoma (*K&C*, p. 290)

- Mucosa-associated lymphoid tissue lymphoma
- Associated with *H. pylori*
- 80% are cured by eradication of the infection

SMALL BOWEL DISEASE

Coeliac disease (*K&C*, p. 301)

- Hypersensitivity to gliadin in wheat, barley, rye → small intestinal disease

Table 10.8 Causes of villous atrophy

Coeliac disease	Infection enteritis in children
Whipple's disease	Kwashiorkor
Small bowel lymphoma	Cow's milk protein intolerance
Primary hypogammaglobulinaemia	Zollinger–Ellison syndrome

Table 10.9 Causes of small bowel malabsorption

Coeliac disease	Crohn's disease
Dermatitis herpetiformis	Whipple's disease
Tropical sprue	Radiation enteritis
Bacterial overgrowth	Giardia intestinalis
Intestinal resection	Lymphoma

Epidemiology

- England 1:300; Ireland 1:100
- Caucasians mainly
- Positive family history

Pathology

- → Subtotal villous atrophy (Table 10.8)
  - Loss of villi
  - Crypt hyperplasia
- → Malabsorption (see Table 10.9)

Clinical features

- Abdominal pain
- Diarrhoea
- Steatorrhoea/malabsorption
- Weight loss
- Symptoms of anaemia
- Mouth ulceration
- Anaemia → pale conjunctivae (50% iron deficiency)
- Dermatitis herpetiformis (blistering rash on extensor surfaces)

Investigations

- Anti-endomysial antibodies ⎫ Negative after
- Tissue transglutaminase ⎭ gluten-free diet
- Antigliadin antibodies
- Antireticulin antibodies
- Endoscopy and duodenal biopsy

I Full blood count
- Anaemia (macrocytic or microcytic)
- Hyposplenism, Howell–Jolly bodies

Disease associations

I Thyroid disease/diabetes
I Primary biliary cirrhosis
I Autoimmune hepatitis

Complications

I Ulcerative jejunitis
I Small bowel lymphoma
I Oesophageal carcinoma
I Osteomalacia

Management

I Gluten-free diet
I Iron/folate supplementation

Bacterial overgrowth (*K&C*, p. 304)

I Bacterial colonisation of the small bowel
I Commonly *Escherichia* or *Bacteroides*
I → Bacterial consumption of vitamin B_{12}
I → Breakdown of bile salts
I → Bacterial synthesis of folate

Aetiology

I Small bowel structural abnormalities
I Strictures

Clinical features

I Diarrhoea
I Steatorrhoea

Investigations

I Lactose hydrogen breath tests
I Low vitamin B_{12}
I High folate

Management

I Correct structural cause
I Tetracyclines
I Ciprofloxacin
I Metronidazole

Whipple's disease (*K&C*, p. 305)

I Due to *Tropheryma whippeii*
I → Villous atrophy

| Diarrhoea and steatorrhoea
| Rare

Management

| Antibiotics

Small bowel tumours (*K&C*, p. 308)

| Lymphomas
| Adenocarcinomas (rare)
| Carcinoids

Carcinoid syndrome (*K&C*, p. 309)

| Associated with metastatic carcinoid tumours
| Due to serotonin (5-hydroxytryptamine, 5-HT), bradykinin and histamine secretion by metastases
| Only symptomatic after hepatic involvement

Clinical features

| Flushing
| Diarrhoea
| Right heart failure
| Hepatomegaly
| Pulmonary valve stenosis
| Tricuspid regurgitation

Investigations

| 24-hour urinary 5-hydroxyindoleacetic acid (5-HIAA)
| CT or ultrasound of liver
| Octreotide-labelled scan

Management

| Octreotide to reduce symptoms
| Embolisation of hepatic secondaries

INFLAMMATORY BOWEL DISEASE (*K&C*, P. 309)

Inflammatory diseases of the GI tract, of unknown aetiology. Both Crohn's disease and ulcerative colitis demonstrate uncontrolled inflammation.

Crohn's disease
Epidemiology

| Prevalence = 50–60/100 000
| More common in Caucasian races

- Familial association
- Genetic predisposition

Pathology

- Any part of gut from mouth to anus
- Skip lesions – patchy disease with normal mucosa in between
- Commonly terminal ileum and ascending colon
- → Inflammation, ulceration, abscesses and fistulae
- Full bowel wall thickness involved
- Inflammatory infiltrates
- Non-caseating granulomata

Clinical features

- Depend on the area of bowel involved
- Mouth ulcers
- Diarrhoea
- Abdominal pain – colicky
- Nausea/vomiting
- Low-grade pyrexia
- Generally unwell, lethargy, weight loss
- Cutaneous fistulae (often perianal)

Disease associations (Fig. 10.3)

- Small joint arthritis
- Sacroiliitis
- Ankylosing spondylitis
- Iritis/uveitis/conjunctivitis
- Erythema nodosum – tender lower leg lesions
- Pyoderma gangrenosum – skin ulceration
- Sclerosing cholangitis

Investigations

- Barium follow-through may show strictures, ulceration and thickened small bowel wall
- Colonoscopy and terminal ileal biopsy
- Proctoscopy and rectal biopsy

Management

- 5-aminosalicylic acid (5-ASA), e.g. mesalazine
- Steroids, e.g. prednisolone
- Azathioprine, methotrexate
- Anti-TNF-a antibodies (infliximab)
- Antibiotics for perianal disease
- Surgery for resistant disease

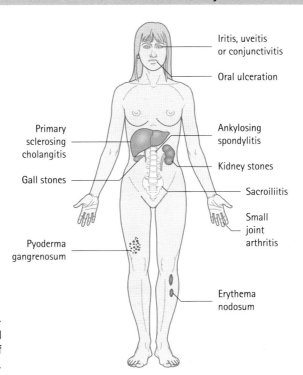

Fig. 10.3 Extra-gastrointestinal manifestations of Crohn's disease.

Complications

- Vitamin B$_{12}$ deficiency after surgery
- Short bowel syndrome after surgery
- Toxic megacolon in colitis
- Kidney stones
- Gallstones
- Malnutrition
- Colonic cancer
- Venous and arterial thromboembolism

Ulcerative colitis (*K&C*, p. 316)
Epidemiology

- Prevalence = 80–120/100 000
- Uncommon in smokers

Pathology

- Limited to colon
- Inflammation spreads proximally from the rectum
- Mucosal inflammation
- → erythema, oedema and ulceration
- Inflammatory infiltrate
- Crypt abscesses
- Goblet cell depletion

Clinical features

- Diarrhoea
- Blood or mucus per rectum
- Mouth ulcers

Disease associations

- Uveitis/iritis/conjunctivitis
- Erythema nodosum/pyoderma gangrenosum
- Arthritis/sacroiliitis/ankylosing spondylitis
- Sclerosing cholangitis

Investigations

- Colonoscopy and biopsy

Indicators of acute severe colitis urgent treatment

- >Six stools per day
- Fever $> 37.5°C$
- Tachycardia $> 90\,bpm$
- ESR $> 30\,mm/hr$
- Haemoglobin $< 10\,g/dL$
- Albumin $< 30\,g/L$

Management

- 5-ASA, e.g. mesalazine
- Steroids, e.g. prednisolone
- Azathioprine
- Surgery
- Topical 5-ASA or steroids (enemas)

Complications

- Toxic megacolon
- Iron deficiency anaemia
- Increased risk of colorectal cancer
- Thromboembolism

COLONIC DISEASE

Colorectal cancer (*K&C*, p. 328)
Epidemiology

- 1 in 27 of the population
- Associated with 'Western' diet
- Risk reduced by taking aspirin
- 10% are familial

Aetiology

- Genetic predisposition
  - *apc* gene mutation
  - *p53* gene mutation
  - Microsatellite instability (failure of DNA repair)

BOX 10.2 TOXIC MEGACOLON

Dilatation of the (transverse) colon with a high risk of perforation
Signs: fever, abdominal pain, bloody diarrhoea, tachycardia, hypotension

I.v. access and fluid resuscitation
Plain abdominal film to monitor colon diameter
Erect chest X-ray to rule out perforation
I.v. steroids and s.c. heparin
Early surgical involvement

Daily plain abdominal film
Intravenous antibiotics

If poor response to treatment → consider colectomy

Pathology

Adenomatous polyps →
adenocarcinoma
- Most commonly in sigmoid colon or rectum

Microsatellite instability tumours
- Not associated with polyp formation
- More common in ascending colon and caecum

Familial cancers

Familial adenomatous polyposis (FAP)
- *apc* gene mutation
- → Multiple adenomatous polyps
- → Very high risk of malignant change

Hereditary non-polyposis colorectal cancer (HNPCC)
- Associated with microsatellite instability
- Associated increased risk of upper GI and gynaecological cancers

Clinical features
- Change in bowel habit to diarrhoea
- Rectal blood/mucus
- Weight loss

Investigations
- Full blood count – iron deficiency anaemia
- Colonoscopy or
- Barium enema
- CT to stage the cancer (Table 10.10)
- MRI for rectal cancers

Management
- Surgical resection
- Adjuvant chemotherapy

Table 10.10 Staging and survival of colorectal cancers

TNM classification	Modified Dukes' classification	5-year survival (%)
Stage 0 – carcinoma in situ Stage I – no nodal involvement no metastases: tumour invades submucosa (T1, N0, M0); tumour invades muscularis propria (T2, N0, M0)	A	90–100
Stage II – no nodal involvement, no metastases: tumour invades into subserosa (T3, N0, M0); tumour invades other organs (T4, N0, M0)	B	75–85
Stage III – regional lymph nodes involved (any T, N1, M0)	C	30–40
Stage IV – distant metastases (T any, N any, M1)	D	<5

Complications

■ Bowel obstruction
■ Iron deficiency anaemia
■ Hepatic metastases

Screening

■ High risk individuals (family history)
■ Population screening
  – Faecal occult blood
  – Colonoscopy if positive

Diverticular disease (*K&C*, p. 324)

■ Presence of mucosal pouches protruding outside the bowel
■ Very common: 50% of those > 50 years old

Clinical features

■ 90% asymptomatic
■ Change in bowel habit
■ Left iliac fossa pain (diverticulitis)

Investigations

■ Barium enema
■ Colonoscopy
■ CT

Management

■ High-fibre diet
■ Antibiotics for diverticulitis

Complications

- Diverticulitis – inflammation/infection
- Diverticular abscess
- Lower GI bleeding
- Perforation

Functional bowel disease (*K&C*, p. 338)

- Irritable bowel syndrome
- GI symptoms without an identified pathology

Clinical features

- Left iliac fossa pain
- Alternating diarrhoea and constipation
- Bloating
- Rabbit pellet stools
- Sensation of incomplete evacuation

Investigations

- Normal physical examination
- Rule out gynaecological problems
- Full blood count and CRP
- Colonoscopy if atypical symptoms/elderly patients

Management

- Reassurance
- Antispasmodics
- Dietary changes (e.g. increased fibre)
- tricyclic antidepressants or serotonin reuptake inhibitors

CHANGES IN BOWEL HABIT

Diarrhoea (Fig. 10.4) (*K&C*, p. 331)

An increase in stool weight to $> 300\,g$ per day, usually associated with an increase in stool frequency.

Osmotic diarrhoea

- Non-absorbable hypertonic substances in the bowel lumen
- $\rightarrow$ Osmotic pressure draws water into the bowel

Aetiology

- Purgatives, e.g. magnesium sulphate
- Malabsorption $\rightarrow$ solutes in the bowel, e.g. glucose

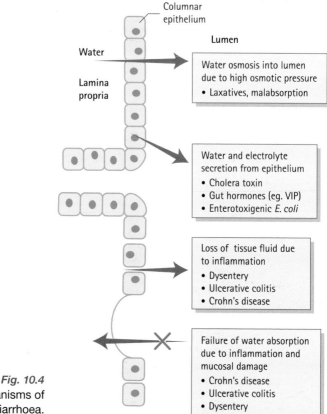

Fig. 10.4
Mechanisms of
diarrhoea.

Columnar
epithelium

Water

Lamina
propria

Lumen

Water osmosis into lumen
due to high osmotic pressure
• Laxatives, malabsorption

Water and electrolyte
secretion from epithelium
• Cholera toxin
• Gut hormones (eg. VIP)
• Enterotoxigenic *E. coli*

Loss of tissue fluid due
to inflammation
• Dysentery
• Ulcerative colitis
• Crohn's disease

Failure of water absorption
due to inflammation and
mucosal damage
• Crohn's disease
• Ulcerative colitis
• Dysentery

❚ Absorptive defects, e.g. lactose deficiency
❚ Diarrhoea stops when the patient stops eating or
taking the purgative

Secretory diarrhoea

❚ Increased secretion and decreased absorption of
fluid and electrolytes

Aetiology

❚ Cholera toxin
❚ *E.coli* heat-labile and stable toxins
❚ Hormones, e.g. vasoactive intestinal peptides
❚ Bile salts following terminal ileal resection
❚ Some laxatives

Inflammatory diarrhoea
- Mucosal inflammation → loss of fluid and blood
- May also → absorptive failure
- e.g. Ulcerative colitis, Crohn's disease, dysentery due to *Shigella*

Increased stool frequency

Abnormal GI tract motility
- Post-vagotomy
- Diabetic autonomic neuropathy
- Hyperthyroidism

Structural abnormalities
- Diverticular disease
- Colorectal carcinoma

Other
- Faecal impaction and overflow

Constipation (*K&C*, p. 320)
Aetiology
- Old age
- Immobility
- Low-volume/fibre diets
- Intestinal obstruction
- Colonic disease, e.g. colorectal carcinoma
- Hypothyroidism
- Hypocalcaemia
- Depression
- Drugs
  - Opiates
  - Iron
  - Antidepressants
  - Aluminium antacids

Management
- Bulking laxatives – fibre/bran
- Stimulants – anthraquinones (senna), bisacodyl
- Osmotics – magnesium sulphate/macrogols
- Suppositories – bisacodyl
- Enemas – phosphate

GASTROINTESTINAL INFECTIONS (*K&C*, P. 67)

A very common cause of morbidity and mortality, notably in the developing world.

Viral infections

Aetiology

- Rotavirus → epidemic diarrhoea in children
- Enteric adenovirus types 40 and 41
- Calicivirus, e.g. Norwalk virus
- Astrovirus → watery diarrhoea and vomiting
- Small round structured viruses (SRSV)

Management

- Supportive

Bacterial infections

Cholera (*K&C*, p. 84)

- *Vibrio cholerae*
- Faecal–oral transmission
- 'Ricewater' high-volume stools
- Secretory diarrhoea due to cAMP activation
- Treat with oral rehydration therapy
- Tetracycline; ciprofloxacin or azithromycin if severe

Salmonella (*K&C*, p. 68)

- *Salmonella enteritidis* and *typhimurium*
- Eggs and poultry products
- 2–3 days of diarrhoea and malaise
- Rarely bloody diarrhoea
- Treat with oral rehydration
- Complications – cholecystitis and chronic carriage with re-infection

Staphylococcus

- *Staphylococcus aureus*
- Toxin-related gastroenteritis
- Short-lived diarrhoea and vomiting
- Treat dehydration

Escherichia coli (*K&C*, p. 69)

- ETEC (enterotoxigenic) → watery diarrhoea
- EIEC (enteroinvasive) → dysentery
- EPEC (enteropathogenic) → diarrhoea
- EAEC (enteroadherent) → diarrhoea
- EHEC (enterohaemorrhagic) → haemorrhagic colitis ± haemolytic uraemic syndrome, associated with serotype O157:H7
- Treat symptoms; if severe, ciprofloxacin

Yersinia

- *Yersina enterocolitica* and *paratuberculosis*
- Enterocolitis, terminal ileitis
- → Fever, diarrhoea and abdominal pain
- May → arthritis and Reiter's syndrome

Campylobacter (*K&C*, p. 68)

- *Campylobacter jejuni*
- Mucosal ulcer and inflammation, colitis
- → Diarrhoea ± blood, fever
- Cramping abdominal pains
- Management: supportive only
- Complications – Guillian–Barré syndrome

Shigellosis (*K&C*, p. 69)

- *Shigella dysenteriae, flexneri, sonnei, boydii*
- Usually affects children
- → Fever, abdominal pain, watery diarrhoea
- → Bloody diarrhoea and abdominal cramps
- Treat symptoms; ciprofloxacin for severe cases

Bacillus cereus

- Toxin-mediated
- Short-lived vomiting
- Often contaminates rice

Clostridium

- *Clostridium perfringens*
- Spores in food
- Watery diarrhoea and pain
- Treat symptoms

Pseudo-membranous colitis

- *Clostridium difficile* A and B toxins
- After antibiotic therapy, e.g. cephalosporins
- → Colitis with ulceration and grey membrane
- → Bloody diarrhoea
- Treat by stopping antibiotics; oral metronidazole or vancomycin

Botulism

- *Clostridium botulinum*
- Preserved canned food

- → Nausea, vomiting and diarrhoea
- Neurotoxin → progressive paralysis
- Supportive treatment and antitoxin
- 50–70% mortality

Protozoal infection (*K&C*, pp. 104–106)

Amoeba

- *Entamoeba histolytica*
- → Dysentery and colitis, liver abscess
- Treat with metronidazole

Giardia

- *Giardia intestinalis (lamblia)*
- Diarrhoea and malabsorption
- Treat with metronidazole

Cryptosporidium

- *Cryptosporidium parvum*
- Water-borne
- Fever and diarrhoea

Helminths (*K&C*, p. 106)

Nematodes

- *Strongyloides stercoralis*
- Hookworm *(Ancylostoma duodenale)*
- Roundworm *(Ascaris lumbricoides)*
- Threadworm *(Enterobius vermicularis)*

Cestodes

- Tapeworms *(Taenia saginata/solium)*

PANCREATIC DISEASE

Acute pancreatitis (*K&C*, p. 409)

- Acute inflammation of the pancreas

Aetiology

- Alcohol
- Gallstones
- Trauma
- ERCP
- Drugs
  - Azathioprine

- Steroids
- Oral contraceptive

▌ Infections
- Mumps virus
- Coxsackie
- *Klebsiella*

▌ Metabolic
- Hypercalcaemia
- Hyperlipidaemia
- Renal failure

▌ Other
- Hypothermia
- Malnutrition
- Scorpion bites

Clinical features

▌ Abdominal pain radiating to back
▌ Nausea and vomiting
▌ Anorexia
▌ Abdominal tenderness and guarding
▌ Flank bruising (Grey–Turner sign)
▌ Basal pulmonary crackles

Investigations

▌ Plain abdominal X-ray – pancreatic calcification if chronic
▌ Blood count – elevated neutrophils
▌ Urea and electrolytes – renal failure
▌ Calcium/glucose
▌ Amylase – elevated (Table 10.11)

Table 10.11 Causes of a raised serum amylase

Pancreatic	**Salivary**
Acute/chronic pancreatitis	Adenitis, tumours, mumps
Pseudocysts	
Carcinoma	**Others**
	Diabetic ketoacidosis
Abdominal	Alcohol
Perforation, duodenal ulcer	Anorexia
Ectopic pregnancy	Burns
Ovarian tumours	
Hepatic	
Gallstones	
Acute hepatitis	

■ Blood gases – hypoxia and acidosis
■ Liver function tests
■ Ultrasound – gallstones
■ CT – for complications

Management

■ Oxygen
■ I.v. access and fluids
■ Supportive management
■ Analgesia
■ Early ERCP for obstructing gallstones
■ High-dependency nursing

Complications

■ Hypoxia (respiratory distress syndrome)
■ Hypocalcaemia (fat saponification)
■ Renal failure
■ Pseudocyst formation
■ Sepsis

Prognosis

■ See Table 10.12

Chronic pancreatitis (*K&C*, p. 411)

■ Long-standing or repeated attacks of pancreatitis resulting in fibrosis

Aetiology

■ Alcohol
■ Autoimmune pancreatitis

Table 10.12 Poor prognostic indicators in acute pancreatitis in the first 48 hours

Age	>55 years
WCC	>15 × 10^9/mL
Glucose	>10 mmol/L
Urea	>16 mmol/L
Albumin	<30 g/L
ALT	>200 IU
Calcium	<2 mmol/L
LDH	>600 IU
PaO_2	<8 kPa

Clinical features

- Chronic abdominal pain
- Weight loss
- Steatorrhoea

Investigations

- Plain abdominal X-ray shows pancreatic calcification
- Amylase is often normal
- Ultrasound – calcification
- Pancreatic function – reduced
- Blood sugar – elevated due to diabetes
- CT scan

Management

- Pancreatic supplements
- Analgesia

Pancreatic malignancy (*K&C*, p. 414)

- Majority are adenocarcinomas
- Often present late
- Poor prognosis

Clinical features

- Painless jaundice – bile duct compression
- Anorexia
- Weight loss

Investigations

- Ultrasound/CT/MRI to identify primary
- ERCP/endoscopic ultrasound

Management

- ERCP stenting to relieve jaundice
- Surgical resection of primary (rarely possible)
- Palliative care

Pancreatic endocrine tumours

- Gastrinomas and rarely other hormone-secreting tumours (e.g. insulinomas)
- Symptoms depend on hormone secreted

Zollinger–Ellison syndrome

- Gastrin-secreting tumour
- → High gastric acid secretion
- → Multiple gastroduodenal ulcers
- Diarrhoea

Table 10.13 Classification of hyperbilirubinaemia

Unconjugated	Conjugated
Water-insoluble	Water-soluble
Not excreted by kidney	Renal excretion
Pre-hepatic jaundice	Post-hepatic jaundice
Gilbert's syndrome	Some inherited jaundice
Crigler–Najjar syndrome	Hepatitis and cirrhosis

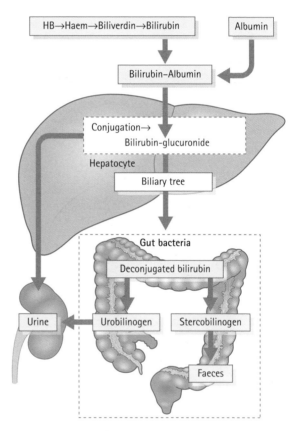

Fig. 10.5
Bilirubin
metabolism.

JAUNDICE (TABLE 10.13 AND FIG. 10.5)
(*K&C*, P. 358)

Pre-hepatic
Increased red cell breakdown

▮ Autoimmune haemolytic anaemia
▮ Malaria

Table 10.14 Causes of chronic hepatitis

Viruses	**Hereditary**
Hepatitis B $\pm$ D	α_1-antitrypsin disease
Hepatitis C	Wilson's disease
Autoimmune hepatitis	**Others**
drugs	Alcohol (rare)
Methyldopa	
Isoniazid	

Hepatic

Failure of bilirubin metabolism or excretion

Congenital defects
- Gilbert's syndrome
- Crigler–Najjar syndrome

Hepatic inflammation (hepatitis)
- Viral hepatitis
- Drugs (see Table 10.14)
- Autoimmune hepatitis
- Alcohol
- Haemochromatosis
- Wilson's disease

Cirrhosis
- Alcohol
- Chronic hepatitis
- Metabolic disorders

Hepatic tumours
- Hepatocellular carcinoma
- Hepatic metastases

Post-hepatic

Biliary obstruction
- Gallstones
- Cholangiocarcinoma
- Pancreatic carcinoma
- Primary biliary cirrhosis
- Sclerosing cholangitis

HEPATITIS (TABLE 10.14) (*K&C*, P. 361)

Acute hepatocyte breakdown leading to release of aminotransferases (ALT, AST) and jaundice. Prolonged or severe damage results in synthetic failure, leading to a reduction in the synthesis of albumin and clotting factors (causing an elevated prothrombin time).

Viral hepatitis (*K&C*, p. 362)

Hepatitis A (HAV) RNA virus

- Faecal–oral spread (e.g. shellfish)
- Incubation 2–3 weeks
- No progression → chronic liver disease

Clinical features

- Nausea
- Anorexia
- Jaundice ± hepatomegaly/rash

Investigations

- Anti-HAV IgM
- Elevated ALT/aspartate aminotransferase (AST)
- Elevated bilirubin (may be subclinical)

Management

- Supportive

Hepatitis B (HBV) DNA virus (*K&C*, p. 364) (Figs. 10.6, 10.7)

- Blood/saliva/sexual/vertical spread
- Incubation 1–5 months
- 10–15% carriage in Africa and Far East

Clinical features

- Jaundice/malaise ± rash
- May be asymptomatic

Investigations (Fig. 10.6)

- Liver biochemistry – ALT elevated first then bilirubin

Acute infection
- Surface antigen (HBsAg) first marker
- e antigen (HBeAg)

Seroconversion
- Anti-HBs antibody
- Anti-HBe antibody
- Anti-HBc antibody (IgM)

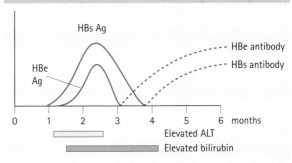

(a) HBV serology and liver function tests in acute hepatitis B

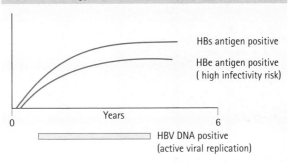

(b) HBV serology in chronic infection with hepatitis

Fig. 10.6 Hepatitis B. A. HBV serology and liver biochemistry in acute hepatitis B. B. HBV serology in chronic infection with hepatitis.

Successful clearance of virus or post vaccine

▌ Anti-HBs antibody

Chronic carrier state

▌ HBs antigen (chronic infection)
▌ HBe antigen (infectious carrier)
▌ Positive HBV DNA (active viral replication)

Management

▌ Treat symptoms
▌ Interferon, lamivudine, adefovir for chronic infection

Complications

▌ Chronic infection → chronic liver disease
▌ Hepatocellular carcinoma
▌ 1% → fulminant hepatitis → death

Hepatitis D

▌ Only causes hepatitis when it coinfects with hepatitis B
▌ Commonest in i.v. drug abusers
▌ Diagnosis by detection of specific antibodies

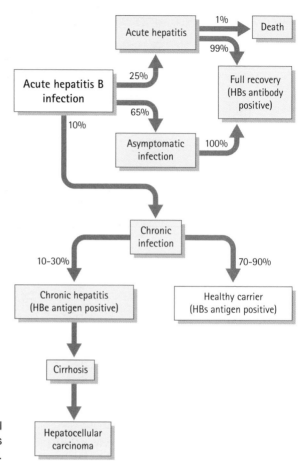

Fig. 10.7 Clinical course of hepatitis B infection.

Hepatitis C (HCV; Fig. 10.8) (*K&C*, p. 367)

▌ RNA virus
▌ Blood spread (rarely sex/saliva)
▌ Acute infection often asymptomatic
▌ 50% → chronic liver disease
▌ 30% of these → cirrhosis
▌ 5% of these → hepatocellular carcinoma

Investigations

▌ Anti-HCV antibodies
▌ HCV RNA in blood
▌ Abnormal liver function in chronic infection
▌ Ultrasound and a-fetoprotein to detect hepatocellular carcinoma

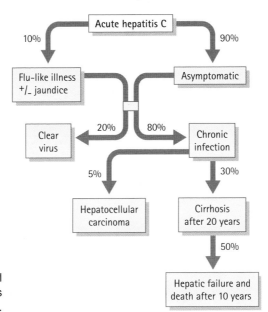

Fig. 10.8 Clinical course of hepatitis C infection.

Management

❚ Interferon and ribavirin give the best chance of clearance of the virus (in 60–70%)

Others

❚ Hepatitis E (1–2% mortality in pregnancy)
❚ Epstein–Barr virus (EBV)
❚ Cytomegalovirus (CMV)
❚ Yellow fever

Autoimmune hepatitis (*K&C*, p. 373)
Epidemiology

❚ ♀ > ♂
❚ Associated with other autoimmune disease

Clinical features

❚ May be asymptomatic
❚ Jaundice
❚ Bruising
❚ Signs of acute or chronic liver disease

Investigations

❚ Antinuclear antibodies ⎱
❚ Anti-smooth muscle antibodies ⎰ Type I
❚ Antimitochondrial antibodies ⎰

Anti-liver/kidney microsomal
antibodies } Type II
Anti-liver cytosol antibodies

Management

▌ Steroids/azathioprine

Fulminant hepatic failure
Aetiology

▌ Hepatitis A/D/E
▌ Drugs
  – Paracetamol
  – Volatile liquid anaesthetics
  – Isoniazid
  – Ecstasy
▌ Wilson's disease
▌ Pregnancy
▌ Reye's syndrome

Clinical features

▌ Jaundice
▌ Encephalopathy
▌ Drowsiness → coma
▌ Hypoglycaemia
▌ Low potassium or calcium
▌ Haemorrhage

Management

▌ Treat on a specialist unit
▌ Supportive therapy
▌ Liver transplant

CIRRHOSIS (*K&C*, P. 374)

Liver cell necrosis followed by nodular regeneration
and fibrosis, resulting in increased resistance to
blood flow and deranged liver function.

Aetiology

▌ Alcohol
▌ Hepatitis B or C
▌ Biliary cirrhosis
▌ Autoimmune hepatitis
▌ Haemochromatosis
▌ Wilson's disease

Table 10.15 Liver function tests

Hepatocellular damage (hepatitis)	Synthetic function
Aminotransferases (ALT/AST)	Albumin
γ-Glutamyl transpeptidase (γ-GT)	Prothrombin time
Cholestasis (bile ducts)	
Bilirubin	
Alkaline phosphatase	

- α 1-antitrypsin disease
- Cystic fibrosis
- Non-alcoholic steatohepatitis (NASH)

Clinical features

Chronic liver dysfunction
- Jaundice
- Anaemia
- Bruising
- Palmar erythema
- Dupuytren's contracture

Portal hypertension
- Splenomegaly
- Ascites
- Spider naevi
- Caput medusae
- Oesophageal/rectal varices

Investigations (Table 10.15)
- ALT/AST may be high or normal
- Alkaline phosphatase is usually high
- Bilirubin is usually high
- Albumin falls as cirrhosis worsens
- Prothrombin time often prolonged
- Sodium low in severe disease
- α-fetoprotein – hepatocellular carcinoma
- Ultrasound – liver may be large, normal or small; splenomegaly
- Endoscopy for oesophageal varices

Management
- Stop drinking
- Treat complications
- Transplantation

Complications (Table 10.16)

Ascites ▌ Transudate (protein < 30 g/L in fluid)

Table 10.16 Indicators of poor prognosis in cirrhosis

Albumin < 25 g/L	Persistent jaundice
Sodium < 120 mmol/L	Ascites
Prolonged prothrombin time	Variceal bleeding

Table 10.17 Causes of ascites

Transudate (protein < 30 g/L)	**Exudate (protein > 30 g/L)**
Portal hypertension	Infections
Cirrhosis of the liver	Peritoneal tuberculosis
Portal vein thrombosis	Malignancy
Low serum protein	Ovarian carcinoma
Liver disease	Peritoneal metastases
Nephrotic syndrome	Inflammatory
Malnutrition	Pancreatitis
Others	
Right ventricular failure	
Myxoedema	

(Table 10.17) ▮ Treatment
- Water and salt restriction
- Spironolactone + loop diuretics
- Ascitic drainage

Serum-ascites ▮ *>11 g suggests transudate*
albumin gradient ▮ More sensitive than absolute protein

Spontaneous ▮ → Worsening of clinical state
bacterial ▮ Diagnosis: ascitic tap
peritonitis ▮ Treatment: parenteral antibiotics

Variceal bleeding ▮ See page 261

Encephalopathy ▮ See page 91

Hepatorenal ▮ Advanced cirrhosis with ascites and jaundice
syndrome ▮ Low urine volume
▮ Low urinary sodium
▮ Hepatocellular carcinoma – see page 293

Specific causes of cirrhosis

Primary biliary cirrhosis (*K&C*, p. 385)
▮ Chronic destruction of bile ducts
▮ ♀ > ♂

Clinical features
▮ Jaundice
▮ Itching
▮ Xanthelasma
▮ Hepatosplenomegaly

Investigations

- Antimitochondrial (M2) antibodies
- High alkaline phosphatase
- Relatively normal ALT
- Ultrasound
- Liver biopsy

Management

- Ursodeoxycholic acid may normalise liver biochemistry
- Supplement fat-soluble vitamins (A, D, E, K)
- Colestyramine for itching
- Consider liver transplant when bilirubin > 100 mmol/L

Hereditary haemochromatosis (*K&C*, p. 386)

- Autosomal recessive
- 1:400 homozygous
- → Abnormalities of iron transportation
- → Accumulation of iron in epithelial cells
- ♂ = ♀ but women less severely affected due to menstruation

Clinical features

- Heart: cardiomyopathy
- Pancreas: diabetes
- Pituitary hypogonadism
- Liver: hepatitis and cirrhosis, hepatocellular carcinoma
- Skin: pigmentation
- Testes: infertility

Investigations

- Ferritin > 500 μg/L
- Serum iron > 30 μmol/L
- Transferrin saturation > 60%
- Liver biopsy
- Screen family for genetic mutation (HFe gene)

Management

- Venesection to normalise ferritin

Wilson's disease (*K&C*, p. 387)

- Autosomal recessive
- Defect of copper transport
- → Failure of biliary copper excretion

Clinical features

- Liver: chronic hepatitis → cirrhosis
- Basal ganglia: tremor, dysarthria, dementia
- Kidneys: tubular degeneration
- Eyes: Kayser–Fleischer rings

Investigations

- Reduced serum copper and caeruloplasmin
- Elevated urinary copper
- Liver biopsy

Management

- Penicillamine – chelates copper

α_1-antitrypsin deficiency (*K&C*, p. 388)

- Inherited deficiency of α_1-antitrypsin
- Autosomal dominant
- Liver cirrhosis
- Early emphysema in smokers

Alcohol-related liver disease and alcoholism (*K&C*, p. 389)

Pathology

- Fatty change
- Alcoholic hepatitis
- Cirrhosis

Clinical features

- Those of the stage of liver disease (see above)

Investigations

- Abnormal liver function
- γ-GT elevation. AST:ALT > 1
- Liver biopsy
- Ultrasound
- α-fetoprotein for hepatocellular carcinoma
- CAGE questionnaire
  - Are you **C**oncerned about your alcohol intake?
  - Are others **A**nxious about your drinking?
  - Do you feel **G**uilty about drinking?
  - Do you need an '**E**ye opener' to avoid withdrawal?

Management

- Cessation of alcohol consumption
- Support during physical withdrawal (Table 10.18)
- Psychological support

Table 10.18 Alcohol withdrawal

Clinical features	Management
Morning shakes	Benzodiazepines to help
Tremor	with symptoms
Delirium tremens: tremor,	Nutritional support
hallucinations	
Convulsions	

Complications

- Hepatocellular carcinoma (10–15%)
- End-stage liver disease
- Wernicke–Korsakoff syndrome (see below)
- Encephalopathy
- Dementia
- Epilepsy (5–10%)

Wernicke–
Korsakoff
syndrome
- Thiamine deficiency
- → Acute Wernicke's syndrome
  - Nystagmus, ataxia, confusion
- → Chronic Korsakoff's syndrome
  - Dementia, chronic amnesia, confabulation
- Investigations: red cell transketolase
- Management: parenteral thiamine

Hepatic encephalopathy

- Reversible neuropsychiatric deficit

Clinical features

- Flapping tremor of hands
- Decreased level of consciousness
- Personality changes
- Intellectual deterioration
- Slow, slurred speech
- Constructional apraxia – unable to copy a drawn five-pointed star

Worsened by
- Sepsis
- Constipation, diarrhoea or vomiting
- Diuretics
- GI bleeding
- Alcohol withdrawal

Investigations

- Urea and electrolytes
- Full blood count
- Liver function tests

- EEG
- Blood cultures to detect sepsis
- Ascitic tap for spontaneous bacterial peritonitis

Management

- Laxatives to reduce constipation
- Treat sepsis
- Careful fluid balance
- Supportive treatment

OTHER DISEASES OF THE LIVER

Liver abscess (*K&C*, p. 391)

- Single or multiple abscesses
- *E. coli*
- *Enterococcus faecalis*
- *Staphylococcus aureus*
- *Entamoeba histolytica* (amoeba)
- → Fever, rigors, vomiting, weight loss, shock

Investigations

- Blood count – anaemia and leucocytosis
- Blood cultures
- Amoeba serology
- Ultrasound

Management

- Broad-spectrum antibiotics
- Ultrasound-guided drainage

Budd–Chiari syndrome (*K&C*, p. 390)

- Hepatic vein thrombosis
- → Hepatic failure
- Clinical ascites, abdominal pain and vomiting
- Hepatomegaly

Pregnancy related liver disease (*K&C*, p. 393)

- Fatty liver
- Hepatitis
- Cholestasis
- Eclampsia → hepatic necrosis
- HELLP syndrome (haemolysis, elevated liver enzymes, low platelets)

Hepatocellular carcinoma (*K&C*, p. 394)

- Common worldwide
- Alcohol, hepatitis B or C-related
- Investigations: ultrasound and α-fetoprotein
- Local treatment or transplantation

Hepatic metastases

- Commonest hepatic tumours
- GI tract, breast and lung carcinomas

Hepatic steatosis (*K&C*, p. 374)

- 'Fatty liver'
- ALT usually elevated
- Commonly asymptomatic
- Commonly associated with alcohol
- Hyperlipidaemia
- Obesity
- Diabetes mellitus

NASH

- Non-alcoholic steatohepatitis
- Fat deposition and inflammation in the liver

NAFLD

- Non-alcoholic fatty liver disease
- Fat deposition
- Does not require inflammation for the diagnosis
- Excludes alcohol as a cause

DISEASES OF THE BILIARY TREE

Gallstones (Table 10.19) (*K&C*, p. 399)

- 10–20% of the population
- Often an incidental finding at ultrasound

Table 10.19 Risk factors for gallstones	
Increasing age	Weight loss
♀ > ♂	Contraceptive pill
Multiparity	Ileal resection/disease
Obesity	Diabetes
Diet high in animal fat	

Table 10.20 Drugs and the liver

Drugs causing hepatitis
Isoniazid
Methyldopa
Enalapril
Nifedipine
Ketoconazole
Volatile anaesthetics
Rifampicin
Atenolol
Verapamil
Amiodarone
Cytotoxics

Amoxicillin
Flucloxacillin
NSAIDs
   Salicylates
   Diclofenac
Allopurinol
Phenytoin
Diltiazem
Antithyroid
   Carbimazole
   Propylthiouracil

Drugs causing cholestasis
Oestrogens
Ciclosporin
Chlorpromazine
Cimetidine
Erythromycin
Imipramine
Azathioprine
Haloperidol
Ranitidine
Nitrofurantoin
Hypoglycaemics

Hypersensitivity-mediated damage
Sulphonamides
Penicillins

Miscellaneous
Necrosis
   Carbon tetrachloride
   Paracetamol
   Salicylates
   Cocaine
Fibrosis
   Methotrexate
   Retinoids
Tumours
   High-oestrogen OCP
Chronic hepatitis
   Methyldopa
   Isoniazid
   Nitrofurantoin

Types

▌ Cholesterol stones
▌ Bile pigment stones

Clinical features

▌ 80% asymptomatic
▌ Acute cholecystitis – impacted stone leading to inflammation → right hypochondrial and shoulder tip pain, fever, vomiting ± jaundice
▌ Biliary obstruction by a gallstone → pain and jaundice; ERCP may be required to remove stone

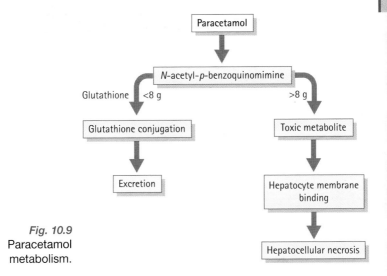

Fig. 10.9
Paracetamol
metabolism.

Complications

▌ Pancreatitis
▌ Biliary – enteric fistula
▌ Gallstone ileus

Cholangio-carcinoma (*K&C*, p. 405)

▌ Primary tumour of bile ducts
▌ → Obstructive jaundice

Primary sclerosing cholangitis (*K&C*, p. 404)

▌ Multiple bile duct strictures
▌ Associated with ulcerative colitis
▌ Increased risk of cholangiocarcinoma
▌ Investigations: ERCP

DRUGS AND THE LIVER (*K&C*, P. 396)

The liver is responsible for the initial metabolism of
oral drugs (first-pass metabolism) prior to the drug
reaching the systemic circulation. Many drugs are
also metabolised or excreted by the liver after reaching the systemic circulation. As a result, drugs can
be responsible for hepatic disease (Table 10.20 and
Fig. 10.9).

BOX 10.3 ASSESSING HEPATIC ENCEPHALOPATHY

Presence of 'liver flap'
Straight arms and hyperextended wrist with fingers splayed
Slow wrist flexion

Assessment of conscious level
Glasgow coma score

Assessment of cognition
Mini-mental test

Assessment of apraxia
Ask patient to copy a five-pointed star
Repeat on a daily basis to demonstrate changes in encephalopathy

SELF-ASSESSMENT QUESTIONS

Best one of five questions

1. Which of the following is the likeliest cause of jaundice in a 24-year-old man in the UK?
   A. Cancer of the head of the pancreas
   B. Sulphonamide antibiotics
   C. Malaria
   D. Iron deficiency anaemia
   E. Epstein–Barr virus

2. Exudative ascites occurs secondary to:
   A. Ovarian cancer
   B. Alcohol misuse
   C. Anaemia
   D. Coeliac disease
   E. Hypoalbuminaemia

3. Which of the following is the most sensitive method of diagnosing *Helicobacter pylori* infection?
   A. Blood urease test
   B. Endoscopy and biopsy
   C. *H. pylori* antigen in stool
   D. ^{13}C urea breath test
   E. Serum *H. pylori* antibodies

4. Which one of the following is most likely to cause hepatomegaly?
   A. Portal vein thrombosis
   B. Carcinoma of the head of the pancreas
   C. Burkitt's lymphoma
   D. Primary biliary cirrhosis
   E. Right heart failure

5. Which one of the following is the commonest complication of chronic gastro-oesophageal reflux disease?
   A. Bronchospasm
   B. Headache

C. Gastric ulcer
D. Achalasia
E. Squamous metaplasia

6. Which one of the following increases the risk of oesophageal carcinoma:
   A. Omeprazole
   B. Aspirin
   C. Acid reflux
   D. Ascorbic acid
   E. *H. pylori*

7. Which one of the following is a characteristic finding in Barrett's oesophagus?
   A. The presence of goblet cells
   B. Transitional cell metaplasia of the oesophageal mucosa
   C. Increased risk of oesophageal squamous cell carcinoma
   D. Villous formation
   E. Mucosal dysplasia

8. Which one of the following is associated with oesophageal varices?
   A. Hyposplenism
   B. Acute viral hepatitis
   C. Nodular regeneration and fibrosis of the liver
   D. Portal hypotension
   E. Increased risk of bleeding with propranolol

9. Which one of the following increases oesophageal sphincter tone?
   A. Alcohol
   B. Nifedipine
   C. Achalasia
   D. Isosorbide mononitrate
   E. Botulinum toxin

10. Which of the following is the commonest cause of gastric ulcer?
  - **A.** Ibuprofen
  - **B.** Proton pump inhibitors
  - **C.** Gastric lymphoma
  - **D.** *H. pylori*
  - **E.** Alendronate

11. Which of the following is associated with gastritis?
  - **A.** *Salmonella enteritidis*
  - **B.** Chlorpromazine
  - **C.** Pantoprazole
  - **D.** Renal failure
  - **E.** Thyrotoxicosis

12. Which one of the following is true of Gastric MALT lymphoma?
  - **A.** Is a tumour arising from basophils in the gastric mucosa
  - **B.** May be effectively treated by omeprazole, clarithromycin and amoxicillin
  - **C.** Frequently metastasises
  - **D.** Can arise anywhere in the gastrointestinal tract
  - **E.** Is a Hodgkin's lymphoma

13. Which one of the following is associated with a decreased risk of gastric adenocarcinoma?
  - **A.** High dietary ascorbic acid
  - **B.** Active *H. pylori* infection
  - **C.** Gastric intestinal metaplasia
  - **D.** Smoking
  - **E.** Coeliac disease

14. Which one of the following is useful in the management of peptic duodenal ulcers?
  - **A.** Omeprazole
  - **B.** Aspirin
  - **C.** Gluten free diet
  - **D.** Iron sulphate
  - **E.** Mesalazine

15. Which one of the following is associated with coeliac disease?
  - **A.** Steatohepatitis
  - **B.** Hypothyroidism
  - **C.** Hypersplenism
  - **D.** Dermatitis herpetiformis
  - **E.** Thiamine deficiency

16. Which one of the following is characteristic of coeliac disease?
  - **A.** Crypt shortening
  - **B.** Decreased lamina propria lymphocytes
  - **C.** Villus shortening
  - **D.** Crypt abscesses
  - **E.** Jejunal ulceration

17. Which one of the following is true of carcinoid syndrome?
  - **A.** Lung metastases result in right-sided cardiac valve lesions
  - **B.** Flushing and diarrhoea usually occurs
  - **C.** Octreotide is of little therapeutic use
  - **D.** The primary tumour is commonly in the liver
  - **E.** Elevated Serum 5-HIAA is diagnostic

18. Which one of the following would favour the diagnosis of ulcerative colitis rather than Crohn's disease?
  - **A.** Non-caseating granulomata
  - **B.** Crypt abscesses
  - **C.** Enterovesical fistula formation
  - **D.** Oral ulceration
  - **E.** Failure to respond to oral methotrexate

19. Which one of the following is a recognised manifestations of Crohn's disease?
   A. Retinitis pigmentosa
   B. Erythema multiforme
   C. Discoid lupus erythematosis
   D. Dermatitis herpetiformis
   E. Uveitis

20. Which one of the following is a risk factor for the development of colorectal cancer?
   A. NSAID consumption
   B. Chronic idiopathic constipation
   C. Alcohol consumption
   D. Ulcerative colitis
   E. Diverticulosis

21. A 28-year-old man presents with increased stool frequency and rectal mucus. What is the most likely diagnosis?
   A. Diverticular disease
   B. Irritable bowel syndrome
   C. Tubulovillous adenoma of the rectum
   D. Colorectal cancer
   E. Thyrotoxicosis

22. Which one of the following symptoms is more suggestive of colonic carcinoma than irritable bowel syndrome?
   A. Rectal bleeding
   B. Weight loss
   C. Alternating diarrhoea and constipation
   D. Sensation of incomplete evacuation of stool
   E. Bloating

23. Which one of the following is most useful in the management of irritable bowel?
   A. Mebeverine
   B. Ibuprofen
   C. Phenelzine
   D. Prednisolone
   E. Mesalazine

24. Which one of the following causes diarrhoea?
   A. Iron sulphate
   B. Octreotide
   C. Vasoactive intestinal peptide (VIP)
   D. Loperamide
   E. Hypothyroidism

25. Which one of the following may cause increased stool frequency?
   A. Vagotomy
   B. Diabetes insipidus
   C. Smoking
   D. Hypercalcaemia
   E. Hyperparathyroidism

26. The following are clinical features of cirrhosis of the liver except:
   A. Palmar erythema
   B. Caput medusae
   C. Macrocytosis
   D. Portal hypotension
   E. Bruising

27. Which one of the following drugs cause abnormalities of liver function?
   A. Ursodeoxycholic acid
   B. Flucloxacillin
   C. Folic acid
   D. Verapamil
   E. Thyroxine

Multiple choice questions

28. The following organisms cause diarrhoea mainly via the mechanism given:
   A. Cholera – mucosal inflammation

B. *E. coli* – enterotoxin
production
C. *Campylobacter* – mucosal
inflammation
D. *Bacillus cereus* – colonic
ulceration
E. Giardia – malabsorption of
water

29. The following are true of
pseudomembranous colitis:
    A. Diagnosis is based on the
    presence of *Clostridium
    difficile* in stool
    B. It is best treated with
    intravenous vancomycin
    C. Risk of the disease is
    increased by intravenous
    cephalosporins
    D. It may result in bloody
    diarrhoea
    E. The causal bacterium is a
    normal commensal gut
    organism

30. The following are recognised
causes of acute pancreatitis:
    A. Gallstones
    B. Prednisolone
    C. Thyroxine
    D. Coxsackie virus infection
    E. Hyperlipidaemia

31. The following are indicators of
poor prognosis in acute
pancreatitis:
    A. Glucose < 6 mmol/L
    B. Hypocalcaemia
    C. Hypoxia
    D. Albumin > 30 g/L
    E. $P_aCO_2 < 5$ kPa

32. The following favour a diagnosis
of pancreatic carcinoma over
acute viral hepatitis in painless
jaundice:
    A. Weight loss

B. Dilated bile ducts on
ultrasound scanning
C. Elevated alkaline
phosphatase
D. Unconjugated
hyperbilirubinaemia
E. Bilirubin > 300 μmol/L

33. The following are associated
with an elevated serum gastrin:
    A. Omeprazole therapy
    B. Zollinger–Ellison syndrome
    C. Hyperchlorhydria
    D. Vagotomy
    E. Hypoglycaemia

34. The following are causes of a
conjugated hyperbilirubinaemia:
    A. Gilbert's syndrome
    B. Carcinoma of the head of the
    pancreas
    C. Cholangiocarcinoma
    D. Viral hepatitis
    E. Haemolytic anaemia

35. The following are associated
with acute hepatitis A
infection:
    A. Elevated alanine
    transaminase
    B. Nausea and vomiting
    C. Bilirubin level always greater
    than 100 μmol/L
    D. Progression to chronic
    hepatitis
    E. Food-related outbreaks

36. The following statements are
correct in the interpretation of
hepatitis B serology:
    A. HBs (surface) antibody
    positive – previous exposure
    to infection
    B. HBe antigen positive – high
    infectivity risk
    C. HBc (core) antibody positive
    – seroconversion

D. HBs antigen positive –
successful immunisation
E. HBe antibody positive –
seroconversion after acute
infection

37. The following are associated
with hepatitis C infection:
   A. Cryoglobulinaemia
   B. Hepatocellular carcinoma
   C. Primary sclerosing
   cholangitis
   D. Hepatic cirrhosis
   E. Ascites

38. The following are causes of viral
hepatitis:
   A. Epstein–Barr virus
   B. Isolated hepatitis D virus
   C. Cytomegalovirus in
   immunosuppressed patients
   D. Coxsackie virus
   E. Adenovirus

39. The following are causes of
fulminant hepatic failure:
   A. Paracetamol
   B. Hepatitis A
   C. Aspirin in childhood
   D. Halothane
   E. Haemochromatosis

40. The following are causes of
transudative ascites:
   A. Right heart failure
   B. Peritoneal tuberculosis
   C. Ovarian malignancy
   D. Nephrotic syndrome
   E. Liver cirrhosis

Extended matching questions

Question 1 *Theme: diarrhoea*
A. *E. coli*
B. Thyrotoxicosis
C. Hypercalcaemia
D. Autonomic neuropathy

E. Laxative abuse
F. Osmotic diarrhoea
G. Ulcerative colitis
H. Tubulovillous adenoma
I. Diverticular disease
J. Coeliac disease
K. Giardiasis
L. Pseudomembranous colitis

For each of the following questions,
select the best answer from the list
above:

I. A 65-year-old man with known
diabetes mellitus is reviewed as
he has worsening diarrhoea.
Upper gastrointestinal
endoscopy, duodenal biopsy
and barium enema were all
normal. Stool culture carried
out on three occasions did not
reveal any abnormality. Blood
testing revealed normal urea
and electrolytes, calcium and
liver function. What is the most
likely cause for his diarrhoea?

II. A 38-year-old man is admitted
with profuse mucus per rectum
and generalised weakness. His
potassium is noted to be
2.9 mmol/L. What is the most
likely diagnosis?

III. A 27-year-old woman is
admitted with abdominal
discomfort, profuse bloody
diarrhoea and a low-grade
fever. Investigations reveal an
iron deficiency anaemia. What
is the most likely reason for her
diarrhoea?

Question 2 *Theme:
abdominal pain*
A. Sigmoid volvulus
B. Acute appendicitis

C. Cholecystitis
D. Duodenal ulceration
E. Bowel ischaemia
F. Diverticulosis
G. Crohn's disease
H. Irritable bowel syndrome
I. Acute pancreatitis
J. Colorectal carcinoma
K. Carcinoid syndrome
L. Ovarian cysts
M. Ectopic pregnancy

For each of the following questions, select the best answer from the list above:

I. A 76-year-old man complains of pain in the abdomen after eating. This is associated with mild diarrhoea. In the past he has had a myocardial infarction and several episodes of angina. He has type II diabetes mellitus. He smokes 20 cigarettes a day and drinks 10 units of alcohol a week. Suggest a likely cause for his pain.

II. A 32-year-old woman is referred by her GP with abdominal pain, nausea, weight loss and diarrhoea. She is also complaining of a bruise-like rash on her lower legs and mild joint pains. On examination she has multiple oral aphthous ulcers and tender bruise-like lesions over her shins. What is the cause of her abdominal pain?

III. A 47-year-old woman is referred with left iliac fossa pain, bloating and alternating diarrhoea and constipation. Her weight is gradually increasing. The discomfort comes and goes but is relieved by defaecation. What is the most likely diagnosis?

Question 3 *Theme: malabsorption*
A. Pernicious anaemia
B. Coeliac disease
C. Whipple's disease
D. Primary biliary cirrhosis
E. Chronic pancreatitis
F. Cystic fibrosis
G. Bacterial overgrowth
H. Surgery for ileal Crohn's disease
I. Partial gastrectomy
J. Chronic alcohol-related liver disease
K. Carcinoma of the head of the pancreas

For each of the following questions, select the best answer from the list above:

I. A 15-year-old man is referred with a 6-year history of abdominal pain, bloating and weight loss. He is 1.78 m (5 feet 2 inches) tall and weighs 47 kg (7 stones 6 pounds). He has diarrhoea 2–3 times a day. What is the most likely diagnosis?

II. A 56-year-old woman is noted to be vitamin B_{12}-deficient and anaemic. She has known autoimmune hypothyroidism but is otherwise well. What is causing her B_{12} deficiency?

III. A 49-year-old man with a long history of alcohol abuse is reviewed due to worsening diarrhoea and abdominal pain. The stools are reported as foul-smelling and difficult to flush. His liver function tests are mildly deranged. What is the cause of his symptoms?

Question 4 *Theme: intestinal bleeding*

A. Oesophageal varices
B. Gastric ulcer
C. Duodenal ulcer
D. Coeliac disease
E. Small bowel angiodysplasia
F. Meckel's diverticulum
G. Terminal ileal Crohn's disease
H. Caecal carcinoma
I. Diverticular bleeding
J. Haemorrhoids

I. A 56-year-old man was admitted with haematemesis, melaena, hypotension and a tachycardia. He had recently been taking indometacin for joint pains. What is the likeliest cause for his symptoms?

II. A 76-year-old woman was seen with 3 months of diarrhoea and weight loss. What is the most likely diagnosis?

III. A 32-year-old woman was seen with bright red bleeding. What is the likeliest diagnosis?

Rheumatology **11**

If you need more detailed explanation refer to Kumar & Clark, *Clinical Medicine*, Chapter 10.

STRUCTURE & FUNCTION (*K&C*, P. 529)

Extracellular matrix
- Macromolecule matrix contained in all connective tissues
- Components:
  - Collagens
  - Elastin
  - Glycoproteins
  - Proteoglycans

Synovial joints (see Fig 11.1 for the components)
- Ball & socket joints, e.g. hip joint
- Hinge joints, e.g. interphalangeal

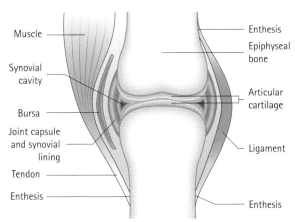

Fig. 11.1 The synovial joint (*K&C*, p. 529).

Fibrocartilaginous joints

I Intervertebral discs
I Sacroiliac joints
I Pubic symphysis
I Costochondral joints

EXAMINING THE MUSCULOSKELETAL SYSTEM

Examination should include all of the following and be done in roughly this order:

Examination of individual joints (K&C, p. 532)

I Ask the patient if the joint is painful; proceed with care if it is

Look for

I Swelling
I Erythema/rash
I Deformity
I Muscle-wasting

Feel for

I Tenderness
I Warmth
I Swelling
   – Hard swelling = bony
   – Fluctuant swelling = fluid/effusion
   – Boggy swelling = synovial swelling

Move the joint

I Passively first
I Assess for crepitus

Examination of the hands

I Expose both arms to the shoulders
I Ask if they are painful
I Describe particular features of osteoarthritis or rheumatoid arthritis if present (Table 11.1 and Fig.11.2)
I Then proceed as for individual joints above
I Also examine the nails and feel for nodules on the forearms

Table 11.1 **Some common particular features of osteoarthritis and rheumatoid arthritis in the hands**

	Hand joints usually affected	Particular features
Osteoarthritis	DIP joints (Heberden's nodes) PIP joints (Bouchard's nodes) Carpometacarpal joint	Square hand
Rheumatoid arthritis	PIP joints MCP joints	Ulnar deviation Palmar subluxation of MCP joints Fixed flexion of PIP joints (Boutonnière deformity) Fixed hyperextension of PIP joints (swan neck deformity)

A
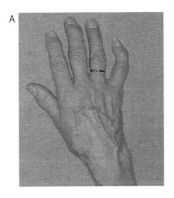

B
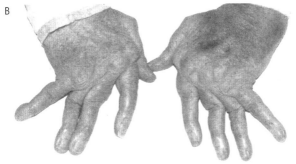

Fig. 11.2 The hands in arthritis. A. Nodal osteoarthritis. Heberden's and Bouchard's nodes and squaring of the thumb bases are seen. B. Rheumatoid arthritis.

Examination of the gait

I Ask the patient to walk a short distance away from you, turn, walk towards you and stand still

ARTHRITIS (*K&C*, P. 550 & 555)

I See Table 11.2 and Figs 11.2 and 11.3.

Septic arthritis (K&C, p. 571)

Aetiology

I Direct injury
I Blood-borne infection
I → Susceptibility in
  – Chronically inflamed joints
  – Immunosuppressed patients
  – Artificial joints

Organisms

I Staphylococcus aureus
I *Streptococcus* and other *staphylococci*
I *Neisseria gonorrhoeae*
I *Haemophilus influenzae*
I Gram-negative organisms

Clinical features

I Joint pain (may be severe)
I Muscle spasm
I Joint hot, red and swollen
I Signs of the source of infection

Investigations

I Urgent joint aspiration
  – Microscopy and culture/gram stain
I Elevated white cell count
I Blood cultures

Management

I Two i.v. antibiotics for 2 weeks (start antibiotics immediately diagnosis suspected)
I Followed by 6 weeks of oral antibiotics
I Initial immobilisation of the joint
I Early physiotherapy
I Consider surgical drainage and washout

Table 11.2 Comparison of osteoarthritis and rheumatoid arthritis

	Osteoarthritis (OA) (K&C, p. 550)	Rheumatoid arthritis (RA) (K&C, p. 555)
Description	Pain and disability associated with;joint space narrowing altered cartilage osteophyte formation	Systemic disease with: chronic, symmetrical polyarthritis synovitis non-articular features
Epidemiology	Most common type of arthritis Prevalence increases with age X-ray OA very common > 60 years	1–3% of the population Presents at all ages Commonly presents 30–50 years ♀ > ♂ before menopause Familial or sporadic HLA-DR4 in 50–70%

Aetiology	Primary idiopathic
	Secondary:
	    Trauma, e.g. previous fracture
	    Chondrocalcinosis
	    Haemochromatosis
	    Acromegaly
	    Haemophilia
	    Avascular necrosis, e.g. steroids
	    Sickle cell disease
		Unexplained
		T cell activation
		Presence of rheumatoid factors

Clinical features	Joint pain/swelling/instability Morning stiffness Joint effusion & crepitus Bony swelling Muscle wasting Limitation of movement & loss of function	Slow onset but progressive Symmetrical peripheral polyarthritis Joint pain & morning stiffness Eased by gentle activity Joints warm and tender Limitation of movement & deformity Joint effusion Muscle-wasting

(Continued)

Table 11.2 (Continued)

	Osteoarthritis (OA) (K&C, p. 550)	Rheumatoid arthritis (RA) (K&C, p. 555)
Clinical subsets	**Nodal OA** Familial ♀ ≫ ♂ Develops in late middle age Polyarticular involvement of the hand Particularly distal interphalangeal joints (Heberden's nodes) Generally good long-term functional outcome Predisposes to OA of the knee, hip and spine X-ray – marginal osteophyte & joint space loss **Erosive OA** Rare DIP and PIP joints Poor functional outcome X-ray – marked subchondral cysts May develop into rheumatoid arthritis **Generalised OA** May occur in combination with nodal OA Hands, knees, first MTP joints and hips Familial ♀ > ♂ May be autoimmune Large joint OA Knees and hips **Crystal-associated OA (chondrocalcinosis)** Calcium pyrophosphate crystal deposition	Lethargy, malaise Non-articular features (Fig. 11.3) **Palindromic** Monoarticular Progresses to other types Transient Self-limiting Usually Rh factor-negative **Remitting** Active for years then remits **Chronic persistent** Most typical form Relapsing and remitting Rapidly progressive Remorseless Progressive Rh factor-positive Associated with non-articular fractures

Investigations	Knees and wrists commonly affected X-ray – may show calcification in the cartilage Inflammatory markers not elevated No autoantibodies X-rays abnormal if damage severe MRI can show early cartilage changes Arthroscopy – early fissuring & cartilage surface erosion	Anaemia ↑ inflammatory markers Rheumatoid factors (in 70%) X-rays – erosions
Management	Treat symptoms and disability, not X-rays Explain diagnosis and reassure Weight loss and exercise Hydrotherapy (particularly lower limb joints) Heat/massage Analgesia Patients often use complementary medicine Joint replacements/other surgery	Explain diagnosis and reassure Multidisciplinary team approach NSAIDs and analgesics Disease-modifying antirheumatic drugs (DMARDs): Sulphasalazine Methotrexate Leflunomide Anti-TNF drugs: Entanercept Infliximab Adalimumab Corticosteroids (see Table 11.4 for side-effects) Less commonly used: Gold Penicillamine Hydroxychloroquine Azathioprine Ciclosporin Anikinra Joint replacements/other surgery

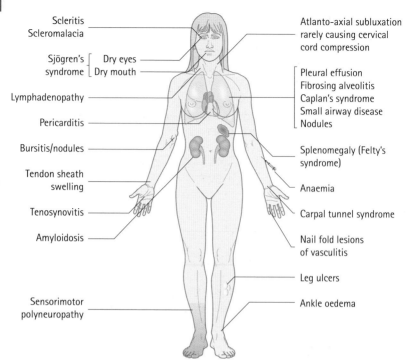

Scleritis
Scleromalacia

Sjögren's [Dry eyes
syndrome [Dry mouth

Lymphadenopathy

Pericarditis

Bursitis/nodules

Tendon sheath
swelling

Tenosynovitis

Amyloidosis

Sensorimotor
polyneuropathy

Atlanto-axial subluxation
rarely causing cervical
cord compression

Pleural effusion
Fibrosing alveolitis
Caplan's syndrome
Small airway disease
Nodules

Splenomegaly (Felty's
syndrome)

Anaemia

Carpal tunnel syndrome

Nail fold lesions
of vasculitis

Leg ulcers

Ankle oedema

Fig. 11.3 Non-articular manifestations of rheumatoid arthritis (*K&C*, Fig. 10.16, p. 559.

Seronegative spondarthropathies (*K&C*, pp. 564–568)

▌ Conditions affecting the spine and peripheral joints which cluster in families and are associated with HLA-B27

Ankylosing spondylitis

▌ Episodic inflammation of spine and sacroiliac joints
▌ Asymmetrical large joint arthritis
▌ HLA-B27 in >90%
▌ Associated with uveitis and costochondritis
▌ Inflammatory markers elevated
▌ X-rays
  – Erosions and sclerosis of affected joints
  – Syndesmophytes
  – Bamboo spine
▌ Treated with preventative exercises and NSAIDs, TNF-α blocking drugs if severe

Psoriatic arthritis
Clinical features

▌ Arthritis in association with psoriasis
▌ May predate skin lesions
▌ DIP most common joints affected
▌ Dactylitis
▌ Erosions on X-rays (centre of joint unlike juxta-articular erosions in RA)
▌ 5% have arthritis mutilans
▌ Nail dystrophy in 85% of cases
▌ HLA-B27 in 50%

Management

▌ Treated with
  – NSAIDs
  – Steroid injections to joints
  – Sulfasalazine
  – Methotrexate/ciclosporin
  – TNF-α blocking drugs, e.g. Infliximab

Reactive arthritis

▌ Sterile synovitis following dysentery or a sexually acquired infection

Aetiology

▌ Trigger organism
  – *Salmonella*
  – *Shigella*
  – *Yersinia*
  – *Chlamydia*
  – *Ureasplasma*

Clinical features

▌ Acute asymmetrical lower limb arthritis
▌ ♂ > ♀
▌ Often also an enthesitis, e.g. plantar fasciitis
▌ Non-articular features
  – Acute anterior uveitis (see above)
  – Circinate balanitis
  – Keratoderma blenorrhagica
  – Nail dystrophy
  – Conjunctivitis
▌ Reiter's disease = urethritis, arthritis and conjunctivitis

Management

- Treatment usually symptomatic with NSAIDs or steroid injections
- Treat underlying infection with antibiotics

Inflammatory bowel disease (IBD)-associated arthritis

- 10–15% of patients with IBD
- Lower limb joints
- In ulcerative colitis treatment of bowel disease may improve arthritis
- In Crohn's disease arthritis persists even when bowel is disease inactive
- 5% have sacroiliitis (independent of activity of IBD)
- Treatment with intra-articular steroids and sulfasalazine

Gout

- Inflammatory arthritis associated with hyperuricaemia and urate crystal deposition

Epidemiology

- 5% of population have hyperuricaemia
- 0.2% of population have gout
- ♂ > ♀
- Commonly presents between 30 and 50 years
- Rare in women before the menopause
- Familial or sporadic
- HLA-DR4 positive in 50–70%

Aetiology

- Causes of hyperuricaemia (Table 11.3)

Clinical features

- Acute onset
- Acute painful, red, swollen joint
- Often affects first MTP joint
- Precipitated by
  - Alcohol
  - Excess food
  - Dehydration
  - Diuretics

Investigations

- Joint fluid microscopy – needle shape crystals
- Serum urate
- Urea and electrolytes

Table 11.3 Causes of hyperuricaemia

Impaired excretion of uric acid
Chronic renal disease (clinical gout unusual)
Drug therapy, e.g. thiazide diuretics, low-dose aspirin
Hypertension
Lead toxicity
Primary hyperparathyroidism
Hypothyroidism
Increased lactic acid production from alcohol, exercise, starvation
Glucose-6-phosphatase deficiency (interferes with renal excretion)

Increased production of uric acid
Increased purine synthesis de novo due to
    Hypoxanthine–guanine–phosphoribosyl transferase (HGPRT) reduction (an X-linked inborn error causing the Lesch–Nyhan syndrome)
Phosphoribosyl-pyrophosphate synthetase overactivity
    Glucose-6-phosphatase deficiency with glycogen storage disease type 1 (patients who survive develop hyperuricaemia due to increased production as well as decreased excretion)
Increased turnover of purines due to
    Myeloproliferative disorders, e.g. polycythaemia vera
    Lymphoproliferative disorders, e.g. leukaemia
    Others, e.g. carcinoma, severe psoriasis

Management

▌ NSAIDs
▌ Colchicine (particularly if NSAIDs cannot be used)
▌ If attacks are frequent give allopurinol to reduce urate 4–6 weeks after acute attack
▌ Lifestyle advice, e.g. diet, reduce alcohol intake

Chronic tophaceous gout

▌ Very high serum urate
▌ White urate deposits (tophi) in skin particularly ear lobes and around joints
▌ Associated with renal failure or use of diuretics

CONNECTIVE TISSUE DISEASE

Systemic lupus erythematosus (SLE) (*K&C*, p. 574)

▌ Inflammatory multisystem disorder with arthralgia and rashes as common symptoms, and cerebral and renal disease as serious problems

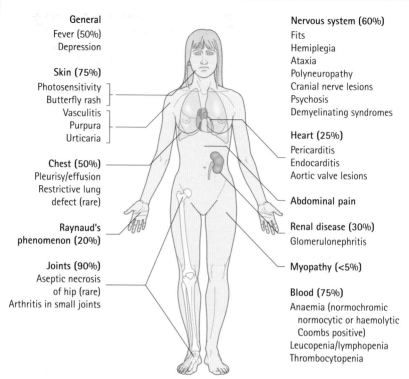

General
Fever (50%)
Depression

Skin (75%)
Photosensitivity
Butterfly rash
Vasculitis
Purpura
Urticaria

Chest (50%)
Pleurisy/effusion
Restrictive lung
defect (rare)

Raynaud's
phenomenon (20%)

Joints (90%)
Aseptic necrosis
of hip (rare)
Arthritis in small joints

Nervous system (60%)
Fits
Hemiplegia
Ataxia
Polyneuropathy
Cranial nerve lesions
Psychosis
Demyelinating syndromes

Heart (25%)
Pericarditis
Endocarditis
Aortic valve lesions

Abdominal pain

Renal disease (30%)
Glomerulonephritis

Myopathy (<5%)

Blood (75%)
Anaemia (normochromic
normocytic or haemolytic
Coombs positive)
Leucopenia/lymphopenia
Thrombocytopenia

Fig. 11.4 Clinical features of systemic lupus erythematosus (*K&C*, Fig. 10.25, p. 575.

Epidemiology

- ♀ > ♂
- Black > Caucasian
- Peak age of onset 20–40 years

Aetiology

- Familial
- ↑ HLA-B8 and DR3 in Caucasians
- Inherited deficiency of complement (C2 and 4)
- ?Related to female sex hormones
- Loss of immunological tolerance
- Environmental triggers
  - Drugs – hydralazine, isoniazid, methyldopa, oral contraceptive pill/HRT
  - Ultraviolet light

Clinical features

- Are the result of vasculitis (Fig. 11.4)

Table 11.4 Side-effects of steroids

General	Cardiovascular
Weight gain	Hypertension
Fluid retention	
	Eyes
Skin	Cataracts
Acne	
Thin skin with easy bruising	**Bones**
	Osteoporosis
Endocrine	
Diabetes	
Cushing's syndrome	

Investigations

Blood tests
- Normochromic normocytic anaemia
- Leucopenia
- Thrombocytopenia
- +/− Autoimmune haemolytic anaemia
- ↑ ESR
- Normal CRP
- Antinuclear antibody (ANA) positive
- Double-stranded DNA positive in 50%, SLE-specific
- Low complement during attacks
- Rh factor-positive in 30–50%
- False positive syphilis serology
- Raised IgG and M

Histology
- e.g. Renal biopsy
- Characteristic histology and immunofluorescence

CT/MRI
- e.g. Brain, may show infarcts/haemorrhage

Management

- Explain diagnosis
- Avoid UV light if photosensitive
- NSAIDs for arthralgia
- Antimalarials (e.g. chloroquine) for skin and joint disease
- Steroids for active disease
- Immunosuppressants
  - azathioprine/cyclophosphamide/ mycophenolate if severe

Course and prognosis

- Episodic
- Periods of complete remission
- 10-year survival 90%

Antiphospholipid syndrome (*K&C*, p. 577)

- A syndrome associated with the presence of antibodies to phospholipids

Clinical features

- Arterial and venous thromboses
- Recurrent miscarriage
- Thrombocytopenia
- Chorea, migraine and epilepsy
- Valvular heart disease
- Skin disease, e.g. livedo reticularis
- A few patients will have SLE

Investigation

- Anticardiolipin antibodies
- Lupus anticoagulant antibodies
- ESR and ANA usually normal
- Prolonged APTT

Management

- Aggressive anticoagulation
  - Aspirin
  - Heparin/warfarin

Systemic sclerosis (*K&C*, p. 577)

- A multisystem disease with widespread obliterative damage to small blood vessels associated with fibrosis of the skin and internal organs

Clinical features

Raynaud's phenomenon
- 97% of cases
- Arterial spasm of hands and feet
- Three phases
  - Pallor
  - Cyanosis
  - Erythema
- Numbness and pain

Skin
- Hands, face, feet, forearms
- Tight, waxy and tethered
- 'Beaking' of nose
- Microstomia
- Digital ulcers
- Telangiectasia
- Nail fold capillary loops

GI Tract ▌ Oesophagus
  – Reflux
  – Poor motility
  – Dilatation
▌ Small bowel
  – Bacterial overgrowth
  – Malabsorption
Renal ▌ Renal failure
▌ Malignant hypertension
Cardiorespiratory ▌ Pulmonary fibrosis (common cause of death)
system ▌ Primary or secondary pulmonary hypertension
▌ Arrhythmias
▌ Conduction defects
▌ Pericarditis

CREST syndrome

▌ **C**alcinosis (calcium deposits in skin and elsewhere)
▌ **R**aynaud's phenomenon
▌ o**E**sophageal involvement
▌ **S**clerodactyly
▌ **T**elangiectasia

Investigations

▌ Normocytic normochromic anaemia
▌ Urea and electrolytes and urinalysis including creatinine clearance
▌ Autoantibodies
  – Speckled/nucleolar/anticentromere – 70–80%
  – Rheumatoid factor – 30%
▌ Chest X-ray – reticulonodular shadowing
▌ Other tests according to organ involved

Management

▌ Education, counselling and family support
▌ Hand-warmers and vasodilators for Raynaud's
▌ Proton pump inhibitors and motility agents
▌ Antibiotics and nutritional supplements
▌ Antihypertensives
▌ I.v. prostacyclin

VASCULITIS (K&C, P. 581)

▌ Inflammation of blood vessel walls (Table 11.5)

Table 11.5 Vasculitides

Name	Type of vessel	Clinical features	Diagnosis	Treatment

Giant cell arteritis (GCA) and polymyalgia rheumatica (PMR)	Large vessel (e.g. temporal artery)	>50 years
		GCA
		  Headache
		  Scalp tenderness
		  Jaw claudication
		  Malaise tiredness
		  Fever
		  Sudden painless vision loss
		PMR
		  Pain and stiffness in shoulders, neck, hips and spine
		  Malaise
		  Tiredness
		  Fever
		  Weight loss
		  Depression
		  Worse in mornings
			Clinical features
			Raised ESR
			Temporal artery biopsy (shows a giant cell arteritis)
				Steroids

Polyarteritis nodosa	Medium-sized vessels	Middle-aged men usually Fever Malaise Weight loss Myalgia Neurological (mononeuritis multiplex) Abdominal (GI bleeding, infarction of viscera)	Clinical features Raised ESR Renal/hepatic/gut microaneurysms ANCA-positive in 20%	Steroids Azathioprine

	Vessels	Clinical features	Investigations	Treatment
		Renal (hypertension and renal failure) Cardiac (myocardial infarction and heart failure) Skin (gangrene, livedo reticularis)		
ANCA-positive vasculitis Wegener's granulomatosis Churg–Strauss syndrome Microscopic polyangiitis	Small vessels	Wegener's and Churg–Strauss polyarteritis Microscopic polyarteritis Crescentic glomerulonephritis Associated with hepatitis B	Clinical features ANCA	Steroids Immunosuppressants
Non-ANCA vasculitis Henoch–Schönlein purpura Cryoglobulinaemic vasculitis	Small vessels	Henoch–Schönlein purpura Children mostly, after upper respiratory tract infection Purpura Polyarthritis Abdominal pain Glomerulonephritis Cryoglobulinaemic Purpura Glomerulonephritis Arthralgia hepatitis C	Clinical features Most self-limiting	Steroids if severe
Behçet's syndrome	Small and large vessels	Japan and countries bordering the Mediterranean Recurrent oral and genital ulceration Uveitis Erythema nodosum Papulopustular and pseudofolliculitis skin lesions Arthritis GI symptoms Neurological symptoms	Clinical features	Steroids Ciclosporin Colchicine

BONE DISEASE (TABLE 11.6) (*K&C*, P. 590)

Osteoporosis (*K&C*, p. 594)

▪ Low bone mass and micro-architectural deterioration of bone leading to bone fragility and increased fracture risk
▪ In osteoporosis the bone is mineralised normally but deficient in quantity and quality including structural integrity

Epidemiology

▪ Common problem
▪ Lifetime risk of hip fracture in
  – ♀ aged 50 years – 15%
  – ♂ aged 50 years – 5%

Risk factors

▪ See Table 11.7

Table 11.6 Biochemical abnormalities in common bone disorders

Disease	Ca^{++}	PO$_4$	Alkaline phosphatase
Osteoporosis	→	→	→
Osteomalacia	↓	↓	↑
Paget's disease	→	→	↑
Bony secondary deposits	↑	↑ or →	↑

Table 11.7 Osteoporosis risk factors, associated disease and drug therapies

Risk factors	Disease
Female sex	Endocrine
Increasing age	Cushing's syndrome
Early menopause (including surgical)	Hyperparathyroidism
White race/Asian	Hypogonadism (including orchidectomy)
Slender habitus	Acromegaly
Lack of exercise/immobility	Type I diabetes mellitus
Smoking	Joints
Family history	Rheumatoid arthritis
Excess alcohol	Other
Nutrition (very low calcium diet, high protein intake for a long time)	Chronic renal failure
	Chronic liver disease
	Mastocytosis
Drug therapy	Anorexia nervosa
Corticosteroids	Inflammatory bowel disease
Heparin	
Ciclosporin	
Cytotoxic therapy	

Clinical features

Vertebral crush fractures
∎ Back pain
∎ Weight loss
∎ Kyphosis

Fractures associated with falls
∎ Colles' fracture
∎ Fractured neck of femur

Investigations

∎ Ca^{++}, PO_4 and alkaline phosphatase normal
∎ X-rays identify fractures
∎ DXA scanning
  – Measurement of bone density in lumbar spine and neck of femur
  – Osteoporosis is defined as bone density $<2.5\,SDs$ below the mean value of age-, sex- and race-matched controls
∎ Bone scan differentiates from bony metastases

Management

∎ Prevention
∎ Identification and monitoring of patients at risk

Non-drug therapies

∎ Diet rich in calcium and vitamin D
∎ Exercise
∎ Stopping smoking
∎ Reducing the risk of falls

Drugs
∎ Calcium and vitamin D supplements
∎ Bisphosphonates
∎ Raloxifene
∎ Recombinant human parathyroid hormone peptide 1–34
∎ Strontium
∎ Androgens in hypogonadal men

Osteomalacia (*K&C*, p. 600)

∎ Defective bone mineralisation associated with low levels of vitamin D
∎ In children the effects on the growth plates lead to rickets

Aetiology

∎ See Table 11.8

Clinical features

Adults
∎ Bone/muscle pain and tenderness
∎ Subclinical fractures

Table 11.8 Causes of rickets and osteomalacia

Vitamin D deficiency
Inadequate synthesis in skin
Low dietary intake
Malabsorption
  Coeliac disease
  Intestinal resection
  Chronic cholestasis,
  e.g. primary biliary cirrhosis

Renal disease
Chronic renal failure
Renal osteodystrophy

Bone disease due to dialysis
Tubular disorders, e.g. renal tubular
  acidosis, Fanconi's syndrome

Miscellaneous
Multiple myeloma
Vitamin D-dependent rickets
  types I and II
X-linked hypophosphataemia
  (vitamin D-resistant rickets)
Mesenchymal tumours

- Proximal myopathy
- Tetany (low calcium)

Children
- Bowed legs
- 'Rickety rosary' costochondritis
- Myopathy

Investigations

- $\downarrow Ca^{++}$, $\downarrow PO_4$, $\uparrow$ alkaline phosphatase, $\downarrow$ 25-hydroxy vitamin D
- X-ray – defective mineralisation
- 'Looser's zones' on X-ray

Management

- Correction of cause
- Replacement of vitamin D

Paget's disease (*K&C*, p. 599)
- Disorder of bone remodelling associated with excessive bone resorption and excess structurally abnormal new bone formation

Epidemiology

- Europe (especially northern England) $\gg$ USA/Africa
- Patients > 40 years
- Asymptomatic X-ray evidence very common
- Patients less commonly have symptoms

Aetiology

- Genetic component
- Geographical/ethnic clusters
- Viral aetiology has been suggested

Clinical features

- Bone pain (spine/pelvis)
- Joint pain (near to involved bone)
- Deformities (tibia and skull)

Complications

Nerve compression
- VIII cranial nerve leads to deafness
- Also II, V and VII cranial nerves

Increased bone blood flow
- → High-output cardiac failure

Pathological fractures
- <1% osteogenic sarcoma

Investigations

- Normal Ca^{++} and PO_4, ↑ alkaline phosphatase
- X-rays – excess abnormal bone

Management

- Simple analgesics for pain
- Bisphosphonates
- Surgery, e.g. joint replacement/osteotomy

DISORDERS OF CALCIUM METABOLISM

Hypercalcaemia (*K&C*, p. 1092)
Aetiology

- See Table 11.9

Clinical features

- Tiredness
- Malaise
- Depression
- Renal stones
- Polyuria
- Bone pains
- Abdominal pain
- Peptic ulcer disease
- Ectopic calcification, e.g. corneal

Investigations

- Ca^{++}, PO_4, alkaline phosphatase
- Urea and electrolytes
- Chest X-ray
- Parathormone (PTH)
- Thyroid-stimulating hormone (TSH)
- Serum electrophoresis

Table 11.9 Causes of hypercalcaemia

Excessive parathormone (PTH) secretion
Primary hyperparathyroidism (commonest by far), adenoma, hyperplasia or carcinoma
Tertiary hyperparathyroidism
Ectopic PTH secretion (very rare indeed)

Excess action of vitamin D
Iatrogenic or self-administered excess
Granulomatous diseases, e.g. sarcoidosis, TB
Lymphoma

Excessive calcium intake
'Milk-alkali' syndrome

Malignant disease (second commonest cause)
Secondary deposits in bone
Production of osteoclastic factors by tumours
PTH-related protein secretion
Myeloma

Other endocrine disease (mild hypercalcaemia only)
Thyrotoxicosis
Addison's disease

Drugs
Thiazide diuretics
Vitamin D analogues
Lithium administration (chronic)
Vitamin A

Miscellaneous
Long-term immobility
Familial hypocalciuric hypercalcaemia

Management

- ❚ Rectify cause
- ❚ I.v. Saline rehydration
- ❚ Bisphosphonates

Hypocalcaemia (*K&C*, p. 1094)
Aetiology

- ❚ See Table 11.10

Clinical features

- ❚ Paraesthesiae
- ❚ Circumoral numbness
- ❚ Cramps
- ❚ Anxiety

Table 11.10 Causes of hypocalcaemia

Increased phosphate levels
Chronic renal failure (common)
Phosphate therapy

Hypoparathyroidism
Surgical – after neck exploration (thyroidectomy parathyroidectomy – common)
Congenital deficiency (DiGeorge syndrome)
Idiopathic hypoparathyroidism (rare)
Severe hypomagnesaemia

Vitamin D deficiency
Osteomalacia
Vitamin D resistance

Resistance to PTH
Pseudohypoparathyroidism

Drugs
Calcitonin
Bisphosphonates

Miscellaneous
Acute pancreatitis (quite common)
Citrated blood in massive transfusion (not uncommon)
Malabsorption e.g. coeliac disease

- Tetany
- Fits
- Dystonia
- Psychosis
- Chvostek's sign – tapping over the facial nerve produces twitching of facial muscles
- Trousseau's sign – compression of the upper arm (e.g. with blood pressure cuff) produces tetany spasms of the hands

Investigations

- Ca^{++}, PO_4, alkaline phosphatase
- Urea and electrolytes
- X-rays
- Parathyroid hormone
- Vitamin D

Management

- Rectify cause
- Calcium/vitamin D

DISORDERS OF COLLAGEN (*K&C*, P. 601)

- Collagen is part of the extracellular matrix
- It consists of three polypeptide chains wound round one another in a triple helical conformation

Ehlers–Danlos syndrome (*K&C*, p. 602)

- Ten different types, mainly autosomal dominant
- Varying degrees of
  - Skin fragility
  - Skin hyperextensibility
  - Joint hypermobility

Clinical features

- Easy bruising
- Extensible velvety skin
- Hypermobile joints

Pseudoxanthoma elasticum (*K&C*, p. 1356)

- Abnormal collagen and elastin

Clinical features

Skin
- Loose, lax, wrinkled ('plucked chicken skin')
- Particularly in the flexures

Other
- GI bleeding
- Angioid streaks in the eye
- Early myocardial infarction
- Claudication

Marfan's syndrome (*K&C*, p. 839)

- Autosomal dominant
- Mutation of the collagen fibrillin
- Chromosome 15

Clinical features

- Tall stature
- Arachnodactyly (long thin digits)
- Long arm span
- High arched palate
- Recurrent joint dislocations
- Inguinal/femoral herniae
- Spontaneous pneumothorax
- Emphysema
- Aortic/mitral incompetence
- Aortic aneurysm
- Dislocation of the lens

SELF-ASSESSMENT QUESTIONS

Best one of five questions

1. The following are features of osteoarthritis but not rheumatoid arthritis:
   - A. Joint swelling
   - B. Heberden's nodes
   - C. More common in women
   - D. Negative rheumatoid factor
   - E. Treatment may include joint replacements

2. In rheumatoid arthritis:
   - A. 90% of patients have positive rheumatoid factors
   - B. Infliximab is used as treatment in all patients
   - C. HLA DR4 is present in 25%
   - D. T cells are activated
   - E. X-rays demonstrate the presence of osteophytes

3. In septic arthritis:
   - A. Artificial joints are not affected
   - B. Gram positive organisms are usually the cause
   - C. The joint is not usually swollen
   - D. Immunosuppressants are used as treatment
   - E. Treatment should wait for results of antibiotic sensitivities

4. Regarding autoantibodies:
   - A. ANA occurs in 90% of cases of antiphospholipid syndrome
   - B. Rheumatoid factor occurs in 40% of cases of systemic lupus erythematosus (SLE)
   - C. Rheumatoid factor occurs in 90% of cases of systemic sclerosis
   - D. Double-stranded DNA is specific for SLE

   - E. Anticentromere antibodies occur in 20% of cases of systemic sclerosis

5. Which of the following is seen in systemic sclerosis:
   - A. Butterfly skin rash
   - B. Pleural effusion
   - C. Thrombocytopenia
   - D. Hemiplegia
   - E. 'Beaking' of the nose

6. In systemic sclerosis:
   - A. Steroids are used
   - B. Malabsorption is caused by villous atrophy
   - C. Pulmonary fibrosis is a common cause of death
   - D. Raynaud's phenomenon occurs in few cases
   - E. Hands are rarely affected

7. In osteoporosis:
   - A. Plasma calcium may be low
   - B. Diagnosis is made when bone density rises 2.5 SDs above the mean for sex- and race-matched controls
   - C. Fracture risk can be reduced by bisphosphonates
   - D. Men and women are equally affected
   - E. Calcaneal fractures are common

8. In polymyalgia rheumatica:
   - A. The ESR is usually low
   - B. There can be an association with giant cell arteritis
   - C. Disease is unresponsive to steroids

D. Weight loss makes the diagnosis unlikely

E. Symptoms are worse at night

9. Osteomalacia:
   A. Is treated with steroids
   B. Is associated with normal bone biochemistry
   C. Does not cause myopathy
   D. Can be caused by inadequate exposure to sunlight
   E. Is rare in primary biliary cirrhosis

10. Causes of hypocalcaemia include:
    A. Secondary deposits in bone
    B. Addison's disease
    C. Hyperparathyroidism
    D. Thiazide diuretics
    E. Massive blood transfusion

11. In hypocalcaemia:
    A. Tapping on the facial nerve may induce twitching of the facial muscles
    B. Tetany does not occur
    C. Treatment with bisphosphonates can be useful
    D. Treatment with calcitonin can be useful
    E. i.v. calcium is contraindicated

12. In relation to serum bone biochemistry which statement is incorrect?
    A. Calcium is normal and alkaline phosphatase elevated in Paget's disease
    B. Phosphate is high in hypocalcaemia associated with chronic renal failure
    C. Calcium is low and alkaline phosphatase elevated in osteomalacia
    D. Calcium is low in hyperparathyroidism
    E. Calcium is high and phosphate low in hyperparathyroidism

Extended matching questions

Question 1 *Theme: back pain*

A. Osteoporosis
B. Osteoarthritis
C. Rheumatoid arthritis
D. Ankylosing spondylitis
E. Gout
F. Reactive arthritis
G. Systemic lupus erythematosus
H. Osteomalacia
I. Paget's disease

For each of the following questions, select the best answers from the list above:

I. A 28-year-old male who has intermittent episodes of back pain has a raised ESR and is HLA-B27-positive. X-rays show syndesmophytes. What is the most likely diagnosis?

II. A 60-year-old male smoker presents with progressive increasing episodes of back pain. His symptoms are worse in the mornings when he has stiffness. X-rays show no erosions. The ESR and alkaline phosphatase are normal. What is the most likely diagnosis?

III. A 72-year-old female presents with an episode of severe back pain. She fractured her wrist recently during a fall and has a long history of asthma. She has normal alkaline phosphatase and calcium. What is the most likely diagnosis?

Question 2 *Theme: painful hands*

A. Systemic sclerosis
B. Osteoarthritis
C. Rheumatoid arthritis
D. Gout
E. Reactive arthritis
F. Systemic lupus erythematosus
G. Septic arthritis
H. Psoriatic arthritis

For each of the following questions, select the best answers from the list above:

I. A 56-year-old businessman has acute episodes of pain in the joints of his hands and feet. The episodes occur particularly in the distal and interphalangeal joints of the hands and first metacarsophalangeal joint of the great toe. His body mass index is 30 and the serum urate is elevated. What is the most likely diagnosis?
II. A 35-year-old female presents with episodes of pain in the metacarpophalangeal joints of the hands. She has a fever and a rash on the face and the following blood results: rheumatoid factor positive, antinuclear antibody positive, ESR 15, CRP 145. What is the most likely diagnosis?
III. A 72-year-old female presents with pains in the joints of her hands and her neck. On examination she has bony

expansion of the distal interphalangeal joints of both hands. ESR is 35. What is the most likely diagnosis?

Question 3 *Theme: autoantibodies*

A. Systemic sclerosis
B. Osteoarthritis
C. Rheumatoid arthritis
D. Gout
E. Reactive arthritis
F. Systemic lupus erythematosus
G. Septic arthritis
H. Antiphospholipid syndrome

For each of the following questions, select the best answers from the list above:

I. 32-year-old female with a previous history of epilepsy presents with a history of recurrent miscarriage. She has a prolonged APTT and a positive anti-cardiolipin antibody. What is the most likely diagnosis?
II. A 35-year-old female presents with episodes of pain in the metacarpophalangeal joints of the hands. She has a fever. There are erosions on hand X-rays. Blood results show: rheumatoid factor negative, antinuclear antibody negative. What is the most likely diagnosis?
III. A 66-year-old retired schoolteacher has numbness and pain in her hands and feet. She has a positive-anticentromere antibody. What is the most likely diagnosis?

Dermatology 12

If you need more detailed explanation refer to Kumar & Clark, *Clinical Medicine*, Chapter 23.

Functions of the skin

- Physical barrier
- Protection against infection, chemicals and UV
- Prevention of excessive water loss or absorption
- UV-induced synthesis of vitamin D
- Temperature regulation
- Sensation
- Antigen presentation/immunological reactions and wound healing

EXAMINING THE SKIN

Examination of a rash (*K&C*, p. 1317)

Look at the rash

- For useful terms see Table 12.1

Note its distribution

Useful terminology
- Flexural/extensor (remember psoriasis is usually extensor and eczema is usually flexural)
- Localised/widespread
- Symmetrical/unilateral
- Facial
- Centripetal (trunk > limbs)
- Acral (hands and feet)
- Linear/annular
- Reticulate (lacy network)

Feel the rash

- Use gloves if necessary

Table 12.1 Useful terms to describe skin lesions

Term	Meaning
Atrophy	Thinning of skin
Bulla	Large fluid-filled blister
Crusted	Dried exudate
Ecchymosis	Large 'bruise'
Erosion	Small denuded area of skin
Excoriation	Scratch mark
Fissure	Deep linear crack
Lichenified	Thickened skin with normal markings
Macule	Flat, circumscribed non-palpable lesion
Nodule	Large papule (>0.5 cm)
Papule	Small palpable circumscribed lesion
Petechia	Pinpoint-sized macule of blood in the skin
Plaque	Large flat-topped palpable lesion
Purpura	Larger macule of blood in the skin which does not blanch on pressure
Pustule	Pus-filled lesion (white/yellow)
Scaly	Visible flakes/shedding of skin surface
Telangiectasia	Abnormal visible dilatation of blood vessels
Ulcer	Larger denuded area of skin
Vesicle	Small fluid-filled blister
Wheal	Raised erythematous swelling (dermal swelling)

Examine the

▌ Nails
▌ Hair
▌ Mouth

INFECTIONS

Bacterial infections (*K&C*, p. 1318)

Impetigo

▌ Weeping exudative areas with honey-coloured crust
▌ Highly infectious
▌ 90% due to *Staphylococcus aureus*

Management

▌ Topical/oral antibiotics

Cellulitis

▌ Hot tender area of confluent erythema
▌ Often on lower legs
▌ Can affect face (erysipelas)
▌ Caused by streptococci
▌ Risk factors
▌ Diabetes mellitus

Management

▌ Oral/i.v. antibiotics

Viral infections (*K&C*, p. 1321)

Herpes simplex

▌ Vesicular lesions
▌ May be recurrent, e.g. cold sores

Management

▌ Topical aciclovir/oral valciclovir

Herpes zoster (shingles)

▌ Reactivation of infection
▌ There may be a prodrome of tingling pain
▌ Unilateral blistering eruption
  – Single dermatomal distribution usually
  – Otoscopy demonstrates vesicles in the external auditory meatus

Management

▌ Analgesia
▌ Oral valciclovir/famciclovir or aciclovir

Complications

▌ Post-herpetic neuralgia (pain)
▌ Ocular involvement (trigeminal nerve)

FUNGAL INFECTIONS (MYCOSES) (*K&C*, P. 1322)

Dermatophyte infections
Tinea corporis

▌ Body ringworm
▌ Slightly itchy asymmetrical scaly patch with central clearing and raised edge

Tinea cruris

▌ Groin ringworm

Tinea pedis

▌ Athlete's foot

Tinea capitis

▌ Scalp ringworm

Management

▌ Antifungal cream
▌ Oral agents for feet/severe infections

Candida albicans
- Flexural areas
- Red areas with ragged edges
- Satellite lesions

Risk factors
- Immunosuppression including steroids
- Diabetes mellitus

Management
- Topical/oral antifungal agents

Infestations (*K&C*, p. 1325)
Scabies
- *Sacoptes scabiei*
- Itchy red papules in web spaces
- Skin burrows visible
- Diagnosis by skin scrapings

Treatment
- Malathion or permethrin
- Treat all skin below neck
- Treat all close contacts

ECZEMA (DERMATITIS) (*K&C*, P. 1326)

- Acute – inflamed weeping skin with vesicles
- Subacute – erythema, dry/flaky skin, crusted
- Chronic – lichenified skin

Epidemiology
- 40% of population have an episode associated with atopy
- Atopic individuals have a tendency to
  - Asthma
  - Eczema
  - Hay fever
  - Allergic rhinitis

Aetiology
- Genetic – polygenic
- Environmental triggers
  - Detergents/chemicals
  - Infection

  – Stress/anxiety
  – Animal fur
  – Foods (dairy products in the very young)

Clinical features

- Itchy erythematous scaly patches
- Often flexural
- May be associated with nail pitting

Investigations

- May have raised IgE or eosinophils
- Skin-patch testing

Management

- Education & explanation
- Avoid irritants
- Emollients, bath oil or soap substitutes
- Topical steroids or immunomodulators (tacrolimus)
- Antibiotics for secondary infection
- Antihistamines
- Second-line agents
  – Ultraviolet (UV) light
  – Oral steroids
  – Ciclosporin/azathioprine

PSORIASIS (*K&C*, P. 1331)

- Common disorder characterised by red scaly plaques

Epidemiology

- 2% of the population

  ♂ = ♀

Aetiology

- T lymphocyte-driven
- Genetic – polygenic
- Environmental triggers
  – Infection
  – Drugs, e.g. lithium
  – UV light
  – Alcohol
  – Stress/anxiety

Clinical features

Chronic plaque psoriasis
- Purplish/red scaly plaques, particularly on extensor surfaces
- Scalp frequently involved
- Can occur in areas of skin trauma (Köbner phenomenon)
- 50% associated with nail changes
  - Nail pitting
  - Distal separation of nail plate (onycholysis)
  - Yellow/brown discoloration
  - Subungual hyperkeratosis
  - If severe, loss of nail plate

Flexural psoriasis
- Occurs in older patients
- Patches in
  - Groin
  - Natal cleft
  - Submammary areas

Guttate psoriasis
- Raindrop-like lesions on trunk
- Occurs in children/young adults 2 weeks after a streptococcal sore throat

Arthritis associated with psoriasis
- See page 313

Management
- Education & explanation
- Avoid irritants
- Topical steroids
- Calcipotriol (vitamin D_3 analogue)
- Coal tar
- Phototherapy, e.g. PUVA (psoralen + UVA)
- Methotrexate if severe

Complications
- Erythroderma – see below

Erythroderma
- Widespread inflammation of the skin

Common causes
- Atopic eczema
- Psoriasis
- Drugs, e.g. sulphonamides, gold
- Seborrhoeic dermatitis

Management
- Bed rest
- Liberal IV fluids
- Keep warm

Table 12.2 Features of the three common skin cancers

Type	Clinical features	Spread	Management
Basal cell carcinoma (rodent ulcer)	Occur in later life Slow-growing nodule May ulcerate Pearly edge Telangiectasia Can erode local structures	No metastases	Surgical excision Radiotherapy
Squamous cell carcinoma	Rapidly growing nodule which ulcerates More common in immunosuppressed patients, e.g. renal transplant patients Also occurs in areas of chronic inflammation	Metastases occur	Surgical excision
Malignant melanoma	Can occur in young patients Transformation of 'moles' Consider in all bleeding pigmented lesions or 'changing moles'	Early metastases	Wide excision Radiotherapy Immunotherapy Chemotherapy for metastases

▐ Emollients
▐ Beware of sepsis
▐ Treat/remove the cause

Complications

▐ High-output cardiac failure
▐ Hypothermia
▐ Dehydration
▐ Hypoalbuminaemia
▐ Increased basal metabolic rate
▐ Capillary leak syndrome

SKIN CANCER (*K&C*, P. 1351)

▐ There are three common types (Table 12.2)
▐ All are related to exposure to sunlight

CUTANEOUS FEATURES OF SYSTEMIC DISEASE (*K&C*, P. 1341–46)

Erythema nodosum

▐ Painful dusky/blue nodules
▐ Commonly on the shins
▐ Associations – see Table 12.3

> ### Table 12.3 Aetiology of erythema nodosum and erythema multiforme
>
> **Erythema nodosum**
> Streptococcal infection
> Drugs (e.g. antibiotics, oral contraceptive pill)
> Tuberculosis
> Inflammatory bowel disease
> Sarcoid
> Leprosy
> Yersinia infection
> Fungal infection e.g. histoplasmosis
> Chlamydia infection
> Idiopathic
>
> **Erythema multiforme**
> Herpes/Epstein–Barr virus infection
> Drugs (e.g. antibiotics, barbiturates)
> Mycoplasma infections
> Connective tissue disease, e.g. SLE
> HIV
> Carcinoma/lymphoma

Erythema multiforme

▌ Erythematous lesion with central pallor (target lesions)
▌ Symmetrical, particularly on limbs
▌ May blister
▌ Mucosal involvement = Stevens–Johnson syndrome
▌ Associations – see Table 12.3

Pyoderma gangrenosum

▌ Erythematous nodules with ulceration
▌ Large areas of ulceration
▌ Bluish/black edge
▌ Purulent surface
▌ Associations
 – Inflammatory bowel disease
 – Rheumatoid arthritis
 – Myeloma/leukaemia/lymphoma
 – Liver disease
 – Idiopathic

Management

▌ Topical/oral steroids
▌ Treatment of underlying condition
▌ Ciclosporin

Acanthosis nigricans

▮ Thickened hyperpigmented skin in the flexures, e.g. axilla
▮ Associations
  – Insulin resistance
  – Malignancy (particularly GI tract)

Chronic discoid lupus

▮ Red scaly atrophic plaques $+/-$ telangiectasia
▮ Face/exposed areas of skin
▮ May be associated with alopecia
▮ Triggered/exacerbated by UV light
▮ 30% antinuclear factor-positive
▮ 5% develop systemic lupus erythematosus (SLE)

Management

▮ Topical steroids
▮ Hydroxychloroquine
▮ Oral steroids/azathioprine/ciclosporin/thalidomide

Systemic lupus erythematosus (skin manifestations)

▮ Macular erythema on cheeks/nose/forehead (butterfly rash)

Pruritus (medical conditions associated with itching)

▮ Iron deficiency
▮ Malignancy, e.g. lymphoma
▮ Diabetes mellitus
▮ Chronic renal failure
▮ Cholestasis
▮ Chronic liver disease
▮ Thyroid disease
▮ HIV
▮ Polycythaemia rubra vera

LEG ULCERS (*K&C*, P. 1353)

Aetiology

▮ Venous hypertension
▮ Arterial insufficiency
▮ Neuropathic (e.g. diabetes mellitus)
▮ Neoplastic (e.g. squamous cell carcinoma)
▮ Vasculitis

- Infection, e.g. syphilis
- Blood disorders, e.g. sickle cell disease
- Trauma

Venous ulcers

- Most common cause
- Associated with venous hypertension or previous thrombosis
- Often recurrent and chronic
- Usually painless
- Medial aspect of leg
- Exclude arterial insufficiency with Doppler

Management

- Topical therapy to ulcer
- Compression bandaging and elevation of legs
- Antibiotics for overt infection
- Diuretics for oedema
- Analgesia if painful
- Skin grafting if resistant to therapy

Arterial ulcers

- Punched out
- Painful
- Leg cold and pale
- Absent pulses
- History of hypertension, claudication, smoking, angina
- Investigate with Doppler studies/angiogram

Management

- Analgesia
- Topical treatment of ulcer
- Vascular reconstruction

Neuropathic ulcer

- Over pressure areas, e.g. metatarsal heads
- Result of trauma
- Polyneuropathy, e.g. diabetes mellitus
- Painless

Management

- Keep clean
- Avoid trauma including good foot care

SELF-ASSESSMENT QUESTIONS

Best one of five questions

1. Which of the following is a risk factor for skin malignancy:
   A. Methotrexate
   B. Diabetes mellitus
   C. Steroids
   D. Phenytoin
   E. Sunlight exposure

2. In dermatology:
   A. A bulla is pus-filled
   B. Acral lesions affect the scalp
   C. An ecchymosis is a large bruise
   D. Purpura blanch on pressure
   E. Ringworm is a viral infection

3. In eczema:
   A. The rash is rarely itchy
   B. The rash is often on the extensor surfaces
   C. Stress can be a trigger factor
   D. Ciclosporin is the usual treatment
   E. 10% of the population experience the condition at some time in their lives

4. Psoriasis:
   A. Is more common in males
   B. Is not triggered by stress
   C. Most commonly affects extensor surfaces
   D. Is easily cured
   E. Is usually treated with topical antibiotics

5. Basal cell carcinoma:
   A. Is associated with early metastases
   B. May have telangiectasia
   C. Never ulcerates
   D. Is treated with chemotherapy
   E. Is most common in young adults

6. Malignant melanoma:
   A. Is not associated with early metastases
   B. Is rarely life-threatening in young people
   C. Is easily distinguished from benign moles
   D. Is treated by wide excision and adjuvant therapy
   E. Only occurs in the skin

7. Erythema nodosum:
   A. Often occurs on the arms
   B. Is not associated with Crohn's disease
   C. Is associated with use of oral contraceptives
   D. Is common in tuberculosis
   E. Is most commonly associated with a viral infection

8. In erythema multiforme:
   A. Uniform red patches occur
   B. Lesions on the feet occur in Stevens–Johnson syndrome
   C. Is not caused by barbiturates
   D. Disease is less likely in immunosuppressed patients
   E. The rash is often asymmetrical

9. Leg ulcers:
   A. Are most commonly caused by arterial insufficiency
   B. Are always painful if venous
   C. Associated with neuropathy occur over metatarsal heads
   D. May need treatment with steroids
   E. Are rarely recurrent

10. Erythroderma:
A. Is not a complication of eczema
B. Is usually treated with fluid restriction
C. Capillary leak syndrome may require intensive care
D. Is treated with induced hypothermia
E. Is localised to the legs

Extended matching questions

Question 1 *Theme: erythematous rash*

A. Eczema
B. Psoriasis
C. Meningococcal septicaemia
D. Squamous cell carcinoma
E. Systemic lupus erythematosus
F. Impetigo
G. Erysipelas
H. Erythema multiforme
I. Erythema nodosum
J. Typhoid fever

For each of the following questions, select the best answer from the list above:

I. A 39-year-old female presents with an erythematous rash on her legs. She has just returned from holiday in North Africa. The lesions are purplish, painful and warm to the touch. She has a medical history of Crohn's disease and at present has a flare-up of her symptoms with diarrhoea. What is the most likely diagnosis?

II. A 12-year-old female presents with an erythematous rash on her arms. She has a history of asthma. She also says that she is having difficulty sleeping because of itching. The rash is flexural in distribution and she has nail pitting. What is the most likely diagnosis?

III. A 28-year-old male presents with a rash on his hands. It is weeping fluid and in parts has yellow crusting areas. His girlfriend has a similar rash. It responds to treatment with antibiotics. What is the most likely diagnosis?

Question 2 *Theme: skin ulcers*

A. Venous ulcers
B. Squamous cell carcinoma
C. Malignant melanoma
D. Erythema multiforme
E. Erythema nodosum
F. Pyoderma gangrenosum
G. Impetigo
H. Erythrasma
I. Leprosy

For each of the following questions, select the best answer from the list above:

I. A 39-year-old female presents with a painless ulcer on her right shin. She recently injured this area whilst on holiday in Africa. She has a medical history of Crohn's disease. She is worried that the ulcer is rapidly increasing in size. What is the most likely diagnosis?

II. An 82-year-old female presents with an ulcer just above the medial malleolus. She has been treated with dressings by the community nurses for 6 weeks without improvement. She has previously had surgery for varicose veins and is on aspirin for angina. The skin around the ulcer is pigmented and brownish. What is the most likely diagnosis?

III. A 48-year-old male presents with an ulcer on his ear. He is a keen gardener. He has had an area of crusting skin there for some time. There is an enlarged hard post-auricular lymph node. What is the most likely diagnosis?

Question 3 *Theme: pruritus*

A. Iron deficiency
B. Squamous cell carcinoma
C. Diabetes mellitus
D. Erythema multiforme
E. Erythema nodosum
F. Cholestasis
G. HIV
H. Erythrasma
I. Polycythaemia rubra vera

For each of the following questions, select the best answer from the list above:

I. A 39 year old male presents with pruritus. A full blood count reveals that he has a low lymphocyte count. What is the most likely cause of his itching?

II. An 82-year-old female presents with itching, weight loss and abdominal pain. Her neighbours have told her that she looks yellow. She has recently been diagnosed with diabetes. An ultrasound suggests a mass in the head of the pancreas. What is the most likely cause of her itching?

III. A 48-year-old male presents with itching. He has also noted a change in his bowel habit and is awaiting colonoscopy. His full blood count shows a haemoglobin of 8.9 g/dl with an MCV of 69 fL What is the most likely cause of his itching?

Endocrinology 13

Hormones
- Transmit information between cells or organs
- Allow adjustment to internal and external environment

Endocrine organs
- Synthesis and release hormones
- Maintain homeostatic mechanisms

Endocrine disorders
- Caused by abnormalities in hormone
  - Synthesis
  - Secretion
  - Control
  - Function
- Common disorders are shown in Table 13.1
- Rarer conditions, however, provide classical cases for both written and clinical examinations and will be included in this chapter

Common pathologies
- Affect endocrine glands or their target organs
- Organ-specific autoimmune disorders
- Endocrine tumours

Table 13.1 Common endocrine disorders

Diabetes mellitus	Osteoporosis
Thyroid disease	Primary hyperparathyroidism
Subfertility	Short stature
Menstrual disorders	Delayed puberty
Excess hair growth	

CLINICAL HISTORY IN ENDOCRINE DISEASE

▌ See Table 13.2

Table 13.2 Points to note in taking an endocrine history

Past medical history
Diabetes mellitus
Hypertension
Previous pregnancies/fertility
Previous surgery – thyroid/parathyroid, ovarian, testicular
Childhood milestones and development
Puberty
Previous radiation exposure – neck (thyroid), gonads

Family history
Autoimmune disorders
Endocrine disorders
Diabetes mellitus

Social history
Alcohol or drug abuse
Diet, e.g. salt/iodine intake

Drug history
Details of *all* drugs taken at present and previous regular medications
Corticosteroids
Sex hormones, e.g. HRT, oral contraceptive pill

EXAMINING THE ENDOCRINE SYSTEM

BOX 1.1 CLINICAL EXAMINATION IN ENDOCRINOLOGY

Overall appearance
Height, weight and nutritional status
Blood pressure (including postural measurements)
Neck – look for goitre
Thyroid status (see Box 13.2, p. 351)
Eyes – look for exophthalmos, Graves' eye disease
Visual fields – pituitary tumours
Secondary sexual characteristics and testicular examination
Skin and hair – pigmentation, bruising, telangiectasia, acne
Urine – check for glucose, protein, β-human chorionic gonadotrophin

---

▌ Overall appearance (i.e. spot diagnosis), e.g. acromegaly, Graves' disease, should be assessed
▌ All clinical 'systems' may be involved in endocrine disorders

- Full examination of all systems is expected
- Certain parts of the examination may be discriminatory in diagnosis

LABORATORY TESTS IN ENDOCRINOLOGY
(*K&C*, P. 1038)

- Hormones may be measured in blood/plasma or urine
- Markers of function
  - Glucose in diabetes
  - Calcium in hyperparathyroidism

Basal levels
Blood or plasma levels

- Useful measurements for hormones with a long half-life, e.g. thyroxine (T_4 and T_3)
- Also applied to certain conditions in which normal values are known, e.g.
  - Time of day – cortisol and adrenocorticotrophic hormone (ACTH)
  - Period of menstrual cycle – follicle stimulating hormone (FSH), oestrogen, progesterone
  - Posture – aldosterone

24-hour urine collections

- Provide an average of a whole day's secretion of a hormone
- Require normal renal function and accurately timed and complete urine collection

Dynamic tests

- Test ability of a gland to respond appropriately to stimulation or suppression
- Failure of normal negative feedback causing uncontrolled hormone secretion
  - From within the gland
  - From an ectopic source
- Failure of a normal positive response to stimulation of a gland

Examples

Stimulation test – Synacthen test

- Normal adrenal response to a dose of synthetic ACTH is an increase in plasma cortisol levels

- Primary adrenal failure – a diminished or absent response
- Adrenal failure secondary to lack of pituitary secretion of ACTH – normal or enhanced cortisol response

Suppression test – dexamethasone suppression test

- Normal response to a dose of synthetic steroid is reduction in pituitary release of ACTH and subsequent fall in adrenal cortisol release and plasma levels
- Uncontrolled endogenous production of ACTH from a pituitary tumour or ectopic source leads to inadequate suppression of plasma cortisol level

THYROID DISORDERS (*K&C, P. 1069*)

Control of thyroxine secretion

- See Figure 13.1 and Table 13.3

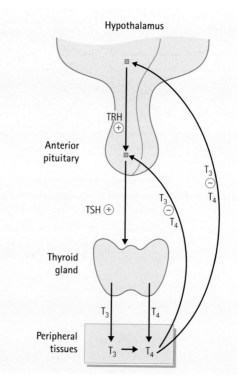

Fig. 13.1 The hypothalamic-pituitary-thyroid axis. TRH: Thyrotrophin releasing hormone. TSH: Thyroid stimulating hormone.

Table 13.3 Biochemistry of thyroid disorders

	Hormone levels		Dynamic and other tests
	T4	TSH	
Hyperthyroidism	↑	↓	Autoantibodies
Primary hypothyroidism	↓	↑	Autoantibodies
Secondary hypothyroidism	↓	↓ or normal	

Examination of thyroid gland and status

❚ See information box and Chapter 3.

BOX 13.2 EXAMINATION OF THYROID GLAND AND STATUS

General inspection
Look for signs of thyroid disease

Examine the neck
Look for a goitre
  Ask the patient to take a sip of water and hold it in the mouth, then ask him or her to swallow while watching the neck – look for movement of goitre with swallowing
  Stand behind the patient and feel the thyroid with both hands, starting in the centre below the thyroid cartilage over the trachea, and moving laterally to the two lobes which extend behind the sternomastoid muscle. Ask the patient to swallow while palpating. Assess the goitre for size, nodularity or diffuse enlargement, discrete nodules and firmness
  Palpate for lymph nodes
  Auscultate – listen over the thyroid for a bruit

Assess thyroid status
Pulse – count the rate and note the presence or absence of atrial fibrillation
Palms – warm and sweaty
Tremor of outstretched arms

Examine the eyes
Exophthalmos
Lid retraction
Lid lag

Examine the reflexes
Slow relaxation in hypothyroidism

Goitre

Aetiology in a euthyroid patient

❚ Simple non-toxic goitre
  – Iodine deficiency
  – Treated Graves' disease
  – Puberty

- Solitary nodule
  - Thyroid adenoma
  - Thyroid cyst
  - Thyroid carcinoma

Aetiology in a hypothyroid patient

- Hashimoto's thyroiditis
- Radioiodine-treated Graves' disease

Aetiology in a hyperthyroid patient

- Graves' disease
- Toxic multinodular goitre

Hypothyroidism (*K&C*, p. 1071)
Aetiology

- Hashimoto's thyroiditis
- Post radioiodine-treated hyperthyroidism
- Thyroidectomy

Clinical features

- Weight gain
- Lethargy
- Depression
- Patient feels the cold
- Constipation
- Poor appetite
- Menstrual disturbances
- Myxoedema facies; thickened skin
- Brittle hair
- Periorbital puffiness
- Bradycardia
- Slow relaxing reflexes

Investigations

- Biochemistry (Table 13.3)
- Haematology
  - Macrocytosis
  - Anaemia
- Anti-thyroid antibodies

Management

- Thyroxine replacement
- Caution in cardiac disease
- Monitor TSH

Hyperthyroidism (*K&C*, p. 1073)
Common causes

- Graves disease
- Toxic multinodular goitre

- Single toxic nodule
- Gestational

Clinical features

- Heat intolerance
- Weight loss
- Increased appetite
- Diarrhoea
- Irritability
- Sleeplessness, tiredness
- Exertional breathlessness
- Goitre
- Tachycardia/atrial fibrillation
- Tremor
- Hyperkinesia
- Proximal muscle wasting
- Cardiac failure
- Pretibial myxoedema

Eye signs
(Graves' disease)
- Exophthalmos
- Lid lag
- Lid retraction
- Ophthalmoplegia

Management
Medical treatment
- Carbimazole
- Propylthiouracil
- Radioiodine

Surgical
treatment for
- Malignancy
- Pressure symptoms
- Failure of medical treatment

PITUITARY DISORDERS

Functions of the anterior pituitary
- See Figure 13.2 and Table 13.4

Control of growth hormone secretion
- See Figure 13.3

Acromegaly (*K&C*, p. 1067)
Aetiology

- Pituitary tumour

Clinical features

- Often insidious non-specific onset

353

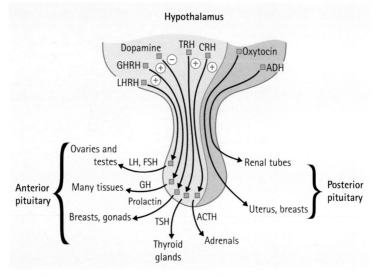

Fig. 13.2 The hypothalamic-pituitary axis. LHRH: Luteinizing hormone releasing hormone. TSH: Thyroid stimulating hormone. FSH: Follicle stimulating hormone. CRH: Corticotrophin releasing hormone. GHRH: Growth hormone releasing hormone. ACTH: Adrenocorticotrophic hormone. TRH: Thyrotrophin releasing hormone. ADH: Antidiuretic hormone.

Table 13.4 Biochemistry of disorders of the hypothalamic-anterior pituitary axis

	Hormone levels	Dynamic and other tests
Acromegaly	Growth hormone ↑	Oral glucose load (growth hormone (GH) fails to suppress)
Prolactinoma	Prolactin ↑	
Panhypopituitarism	Luteinizing hormone (LH)/follicle stimulating hormone (FSH) ↓	Luteinizing hormone releasing hormone (LHRH) test
	GH ↓ TSH ↓ ACTH ↓	Insulin stress test TRH test Synacthen test

▌ Headaches
▌ Polyuria
▌ Erectile dysfunction
▌ Visual field defects, e.g. bitemporal hemianopia

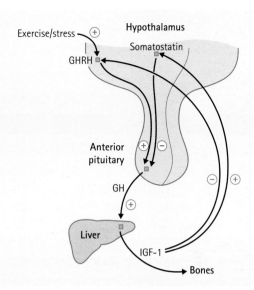

Fig. 13.3 The growth axis. IGF-1: Insulin-like growth factor 1.

- Nerve compression, e.g. carpal tunnel syndrome
- Typical facies, e.g.
  - Thick greasy skin
  - Protrusion of lower jaw
  - Gaps between teeth
- Large 'spade-like' hands
- Cardiac failure
- Diabetes mellitus
- Hypertension

Management

- GH antagonists
- Bromocriptine
- Somatostatin analogues
- Pituitary radiotherapy
- Surgical hypophysectomy

Hypopituitarism (*K&C*, p. 1046)
Aetiology

Congenital
- Kallmann's syndrome

Infective
- Basal meningitis
- Encephalitis
- Syphilis

Vascular
- Sheehan's syndrome

Tumours	▋ Pituitary
	▋ Hypothalamic
	▋ Craniopharyngioma
	▋ Meningioma
	▋ Glioma
	▋ Metastases (especially breast)
	▋ Lymphoma
Infiltration	▋ Sarcoidosis
	▋ Langerhan's histiocytosis
	▋ Haemochromatosis
Others	▋ Radiation
	▋ Anorexia nervosa
	▋ Trauma or previous surgery

Clinical features

▋ Due to progressive loss of anterior pituitary hormones (listed in order of frequency)

Growth hormone ▋ Growth failure
▋ Short stature
Prolactin ▋ Failure of lactation
Gonadotrophins ▋ Delayed puberty
▋ Infertility
▋ Amenorrhoea
▋ Loss of body hair
TSH ▋ Hypothyroidism
ACTH ▋ Adrenal failure (without pigmentation)

Investigations

▋ Determine hormone deficiencies
▋ Pituitary imaging, e.g. CT scan, MRI scan

Management

▋ Treat cause
▋ Hormone replacement

ADRENAL HORMONE ABNORMALITIES

Control of cortisol secretion

▋ See Figure 13.4

Cushing's syndrome (*K&C*, p. 1085)

▋ Overproduction of corticosteroids or excess corticosteroid treatment

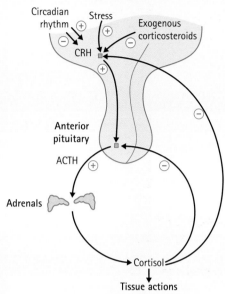

Fig. 13.4 The hypothalamic-pituitary-adrenal axis.

Aetiology

ACTH-dependent	▌ Pituitary adenoma
	▌ Ectopic ACTH-secreting tumours
Non-ACTH-dependent	▌ Adrenal adenoma
	▌ Adrenal carcinoma
	▌ Steroid treatment
Others	▌ Alcohol-induced pseudo-Cushing's syndrome

Clinical features

▌ Weight gain
▌ Thin skin
▌ Striae
▌ Bruising
▌ Menstrual disturbances
▌ Psychosis
▌ Red face
▌ Central obesity
▌ Buffalo hump
▌ Hirsutism
▌ Proximal myopathy
▌ Hypertension
▌ Diabetes mellitus

Table 13.5 Biochemistry of disorders of the pituitary-adrenal axis

	Hormone levels	Dynamic and other tests
ACTH-secreting pituitary adenoma (Cushing's disease)	24-hour urine cortisol ↑ Midnight cortisol ↑	Dexamethasone suppression test
Ectopic ACTH secretion	24-hour urine cortisol ↑ Midnight cortisol ↑	Dexamethasone suppression test
Adrenal adenoma	24-hour urine cortisol ↑ Midnight cortisol ↑	Dexamethasone suppression test
Pituitary failure	9 am cortisol ↓	Synacthen test (normal response)
Primary adrenal failure	9 am cortisol ↓	Synacthen test (diminished response)

Investigations

- Biochemistry See Table 13.5
- Serum electrolytes
  – Sodium ↓
  – Potassium ↑
- Pituitary imaging
- Adrenal imaging
- Chest X-ray

Management

Pituitary-dependent
- Trans-sphenoidal resection of tumour

Adrenal adenomas
- Medical treatment with metyrapone, to induce remission before adrenalectomy

Ectopic ACTH
- Remove tumour if possible
- Control Cushing's with metyrapone

Primary hypoadrenalism – Addison's disease (*K&C*, p. 1082)

- Destruction of adrenal cortex causing reduced production of glucocorticoid, mineralocorticoid and sex steroids

Aetiology

- See Table 13.6

Clinical features

- Tiredness
- Debility
- Nausea, vomiting

Table 13.6 Causes of primary hypoadrenalism
Common
Autoimmune disease (approx 90%)
Tuberculosis (<10% in UK)
Surgical removal
Uncommon
Haemorrhage/infarction
Meningococcal septicaemia
Venography
Malignant destruction
Amyloid

▌ Anorexia, weight loss
▌ Abdominal pain
▌ Diarrhoea
▌ Depression
▌ Menstrual disturbance
▌ Pigmentation – mouth, palmar creases
▌ Postural hypotension
▌ Dehydration
▌ Loss of body hair

Investigations

▌ See Table 13.5

Management

▌ Replacement of glucocorticoids and mineralocorticoids with oral hydrocortisone and fludrocortisone

PARATHYROIDS (SEE ALSO CHAPTER 11)

Hyperparathyroidism (*K&C*, p. 1092)
Aetiology

Primary ▌ Adenoma (80% solitary)
▌ Hyperplasia
▌ Carcinoma

Secondary ▌ Hyperplasia in hypocalcaemia
▌ Chronic renal failure
▌ Osteomalacia

Tertiary ▌ Autonomous secretion after prolonged hypocalcaemia

Table 13.7 Biochemistry of disorders of calcium homeostasis

	Hormone levels	Dynamic and other tests
Osteoporosis	PTH normal	
Primary hyperparathyroidism	PTH ↑	Serum calcium ↑
		Serum phosphate ↓
Tertiary hyperparathyroidism	PTH ↑	Serum calcium ↑
		Serum phosphate ↑
Primary hypoparathyroidism	PTH undetectable	Serum calcium ↓
Pseudohypoparathyroidism	PTH normal	Serum calcium ↓

Clinical features

- Anorexia
- Abdominal pain
- Constipation
- Polydipsia and polyuria
- Renal calculi
- Pain
- Pathological fractures

Due to hypercalcaemia

Investigations

- See Table 13.7

Management

- Treat underlying cause
- Parathyroidectomy if $Ca^{++} > 3$ or symptoms
- Treat hypercalcaemia (page 326)

Hypoparathyroidism (*K&C*, p. 1094)
Aetiology

- Post-surgical
- Post-radiotherapy
- Autoimmune
- Pseudohyperparathyroidism = end organ resistance

Clinical features

- Tetany
- Paraesthesiae
- Cramps
- Fits
- Cataracts

Due to hypocalcaemia

Investigations

- See Table 13.7

Osteoporosis

- Reduction in bone density below normal for age and sex (page 322)

SEX HORMONE AND REPRODUCTIVE DISORDERS

Amenorrhoea – primary or secondary (*K&C*, p. 1056)
Aetiology

Pituitary causes	▌ Hyperprolactinaemia
	▌ Hypopituitarism
	▌ Thyrotoxicosis
	▌ Anorexia nervosa
Ovarian causes	▌ Surgery
(Table 13.8)	▌ Primary ovarian failure
	▌ Polycystic ovary syndrome
	▌ Congenital adrenal hyperplasia
	▌ Chromosomal abnormalities
	▌ Turner's syndrome

SALT AND WATER BALANCE DISORDERS

Control of salt and water homeostasis
▌ See Figure 13.5

Diabetes insipidus (*K&C*, p. 1090)
▌ Deficiency of antidiuretic hormone (ADH) or insensitivity to its action

Aetiology

▌ Cranial causes
- Idiopathic
- Familial (DIDMOAD – diabetes insipidus, diabetes mellitus, optic atrophy, deafness)
- Tumours, e.g. craniopharyngioma, glioma, metastases (breast)
- Infiltration, e.g. sarcoidosis, histiocytosis
- Sheehan's syndrome (pituitary infarction following post– or antepartum haemorrhage)

Table 13.8 **Biochemistry of ovarian disorders**

	Hormone levels	Dynamic and other tests
Polycystic ovary syndrome	Androgens ↑	
Primary ovarian failure	FSH ↑	LHRH test
	LH ↑	Clomiphene stimulation test
	Oestrogen ↓	

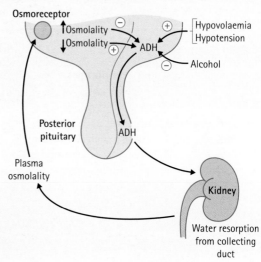

Fig. 13.5 The thirst axis.

- Nephrogenic causes
  - Idiopathic
  - Renal tubular acidosis
  - Hypokalaemia
  - Hypercalcaemia
  - Drugs, e.g lithium, demeclocycline, glibenclamide

Clinical features

- Polyuria urine output (10–15 L/day)
- Thirst
- Nocturia
- Polydipsia
- Dehydration

Differential diagnosis

- Primary polydipsia (excessive water drinking/normal ADH secretion)

Investigations

- See Table 13.9

Management

- Treat underlying cause
- Synthetic vasopressin analogue
- DDAVP

Table 13.9 Biochemistry of the hypothalamic-posterior pituitary axis

	Hormone levels	Dynamic and other tests
Cranial diabetes insipidus	ADH ↓ (not measured routinely)	Water deprivation test High plasma osmolality Low urine osmolality Normal response to DDAVP
Nephrogenic diabetes insipidus	ADH ↑ (not measured routinely)	Water deprivation test High plasma osmolality Low urine osmolality No response to DDAVP
Inappropriate ADH	ADH ↑ (not measured routinely)	Plasma osmolality low Urine osmolality high

- Carbamazepine
- Chlorpropamide

Syndrome of inappropriate ADH secretion (SIADH)
(*K&C*, p. 1091)

- Inappropriate ADH secretion leads to retention of water and hyponatraemia

Aetiology

Tumours
- Small cell carcinoma of lung
- Prostate cancer
- Pancreatic cancer

Lungs
- Pneumonia
- TB

CNS
- Meningitis
- Tumours
- Head injury
- Chronic subdural haematoma
- SLE vasculitis

Drugs
- Chlorpropamide
- Carbamezepine
- Phenothiazines

Clinical features

- Confusion
- Nausea
- Fits
- Coma

Management

- Underlying cause
- Fluid restriction
- Dimethylchlortetracycline

BOX 13.3 WATER DEPRIVATION TEST

Free fluid overnight

08.00 hrs
No access to fluids
Record hourly
  Urine and plasma osmolality
  Urine volume
  Body weight
Stop and allow fluid if body weight loss > 3%

16.00 hrs
2 µg desmopressin injection i.m.
Continue fluid restriction according to urine output

04.00 hrs
Stop

Normal
Normal plasma osmolality maintained up to urine concentration > 800 mosm/kg

Cranial DI
Urine fails to concentrate
Plasma osmolality rises
Abnormality is corrected with desmopressin

Nephrogenic DI
As for cranial DI but not corrected by desmopressin

ENDOCRINE CAUSES OF HYPERTENSION
(*K&C*, P. 1095)

Control of the renin-angiotensin-aldosterone system
▌ See Figure 13.6

Primary hyperaldosteronism (Table 13.10)
▌ Rare (<1% of all hypertension)

Aetiology

▌ Conn's syndrome (adrenal adenoma 60%)
▌ Bilateral adrenal hyperplasia (40%)

Management

▌ Surgery for tumours
▌ Aldosterone antagonists, e.g. spironolactone

Phaeochromocytoma
▌ Very rare
▌ Tumour of the sympathetic nervous system (90% adrenal)

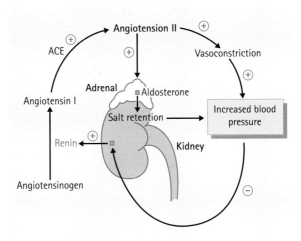

Fig. 13.6 The renin-angiotensin-aldosterone system. ACE: Angiotensin-converting enzyme.

Table 13.10 Biochemistry of hyperaldosteronism

	Hormone levels	Dynamic and other tests
Primary hyperaldosteronism (Conn's syndrome)	Renin ↓ Aldosterone ↑	Serum K ↓ Aldosterone:renin ratio ↑ Metabolic alkalosis
Secondary hyperaldosteronism	Renin ↑ Aldosterone ↑	Serum K ↓ Metabolic alkalosis

❚ Secretion of norepinephrine and epinephrine leading to
 – Peripheral vasoconstriction
 – Inotropic effects
 – Tachycardia
 – High blood pressure

Clinical features

❚ Anxiety, panic attacks
❚ Palpitations
❚ Tremor
❚ Sweating
❚ Headache
❚ Flushing
❚ GI upset
❚ Weight loss
❚ Hypertension (paroxysmal or continuous)
❚ Tachycardia
❚ Arrhythmias
❚ Fever

Investigations

- Raised 24-hour excretion of urinary catecholamines
- CT or MRI adrenal glands
- MIBG scan ^{131}I metaiodobenzylguanidine is specifically taken up in sites of sympathetic activity
  - Positive in 90% of phaeochromocytomas

Management

- Remove tumour
- α- and β-blockade (α first with phenoxybenzamine, then β with propranolol) prior to surgery to prevent dangerous swings in blood pressure

Multiple endocrine neoplasia (MEN)

- Simultaneous or metachronous occurrence of tumours in a number of endocrine glands with autosomal dominant inheritance

Type 1

- Parathyroid – adenomas, hyperplasia
- Pituitary – adenomas
- Pancreas – islet cell tumours (e.g. insulinoma), gastrinoma
- Adrenal adenoma
- Thyroid adenoma

Type 2a

- Adrenal – phaeochromocytoma
- Thyroid – medullary carcinoma
- Parathyroid – adenomas, adenocarcinoma

Type 2b

- Type 2a plus Marfanoid phenotype plus visceral ganglioneuromas

DIABETES MELLITUS (*K&C*, P. 1101)

- Syndrome characterised by chronic hyperglycaemia due to relative insulin deficiency or resistance or both

WHO classification of diabetes

Type 1 (*K&C*, p. 1102)

- β cell destruction usually leading to absolute insulin deficiency
- Autoimmune or idiopathic

Type 2 (*K&C*, p. 1106)

❚ Variable combination of insulin resistance and defects in insulin secretion

Other specific types
Genetic defects

❚ Defects of β cell function or insulin function

Endocrinopathies

❚ Cushing's syndrome
❚ Acromegaly
❚ Phaeochromocytoma
❚ Hyperthyroidism

Diseases of the endocrine pancreas

❚ Trauma
❚ Pancreatectomy
❚ Chronic pancreatitis
❚ Fibrocalculous pancreatic diabetes
❚ Cystic fibrosis
❚ Haemochromatosis
❚ Cancer

Drug-induced

❚ Corticosteroids
❚ Thiazides

WHO criteria for diagnosis of diabetes (*K&C*, p. 1109)

❚ See Table 13.11 and Figure 13.7

Presenting clinical features (*K&C*, p. 1108)

Due to hyperglycaemia

❚ Thirst
❚ Polyuria

Table 13.11 WHO criteria for the diagnosis of diabetes (glucose mmol/L)

	Whole blood	Plasma
Diabetes mellitus		
Fasting	≥6.1	≥7.0
2 hrs after oral glucose load	≥10.0	≥11.1
Impaired glucose tolerance		
Fasting	<6.1	<7.0
2 hrs after oral glucose load	≥6.7 – <10.0	≥7.8 – <11.1
Impaired fasting glucose		
Fasting	≥5.6 – <6.1	≥6.1 – <7.0
2 hrs after oral glucose load	<6.7	<7.8

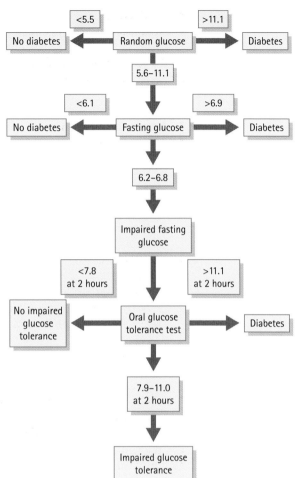

Fig. 13.7
Diagnostic
algorithm for
diabetes mellitus
(glucose mmol/L).

▌ Weight loss
▌ Ketoacidosis
▌ Lack of energy
▌ Visual blurring
▌ *Candida* infections
▌ Asymptomatic, picked up on blood/urine testing

Due to complications

▌ Skin infections
▌ Retinopathy
▌ Polyneuropathy
▌ Erectile dysfunction

❚ Arterial disease
❚ Renal disease

Clinical features of complications (*K&C*, pp. 1123–1131)
Macrovascular and microvascular disease

❚ Atheroma
❚ Strokes
❚ Myocardial ischaemia
❚ Renal disease
❚ Peripheral vascular disease
❚ Retinopathy

Eyes

❚ See Figure 13.8

Kidney

❚ Glomerulosclerosis
❚ Microalbuminuria
❚ Persistent proteinuria
❚ End-stage renal failure (associated with anaemia, raised ESR and hypertension)
❚ Ischaemia
❚ Ascending infection (pyelonephritis)

Neuropathy

❚ Peripheral polyneuropathy (loss of ankle jerks and malleolar vibration sense)
❚ Glove and stocking sensory neuropathy
❚ Mononeuritis multiplex
❚ Peripheral and cranial nerve
❚ Autonomic neuropathy:
  – Diarrhoea
  – Postural hypotension
  – Erectile dysfunction
  – Gastroparesis
❚ Diabetic amyotrophy – painful asymmetrical wasting of quadriceps
❚ Charcot's joints

Diabetic foot (Table 13.12)

❚ Ischaemic and/or neuropathic ulcers

Infections

❚ Only increased in poor glycaemic control
❚ Skin sepsis, e.g. staphylococcal or candida
❚ Urinary tract infection

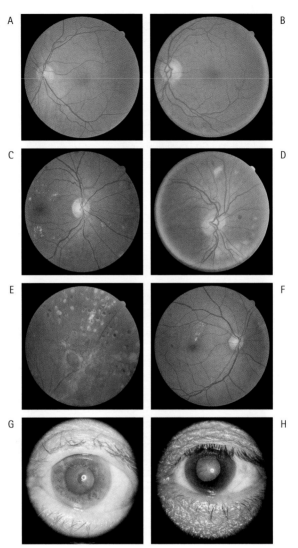

Fig. 13.8 Features of diabetic eye disease. A. The normal macula (centre) and optic disc. B. Dot and blot haemorrhages (early background retinopathy). C. Hard exudates are present in addition in background retinopathy. D. Multiple cotton-wool spots indicate pre-proliferative retinopathy requiring routine ophthalmic referral. E. Multiple frond-like new vessels, the hallmark of proliferative retinopathy. White fibrous tissue is forming near the new vessels, a feature of advanced retinopathy. (This eye also illustrates multiple xenon arc laser burns superiorly.) F. Exudates appearing within a disc width of the macula are a feature of an exudative maculopathy. G and H. Central and cortical cataracts can be seen against the red reflex with the ophthalmoscope. (Reproduced with permission from Kumar and Clark (2002). *Clinical Medicine*: Saunders, Edinburgh.)

Table 13.12 The diabetic foot

	Ischaemic	Neuropathic
Symptoms	Claudication Rest pain	Usually painless
Signs	Trophic changes Cold Pulseless Painful ulcers Ulcers on heels and toes	High arch, clawed toes Warm Bounding pulse Painless ulcers Ulcers on sole and where shoes rub

---

BOX 13.4 HYPOGLYCAEMIA

Clinical features
Sweating
Tremor
Pounding heart
Pallor
Drowsiness
Confusion
Coma
Fits

Management
Mild
    Oral rapidly absorbed carbohydrate, e.g. glucose drink, tea with sugar or sweets
Severe
    i.v. 50% glucose injection 20–50 ml (after taking blood to confirm hypoglycaemia but before waiting for result)
        1 mg i.m. glucagon injection

▌ Pneumonia
▌ TB

Management of diabetes mellitus (K&C, p. 1109)

▌ Based on self-monitoring and management by the patient, helped and advised by specialists
▌ Requires good education and understanding of disease by the patient, including
  – Monitoring blood sugar
  – Self-injection of insulin
  – Managing hypoglycaemic events
  – How to recognise complications
  – When to contact specialists for help

Table 13.13 Indications for insulin treatment

Anyone who has been in ketoacidosis
Patients presenting under 40 years old
Failure of oral therapy

Glycaemic control

Diet

▮ All patients need education regarding a diabetic diet

Insulin

▮ See Table 13.13

Drugs

Sulphonylureas, e.g. gliclazide
▮ May cause hypoglycaemia and weight gain

Biguanides, e.g. metformin
▮ Do not cause hypoglycaemia
▮ May aid weight loss

α-glucosidase inhibitors, e.g. acarbose
▮ Do not cause hypoglycaemia

Insulin sensitisers, e.g. rosiglitazone
▮ May cause hepatotoxicity
▮ May cause drop in haemoglobin

Insulin formulations (*K&C*, p. 1112)

▮ Synthetic human insulins are almost exclusively used
▮ Insulin is given regularly by subcutaneous injection
▮ Insulin regimes are developed to suit individual patients and may be tailored according to specific needs for certain situations, e.g. missing meals, heavy exercise

Soluble insulin

▮ Fast-acting and short duration of action
▮ Good for fine control
▮ Needs frequent administration

Prolonged acting insulin

▮ Mixed in varying degrees with soluble insulin to give a prolonged duration of action but with less accuracy and slower onset of action

Insulin analogues

Long acting ▮ Insulin glargine; longer duration of action and less peaked concentration

Short acting

▌ Enter and leave circulation more rapidly

Complications of insulin treatment (*K&C*, p. 1115)

▌ Lipoatrophy and lipohypertrophy at injection site
▌ Weight gain
▌ Hypoglycaemia

Monitoring diabetic control (*K&C*, p. 1116)
Home monitoring

▌ Urine reagent strips – simple but not very accurate
▌ Blood glucose reagent strips – more immediately accurate

Hospital blood tests

▌ HbA_{1c} (glycosylated haemoglobin)
▌ Fructosamine (glycosylated plasma protein)
▌ Both give an index of average blood glucose concentration over the past 6 weeks

Diabetes clinic checkup visits

▌ Every visit
  – Review self-monitoring
  – Review current treatment (including diet)
  – Ongoing patient education
▌ Annual review
  – Weight
  – Blood pressure
  – Biochemical assessment of control
  – Visual acuity and retinal examination
  – Check feet for condition, pulses, sensation and ankle jerks
  – Urinalysis for proteinuria
  – Blood lipids
  – Renal function

Diabetic emergencies

Diabetic ketoacidosis (*K&C*, p. 1119)

▌ Uncontrolled diabetes with acidosis and ketosis due to insulin deficiency (Box 13.5)

Hyperglycaemic hyperosmolar state (*K&C*, p. 1122)

▌ Severe hyperglycaemia without ketosis usually in type II diabetes

BOX 13.5 DIABETIC KETOACIDOSIS

Clinical features
Prostration
Hyperventilation (Kussmaul's breathing)
Nausea and vomiting
Abdominal pain
Confusion
Coma
Dehydration
Ketones on breath
Hyperglycaemia
Ketonuria or ketonaemia
Acidosis

Principles of management
Replace fluid loss
Replace electrolyte loss
Restore acid–base balance (usually achieved by correcting circulating volume and stopping ketone production with insulin)
Replace deficient insulin
Continuous i.v. infusion of soluble insulin
Monitor blood glucose
I.v. glucose in i.v. fluids to prevent hypoglycaemia
(Do not stop insulin)
Seek underlying cause and treat appropriately

Emergency treatment
Insulin
  Intravenous insulin 6 units stat then
  6 units/hour by continuous infusion with blood glucose monitoring
Fluid
  0.9% saline
  1 L in 30 minutes then
  1 L in 1 hour then
  1 L in 2 hours then
  1 L in 4 hours then
  1 L every 6 hours for 24 hours
  i.e. at least 4 L in first 24 hours
Check serum potassium hourly initially and add 20 mmol/L of i.v. fluid when < 4 mmol
Monitor central venous pressure if shocked at presentation
Insert urinary catheter if anuric for > 2 hours
Antibiotics if septic
Subcutaneous heparin to prevent thrombosis

Clinical features

▌ Severe dehydration
▌ Stupor
▌ Coma
▌ Underlying illness (e.g. pneumonia)

Investigations

- High plasma osmolarity
- High serum sodium
- Very high plasma glucose
- High urea
- Normal arterial pH

Management

- Treat underlying cause
- Intravenous insulin to correct hyperglycaemia
- 0.9% saline to correct fluid depletion – beware rapid changes of osmolality due to reducing plasma sodium or glucose levels too fast
- Subcutaneous prophylactic heparin
- Mortality is up to 25%

SELF-ASSESSMENT QUESTIONS

Best of five questions

1. TSH:
   A. Is produced by the parathyroid glands
   B. Is reduced in primary hypothyroidism
   C. Is a sensitive marker of under-treatment during thyroxine replacement
   D. Secretion should be inhibited in a normal TRH stimulation test
   E. Levels are high in Graves' disease

2. The following are common features of Graves' disease:
   A. Atrial fibrillation
   B. Multinodular goitre
   C. Oedema
   D. Anorexia
   E. Weight gain

3. The following are common features of hypothyroidism:
   A. Heat intolerance
   B. Pretibial myxoedema
   C. Hoarse voice
   D. Weight loss
   E. Suicide

4. The following statements about pituitary function are correct:
   A. Suspected diabetes insipidus is investigated with a fluid challenge
   B. Prolactin production, unlike that of other pituitary hormones, is principally controlled by an stimulatory factor
   C. ACTH and cortisol production display a circadian rhythm
   D. Sheehan's syndrome is commoner in men than women
   E. TSH is secreted from the posterior pituitary

5. In patients with untreated active acromegaly:
   A. About 25% of patients have impaired glucose tolerance
   B. Arthritis is a common feature
   C. An oral glucose tolerance test is used to confirm the diagnosis
   D. The incidence of carcinoma of the colon is increased
   E. All of the above

6. The following are common features of panhypopituitarism:
   A. Diabetes mellitus
   B. Galactorrhoea
   C. Infertility
   D. Pigmentation
   E. Increased urinary catecholamines

7. The following biochemical findings are often seen in an acutely unwell patient presenting with an Addisonian crisis:
   A. Hypernatraemia
   B. Hyperkalaemia
   C. A low ACTH
   D. Hypocalcaemia
   E. A raised glucose

8. The following statements about Cushing's syndrome are correct:
   A. The commonest cause is an ACTH-secreting tumour of the pituitary
   B. There is impaired glucose tolerance in 75% of cases

C. Severe hypokalaemia may be indicative of ectopic ACTH production

D. Proximal myopathy is a common feature

E. C and D

9. The following are true of ectopic ACTH secretion:
A. There is failure of suppression of cortisol secretion during a high-dose dexamethasone suppression test
B. It may be caused by a bronchial carcinoma
C. It may cause increased skin pigmentation
D. It is associated with small atrophic adrenal glands
E. A, B and C

10. The following are features of cranial diabetes insipidus:
A. It may be associated with acanthosis nigricans
B. It may be associated with postpartum haemorrhage
C. It is caused by treatment with lithium
D. It responds to treatment with DDT
E. It is treated with fluid restriction

11. The following are causes of nephrogenic diabetes insipidus:
A. Sheehan's syndrome
B. Pancreatic islet cell antibodies
C. Excessive water drinking
D. Hypocalcaemia
E. Hypokalaemia

12. The following are features of SIADH:
A. Hypernatraemia
B. Low urine osmolality

C. Diagnosis requires serum ADH measurement
D. It often present with fits
E. Treatment includes fluid restriction

13. The following are true of phaeochromocytoma:
A. It is the cause of 10% of all hypertension
B. It is caused by a tumour of adrenal cortex in 90% of cases
C. alpha- and β-adrenergic blockers are used prior to surgery to prevent swings in blood pressure
D. It is seen in MEN type 1
E. It is associated with coarctation of the aorta

14. The following are seen in MEN type 2a:
A. Marfanoid phenotype
B. Phaeochromocytoma
C. Pancreatic islet cell tumours
D. Pituitary tumours
E. Papillary carcinoma of the thyroid

15. The following statements about diabetes mellitus are correct:
A. The diagnosis is made on the basis of a fasting glucose $> 7.8\,mmol/L$
B. When it presents in pregnancy (gestational diabetes) it usually continues after delivery
C. In patients with proliferative diabetic nephropathy, thrombolysis is contraindicated in the event of a myocardial infarction

D. The glycated haemoglobin (HbA_{1c}) level is used to diagnose diabetes

E. The mortality following anterior myocardial infarction is twice as high in diabetic as in non-diabetic patients

16. Regarding type II diabetes:
    A. Treatment with metformin works by increasing pancreatic insulin production
    B. Retinopathy is much rarer than in type I diabetes
    C. The thiazolidinediones are a new class of drug for treatment
    D. It only affects adults over the age of 40
    E. The incidence in the UK is falling

17. In type I diabetes:
    A. Patients control their blood glucose by regular self-injection of i.m. insulin
    B. There is a strong genetic association with HLA-B27
    C. The average life expectancy is less than in type II diabetes
    D. There is an association with coeliac disease
    E. Patients on insulin are unable to hold a UK driving licence

18. The following statements about diabetic ketoacidosis are correct:
    A. It does not occur in patients with type II diabetes
    B. The plasma potassium is usually raised at presentation
    C. When treatment is started the arterial pH falls

D. The plasma anion gap is normal

E. It can result in a low plasma phosphate level

19. In diabetic ketoacidosis:
    A. Patients should be treated immediately with subcutaneous insulin
    B. Acid reflux usually corrects with insulin and fluid replacement
    C. Patients should eat normally as soon as possible
    D. A fast respiratory rate indicates concurrent pneumonia
    E. Insulin therapy is no longer needed when the blood glucose returns to normal

Extended matching questions

Question 1 *Theme: polyuria*

A. Diabetes mellitus
B. Diabetes insipidus
C. Chronic renal failure
D. Primary hyperparathyroidism
E. Chronic hypokalaemia
F. Urinary tract infection
G. Diuretic therapy
H. Compulsive water drinking
I. Supraventricular tachycardia

For each of the following questions, select the best answer from the list above:

I. A 48-year-old female with a previous Whipple's operation (pancreatoduodenectomy) for Zollinger–Ellison syndrome presents with a 3-month history of polyuria and constipation. What is the most likely diagnosis?

II. A 27-year-old female presents with polyuria 2 months after home delivery of a healthy 3.2 kg son. She needed urgent hospital admission after the birth for blood transfusion for postpartum haemorrhage. What is the most likely diagnosis?

III. A 16-year-old male presents with a 4-week history of thirst, polyuria, malaise and loss of appetite. Serum urea and electrolytes are normal apart from $HCO_3 = 19$ mmol/L. What is the most likely diagnosis?

Question 2 *Theme: weight loss*

A. Thyrotoxicosis
B. Coeliac disease
C. Carcinoma of the stomach
D. Diabetes mellitus
E. Addison's disease
F. Anorexia nervosa
G. Breast cancer
H. Crohn's disease
I. Amphetamine abuse

For each of the following questions, select the best answer from the list above:

I. A 57-year-old female on B_{12} injections for pernicious anaemia presents with anxiety, palpitations, intermittent diarrhoea and weight loss of 6 kg over 3 months. What is the most likely diagnosis?

II. A 29-year-old male presents with night sweats, fever, abdominal pain and weight loss of 10 kg since he returned from Bangladesh 3 months ago. Examination shows increased pigmentation in the palmar creases and postural hypotension. What is the most likely diagnosis?

III. A 36-year-old female from Galway presents with a 6-month history of weight loss and abdominal cramps. Blood tests show iron deficiency and folate deficiency. What is the most likely diagnosis?

Short answer questions

1. Describe the clinical features of the following
  A. Hyperthyroidism
  B. Acromegaly
  C. Primary hypoadrenalism

2. Write short notes on the following
  A. Multiple endocrine neoplasia
  B. Phaeochromocytoma
  C. Goitre

3. Briefly discuss the causes of the following
  A. Cushing's syndrome
  B. Adrenal failure
  C. Diabetes insipidus

4. Write short notes on the following
  A. Thyroid related eye abnormalities
  B. SIADH
  C. Causes of polyuria

5. List the following
  A. The hormones secreted by the anterior pituitary and their functions
  B. The causes of hypopituitarism
  C. The biochemical changes seen in primary hyperaldosteronism

FUNCTIONS OF THE KIDNEY

Excretory

  ▌ Waste products

Regulatory

  ▌ Control of body fluid volume and composition

Endocrine

  ▌ Erythropoietin
  ▌ Renin-angiotensin
  ▌ Prostaglandins

Metabolic

  ▌ Vitamin D

EXAMINING THE RENAL SYSTEM

  ▌ All systems need to be examined but pay special
    attention to the following

BOX 14.1 PALPATION OF THE KIDNEYS

Place one hand posteriorly on the flank with the other
hand anteriorly
Gently push up from below aiming to 'ballot' the
kidney
Differences between kidney and spleen
• Kidneys are ballotable
• Spleen has a notch
• You cannot get above the spleen
• Spleen is dull to percussion

Kidneys

- Position
- Size
- Shape
- Scars from previous surgery

Urine (*K&C*, p. 612)
Urinalysis

- Chemical (Stix) testing
- Blood
- Protein
- Glucose
- Bacterial nitrites
- Urinary pH
- Specific gravity and osmolality

Microscopy

- White cells
- Red cells
- Bacteria
- Casts

Volume

- Oliguria
- Polyuria

INVESTIGATIONS IN NEPHROLOGY

Imaging (*K&C*, p. 615)

Plain X-rays

- Renal calcification
- Renal calculi

Excretory urography

- Intravenous urogram
- Anatomy of renal tract
- Excretion of contrast

Ultrasound

- Renal masses
- Renal cysts
- Dilatation of renal tract – obstruction
- Renal size
- Bladder emptying
- Renal vessel doppler

CT and MRI

- Detection of calculi/urography
- Renal masses
- Staging tumours
- Renal vessel imaging
- Retroperitoneal masses

Arteriography

- Extrarenal arterial imaging

Dynamic scintigraphy

- DPTA/MAG3/ Hippuran – show perfusion
- Glomerular filtration
- Outflow of urine from collecting system

Static scintigraphy

- DMSA – renal function
- Visualisation of kidney

Renal biopsy (*K&C*, p. 618)

- Transcutaneous under ultrasound control

Indications

- Nephrotic syndrome
- Unexplained renal failure
- Diagnosis of systemic disease

Contraindications

- Single kidney
- Small kidneys
- Haemorrhagic disorders
- Uncontrolled hypertension

Biochemical renal function tests (*K&C*, p. 608)

Serum urea and creatinine

- Increase when glomerular filtration rate (GFR) is reduced by 50–60% (i.e. may be normal in the presence of significant decrease in renal function)

Creatinine clearance

- Estimates GFR

$$= \frac{V \text{ (urine volume)} \times U \text{ (urine creatinine concentration)}}{P \text{ (plasma creatinine concentration)}} \times 100$$

Arterial blood gases

▌ Metabolic acidosis in renal failure due to failure to excrete fixed acid and to renal bicarbonate wasting

GLOMERULONEPHRITIS (*K&C*, P. 619)

▌ A group of disorders
  – With immunologically mediated injury to glomerulus
  – Involving both kidneys
  – With secondary injury after initial immune insult
  – May be part of generalised disease
  – Classified by histology

Pathogenesis

▌ Deposition of immune complexes
▌ Deposition of anti-glomerular basement membrane (anti-GBM) antibody

Aetiology

Immune complex nephritis

▌ Unknown antigen
▌ Viruses
  – Mumps
  – Measles
  – Hepatitis B and C
  – Epstein–Barr virus (EBV)
  – Coxsackie
  – Varicella
  – HIV
▌ Bacteria
  – Group A β-haemolytic streptococci
  – *Streptococcus viridans*
  – Staphylococci
  – *Treponema pallidum*
  – Gonococci
  – Salmonellae
▌ Parasites
  – *Plasmodium malariae*
  – *Schistosoma*
  – Filariasis
▌ Host antigens
  – DNA (systemic lupus erythematosus – SLE)
  – Cryoglobulins
  – Malignant tumours

▌Drugs
  – Penicillamine
Anti-GBM **▌Antibodies to type IV collagen**
antibody

Secondary **▌Complement activation**
mechanisms **▌Fibrin deposition**
  ▌Platelet aggregation
  ▌Neutrophil-driven inflammation
  ▌Kinin activation

Clinical features

▌GN presents in one of four ways
  – Asymptomatic proteinuria $+/-$ microscopic haematuria
  – Acute nephritic syndrome (Fig. 14.1)

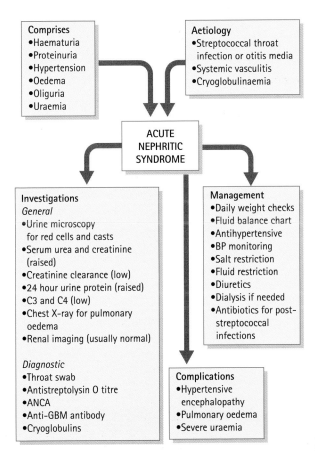

Comprises
•Haematuria
•Proteinuria
•Hypertension
•Oedema
•Oliguria
•Uraemia

Aetiology
•Streptococcal throat infection or otitis media
•Systemic vasculitis
•Cryoglobulinaemia

ACUTE NEPHRITIC SYNDROME

Investigations
General
•Urine microscopy for red cells and casts
•Serum urea and creatinine (raised)
•Creatinine clearance (low)
•24 hour urine protein (raised)
•C3 and C4 (low)
•Chest X-ray for pulmonary oedema
•Renal imaging (usually normal)

Diagnostic
•Throat swab
•Antistreptolysin O titre
•ANCA
•Anti-GBM antibody
•Cryoglobulins

Management
•Daily weight checks
•Fluid balance chart
•Antihypertensive
•BP monitoring
•Salt restriction
•Fluid restriction
•Diuretics
•Dialysis if needed
•Antibiotics for post-streptococcal infections

Complications
•Hypertensive encephalopathy
•Pulmonary oedema
•Severe uraemia

Fig. 14.1 Acute nephritic syndrome.

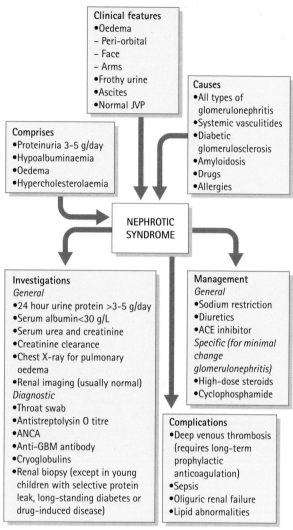

Clinical features
- Oedema
  - Peri-orbital
  - Face
  - Arms
- Frothy urine
- Ascites
- Normal JVP

Causes
- All types of glomerulonephritis
- Systemic vasculitides
- Diabetic glomerulosclerosis
- Amyloidosis
- Drugs
- Allergies

Comprises
- Proteinuria 3-5 g/day
- Hypoalbuminaemia
- Oedema
- Hypercholesterolaemia

NEPHROTIC SYNDROME

Investigations
General
- 24 hour urine protein >3-5 g/day
- Serum albumin<30 g/L
- Serum urea and creatinine
- Creatinine clearance
- Chest X-ray for pulmonary oedema
- Renal imaging (usually normal)
Diagnostic
- Throat swab
- Antistreptolysin O titre
- ANCA
- Anti-GBM antibody
- Cryoglobulins
- Renal biopsy (except in young children with selective protein leak, long-standing diabetes or drug-induced disease)

Management
General
- Sodium restriction
- Diuretics
- ACE inhibitor
Specific (for minimal change glomerulonephritis)
- High-dose steroids
- Cyclophosphamide

Complications
- Deep venous thrombosis (requires long-term prophylactic anticoagulation)
- Sepsis
- Oliguric renal failure
- Lipid abnormalities

Fig. 14.2 Nephrotic syndrome.

- Nephrotic syndrome (Fig. 14.2)
- Chronic renal failure

Investigations

▌ 24-hour urinary protein (measure twice)
▌ Urine microscopy
▌ Renal function
▌ Auto antibodies
▌ Renal biopsy

Specific types of GN (Table 14.1)

IgA nephropathy (*K&C*, p. 630)
Pathology

- Focal proliferative GN
- Mesangial deposits of IgA

Clinical features

- Microscopic haematuria
- Children and young adults

Prognosis

- Usually good
- 20% eventually develop renal failure

Henoch–Schönlein purpura (*K&C*, p. 629)
Pathology

- Focal segmental GN

Clinical features

- Purpuric rash
- Abdominal colic
- Joint pain
- ♂ > ♀ (2:1)
- May follow recent respiratory infection

Prognosis

- Usually good

Goodpasture's syndrome (*K&C*, p. 632)
Pathology

- Severe proliferative crescentic GN

Clinical features

- Haemoptysis
- Progressive renal failure

Prognosis

- Usually progresses to renal failure

Acute nephritic syndrome (*K&C*, p. 629)

- Classically occurs 3 weeks after streptococcal throat infection or otitis media
- See Fig. 14.1

Nephrotic syndrome (*K&C*, p. 620)

- See Fig. 14.2

Table 14.1 Glomerulonephritis

Histology	Example of causes	Clinical presentation
Proliferative glomerulonephritis		
Diffuse	Post-streptococcal	Acute nephritic syndrome
Focal segmental	SLE	Haematuria
	Henoch–Schönlein purpura	Proteinuria
Crescentic	Wegener's granulomatosis	Progressive renal failure
	Goodpasture's syndrome	
Mesangiocapillary		
Type1	Hepatitis B and C	Haematuria
		Proteinuria
Type 2	Measles	Nephrotic syndrome
Membranous	Unknown	Nephrotic syndrome
	Malaria	
Minimal change	Unknown	Nephrotic syndrome (especially in children)
IgA nephropathy	Henoch–Schönlein purpura	Asymptomatic haematuria
Focal glomerulosclerosis	Diabetes mellitus	Proteinuria
		Nephrotic syndrome

Glomerular disorders in systemic disease

Systemic vasculitis

- SLE – all types of glomerulonephritis
- Polyarteritis nodosa (PAN) – renal failure
- Microscopic polyarteritis – crescentic glomerulonephritis
- Wegener's granulomatosis – glomerulonephritis

Cryoglobulinaemia (*K&C*, p. 628)

- Monoclonal or polyclonal expansion of abnormal immunoglobulins which precipitate reversibly in the cold (cryoglobulins)

Aetiology

- Viral infections, e.g. hepatitis B and C, cytomegalovirus (CMV), EBV
- Fungal infections
- Malaria
- Infective endocarditis
- Autoimmune diseases

Clinical features

- Glomerulonephritis
- Purpura
- Raynaud's phenomenon
- Systemic vasculitis
- Polyneuropathy
- Hepatic involvement

Diabetes mellitus

- See Chapter 13

Amyloidosis (*K&C*, p. 625)

- A disorder of protein metabolism with extracellular deposition of insoluble fibrillar proteins in organs and tissues

Types

- AL amyloidosis
- Familial amyloidosis
- Secondary amyloidosis

AL amyloidosis (*K&C*, p. 1147)
Pathology

- Plasma cell production of amyloidogenic immunoglobulin light chains (AL)

- AL chains are excreted in urine (Bence Jones proteins)
- Associated with myeloma and Waldenström's macroglobulinaemia

Clinical features

- Nephrotic syndrome
- Cardiomyopathy
- Autonomic neuropathy
- Sensory neuropathy
- Carpal tunnel syndrome
- Hepatomegaly
- Splenomegaly
- Bruising
- Macroglossia

Familial amyloidosis (*K&C*, p. 1147)
Pathology

- Autosomal dominant inherited mutant protein formation
- Mutant protein forms amyloid fibrils

Mutant proteins
- Transthyretin (commonest)
- Apolipoprotein A-1
- Fibrinogen
- Lysosyme

Clinical features

- Peripheral sensorimotor neuropathy
- Autonomic neuropathy
- Conduction defects in heart

Secondary amyloidosis
Pathology

- Amyloid is formed from acute phase protein serum amyloid A (SAA)

Aetiology

- Rheumatoid arthritis
- Inflammatory bowel disease
- Familial Mediterranean fever
- Tuberculosis
- Bronchiectasis
- Osteomyelitis

Clinical features

- Renal disease
- Hepatosplenomegaly

Diagnosis of amyloidosis
- Rectal or gum biopsy
- Amyloid stains with Congo red with green birefringence in polarised light

Management of amyloidosis
- Treat associated disorder
- Treat nephrotic syndrome or cardiac failure
- Chemotherapy for AL
- Liver transplant for transthyretin-associated amyloidosis

Haemolytic uraemic syndrome (HUS) (*K&C*, p. 636)
- Follows gastroenteritis or respiratory tract infection, *E. coli* 0157
- Comprises
  - Intravascular haemolysis
  - Thrombocytopenia
  - Acute renal failure

Thrombotic thrombocytopenic purpura (*K&C*, p. 636)
- Microangiopathic haemolysis
- Renal failure
- Neurological disturbance

Multiple myeloma
- Monoclonal expansion of B cells which secrete light chains (immunoglobulin fragments)
- Acute renal failure
- Myeloma kidney
- Renal amyloid deposits

URINARY TRACT INFECTION (*K&C*, P. 637)
- Common in women; 90% of attacks are isolated
- Uncommon in men

Bacterial infections
Causative organisms
- *E. coli* – 70%
- *Proteus mirabilis* – 10%
- *Staphylococcus saprophyticus* or *epidermidis* – 10%
- *Klebsiella aerogenes* – 5%
- *Enterococcus faecalis* – 5%

Associated diseases

- Diabetes mellitus
- Sickle cell disease or trait
- Analgesic abuse
- Stones
- Obstruction
- Polycystic kidneys
- Vesico-ureteric reflux

Clinical features

- Cystitis
  - Frequency of micturition
  - Dysuria
  - Suprapubic pain/tenderness
  - Haematuria
  - Offensive urine
- Pyelonephritis
  - Loin pain/tenderness
  - Fever
  - Systemic upset

Investigations

- Symptomatic women
  - Dipstix + for nitrites and leucocytes
  - $> 10^2$ coliforms/mL + pyuria *or* ⎤
  - $>10^5$ any pathogenic organism/mL *or* ⎬ MSU
  - Any growth from suprapubic bladder aspiration ⎦
- Symptomatic men
  - $>10^3$ pathogenic organisms/mL
- Asymptomatic patients
  - $>10^5$ pathogenic organisms/mL (on two occasions)
- Causes of sterile pyuria
  - *Chlamydia*
  - TB
  - partially treatedbacterial UTI

Radiology

- Excretory urography
  - Women with ≥3 attacks
  - All men
  - All children
- Abdominal X-ray and ultrasound
  - Acute pyelonephritis

Management

❚ Oral antibiotics
  – Amoxicillin
  – Nitrofurantoin
  – Trimethoprim
  – Oral cephalosporin
❚ Intravenous antibiotics
  – For acute pyelonephritis with high fever, vomiting or systemic upset
  – Cefuroxime
  – Gentamicin
  – Ciprofloxacin

Tuberculosis of the renal tract (*K&C*, p. 642)

❚ Affects the renal cortex spreading to the papillae and into the urine, ureters and bladder
❚ May cause ureteric obstruction and hydronephrosis

Investigations

❚ Culture of acid-fast bacillae from early morning urine (EMU) samples

RENAL CALCULI (*K&C*, P. 648)

Prevalence

❚ 2% of UK population

Types of urinary stone

❚ See Table 14.2

Aetiology

❚ Dehydration
❚ Hypercalcaemia
❚ Hypercalciuria
❚ Hyperoxaluria
❚ Hyperuricaemia
❚ Infection
❚ Cystinuria
❚ Renal tubular acidosis
❚ Primary renal disease

Clinical features

❚ Asymptomatic
❚ Renal colic
❚ Haematuria

Table 14.2 Types of urinary stone

Type	Frequency
Calcium oxalate	65%
Calcium phosphate	15%
Magnesium ammonium phosphate	10–15%
Uric acid	3–5%
Cystine	1–2%

I Urinary tract infection
I Obstruction

Investigations

I Midstream urine (MSU) and culture
I Serum urea and electrolytes, creatinine
I Serum calcium
I Serum urate
I Plain abdominal X-ray
I Spiral CT
I Excretion urography
I Urinary calcium, oxalate and uric acid
I Sieve urine to trap stones for analysis

Management

I Analgesia (opiates, NSAIDs)
I High fluid intake
I Stones < 0.5 cm pass spontaneously
I Stones > 1 cm require intervention
I Obstruction or infection requires intervention

Intervention

Percutaneous   I Endoscopic extraction of renal pelvis stones
nephrolithotomy   through a percutaneous tract

Extracorporeal   I Fragmentation of stones with shock waves
shock-wave   focused in from an external source
lithotripsy (ESWL)

URINARY TRACT OBSTRUCTION (K&C, P. 654)

I See Table 14.3

Hydronephrosis

I Dilatation of renal pelvis above obstruction

Table 14.3 Causes of urinary tract obstruction	
Within lumen	Neuropathic bladder
Calculus	Urethral stricture
Blood clot	Calculus
Sloughed papilla	Gonococcal infection
Tumour	
	Outside pressure
Within wall	Tumours
Ureteric stricture	Aortic aneurysm
TB	Prostatic obstruction
Calculus	Retroperitoneal fibrosis
Post-surgical	Accidental ligation of ureter
Schistosomiasis	Phimosis

Clinical features

▌ Loin pain/tenderness
▌ Anuria – bilateral obstruction
▌ Polyuria
▌ Bladder outflow obstruction (hesitancy, poor stream, terminal dribbling)
▌ Palpable enlarged kidney(s)

Investigations

▌ Urea and electrolytes
▌ Ultrasound
▌ Excretion urography
▌ Cystoscopy

Management

▌ Relieve obstruction by temporary drainage via nephrostomy or urethral or suprapubic catheter
▌ Treat underlying cause
▌ Prevent and/or treat infection

Surgical drainage ▌ Urinary diversion
▌ Ureteric stents

ACUTE RENAL FAILURE (K&C, P. 659)

▌ Abrupt deterioration in renal function which is usually reversible

Pre-renal uraemia

▌ Impaired perfusion of kidneys

Aetiology

- Hypovolaemia (acute blood loss, dehydration, sepsis)
- Hypotension
- Cardiac failure
- Renal artery stenosis ($+/-$ ACE inhibitors)

Management

- Correct hypovolaemia or hypotension
- Monitor central venous pressure to maintain adequate vascular volume

Acute uraemia due to renal causes
Aetiology

- Acute tubular necrosis (Fig. 14.3)
- Vasculitis

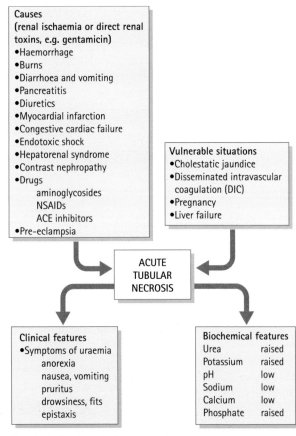

Causes
(renal ischaemia or direct renal toxins, e.g. gentamicin)
- Haemorrhage
- Burns
- Diarrhoea and vomiting
- Pancreatitis
- Diuretics
- Myocardial infarction
- Congestive cardiac failure
- Endotoxic shock
- Hepatorenal syndrome
- Contrast nephropathy
- Drugs
    aminoglycosides
    NSAIDs
    ACE inhibitors
- Pre-eclampsia

Vulnerable situations
- Cholestatic jaundice
- Disseminated intravascular coagulation (DIC)
- Pregnancy
- Liver failure

ACUTE TUBULAR NECROSIS

Clinical features
- Symptoms of uraemia
    anorexia
    nausea, vomiting
    pruritus
    drowsiness, fits
    epistaxis

Biochemical features
Urea	raised
Potassium	raised
pH	low
Sodium	low
Calcium	low
Phosphate	raised

Fig. 14.3 Acute tubular necrosis.

- Pre-eclampsia
- Haemolytic uraemic syndrome
- Rhabdomyolysis

Post-renal uraemia

- Urinary tract obstruction

Investigations in acute renal failure
Determine whether pre-renal, renal or post-renal

- Exclude bladder outflow obstruction – insert urinary catheter
- Ultrasound – to exclude upper urinary tract obstruction
- Fluid challenge – increased urine output will differentiate pre-renal from renal

Urinalysis

- Dipstick for protein and blood
- Myoglobin

Serum biochemistry

- Urea and electrolytes
  - Urea $\uparrow$, K^+ $\uparrow$
- Creatinine $\uparrow$
- Calcium $\downarrow$ and phosphate $\uparrow$
- Albumin
- Alkaline phosphatase
- Urate
- Drug levels

Haematology

- Full blood count and blood film
  - Normal Hb
- ESR
- Coagulation studies

Microbiology

- Urine microscopy and culture
- Blood cultures

Management of acute uraemia
General management

- Admit to renal unit or ITU for support of all systems, with the aim of keeping the patient alive while waiting for renal function to recover

Diet

▮ Sodium and potassium restriction
▮ Protein restriction only if trying to avoid dialysis

Fluid balance

▮ Assessment of input–output chart
▮ Signs of fluid overload
▮ Serum electrolytes
▮ Daily weight check

Treat sepsis

▮ Avoid nephrotoxic drugs and alter dose for renally excreted drugs

Dialysis and haemofiltration in acute renal failure
Indications

▮ Symptomatic uraemia
▮ Complications of uraemia, e.g. pericarditis
▮ Severe biochemical derangement
▮ Uncontrolled hyperkalaemia
▮ Pulmonary oedema
▮ Acidosis
▮ Removal of toxic drugs, e.g. aspirin overdose, gentamicin

Options

▮ Peritoneal dialysis
▮ Continuous haemofiltration

Prognosis

▮ up to 50% mortality

Contrast nephropathy

▮ Caused by iodinated radiological contrast media
▮ Dose-dependent effect

BOX 14.2 HYPERKALAEMIA

Check result is compatible with patient's clinical condition (if not repeat sample)
Do ECG to look for changes of hyperkalaemia (peaked T waves, widened QRS complexes – Fig. 14.4) and put patient on cardiac monitor
For $K^+ > 6.0$ or with symptoms or ECG changes, give:
  i.v. calcium gluconate 10 mL 10%
  i.v. 100 mL 50% dextrose plus 10 units soluble rapid-acting insulin over 30 minutes, monitoring blood glucose for hypoglycaemia
  Nebulised salbutamol 10 mg
  Oral calcium resonium 15–30 g 2–3 times daily *or*
  Rectal calcium resonium retention enema 50 g daily
  Dialysis or haemofiltration if no correction

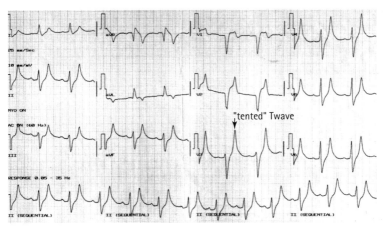

Fig. 14.4 The ECG in hyperkalaemia.

▌ Risk increased with
  - Pre-existing renal impairment
  - Hypovolaemia
  - Low cardiac output
  - Diabetes mellitus
  - Hyperviscosity
▌ Risk reduced by
  - *n*-Acetyl cysteine
  - Pre-hydration with saline

CHRONIC RENAL FAILURE (*K&C*, P. 665)

▌ Long-standing progressive impairment of renal function

Prevalence

▌ 600/million/year in UK
▌ End-stage renal failure – 200/million/year in UK

Aetiology

▌ See Table 14.4

Clinical features
History ▌ Duration of symptoms
▌ Drug ingestion e.g. NSAIDs, analgesics and herbal therapies
▌ Past surgical history
▌ Previous chemotherapy

Table 14.4 Causes of chronic renal failure

Congenital Polycystic kidney disease	**Tubulo-interstitial disease** Nephritis
Glomerular disease Primary glomerulonephritis Secondary glomerulonephritis (SLE, diabetes, amyloidosis)	Idiopathic Drugs Reflux nephropathy TB Schistosomiasis Diabetes
Vascular disease Atherosclerosis Vasculitis SLE Hypertension	**Obstruction** Stones Prostate disease Pelvic tumours Retroperitoneal fibrosis

	∎ Family history of renal disease
Symptoms	∎ Asymptomatic
	∎ Malaise, loss of energy
	∎ Insomnia
	∎ Nocturia, polyuria
	∎ Itching
	∎ Nausea, vomiting, diarrhoea
	∎ Paraesthesiae
	∎ 'Restless legs' syndrome
	∎ Bone pain
	∎ Peripheral or pulmonary oedema
	∎ Anaemia
	∎ Amenorrhoea and erectile dysfunction
Signs	∎ Short stature
	∎ Anaemia
	∎ Pigmentation on sun-exposed areas
	∎ Brown nails
	∎ Fluid overload
	∎ Signs of underlying disease

Investigations

Urine	∎ Urinalysis
	∎ Microscopy
	∎ Culture
	∎ 24-hour creatinine clearance
Biochemistry	∎ Urea and electrolytes
	– Urea ↑
	– normal K^+ or ↑
	∎ Creatinine ↑
	∎ Calcium ↓ and phosphate ↑

Haematology	▌ Full blood count
	– Anaemia
Radiology	▌ Renal tract ultrasound
	▌ Plain abdominal X-ray
	▌ CT scan of abdomen and pelvis
Immunology	▌ Urinary Bence Jones proteins
	▌ Serum electrophoresis and immunoglobulins
	▌ Autoantibodies
	▌ Complement levels
Microbiology	▌ Antistreptolysin O titre – post *Strep.* infection
	▌ Malaria film
	▌ Hepatitis B and C serology
Histology	▌ Renal biopsy

Complications

▌ Anaemia (erythropoietin)
▌ Renal osteodystrophy (osteomalacia, rickets, hyperparathyroidism, osteoporosis, osteosclerosis)
▌ Pruritus
▌ Delayed gastric emptying
▌ Peptic ulceration (↑ gastrin)
▌ Pancreatitis
▌ Constipation
▌ Gout
▌ Hyperlipidaemia
▌ Hyperprolactinaemia
▌ Erectile dysfunction and male infertility
▌ Amenorrhoea and female infertility
▌ Short stature
▌ Cardiovascular disease
▌ Cardiac failure
▌ Sudden death
▌ Pericarditis
▌ Stroke

Management

General ▌ Treat underlying disease if possible
▌ Control hypertension
▌ Early referral to nephrologist when serum creatinine >350 mol/L *or* in diabetics >250 mol/L
Diet ▌ Calcium supplements
▌ Low phosphate diet
▌ Sodium and potassium restriction
▌ Protein restriction
▌ Fluid restriction

Anaemia ▐ Erythropoietin
▐ Iron therapy

RENAL REPLACEMENT THERAPY

Haemodialysis (*K&C*, p. 673)
▐ Blood from the patient is pumped through semipermeable membranes against a dialysate fluid allowing diffusion of molecules along concentration gradients
▐ Requires rapid blood flow through a large-bore double-lumen central venous catheter or arteriovenous fistula

Frequency
▐ Usually 4–5 hours 3 times per week

Complications
▐ Hypotension whilst on dialysis

Haemofiltration
▐ Removal of plasma water and dissolved electrolytes (potassium, sodium, urea and phosphate) by flow across a semipermeable membrane and replacement with a solution of desired biochemical composition
▐ Mostly used in acute renal failure

Frequency
▐ Usually continuous

Peritoneal dialysis (*K&C*, p. 676)
▐ Uses peritoneum as semipermeable membrane
▐ Dialysis fluid is run into peritoneal cavity through a tube in the anterior abdominal wall
▐ Urea, creatinine and phosphate pass into the dialysate from the blood in peritoneal capillaries along a diffusion gradient
▐ Water and electrolytes go in through osmosis

Frequency
▐ Dialysis fluid is exchanged usually 3–5 times per day
▐ Fluid exchange takes about 40 minutes

Renal transplantation (*K&C*, p. 678)

- A kidney, explanted from either a cadaveric or living related donor, is anastomosed to the iliac vessels of the recipient
- The ureter is placed into the bladder
- Immunosuppression is required for the rest of the patient's life

Prognosis

- 80% of grafts survive 5–10 years
- 60% of grafts survive for 10–30 years

CYSTIC RENAL DISEASES

- Solitary or multiple simple renal cysts are common, affecting
- 50% of the population > 50 years old
- Usually asymptomatic

Autosomal dominant polycystic kidney disease (*K&C*, p. 681)

- Inherited disorder
- Presents in adulthood
- Multiple bilateral renal cysts
- Associated with hepatic cysts

Prevalence

- 1:400–1000

Responsible genes

- PKD 1 on chromosome 16
- PKD 2 on chromosome 4

Clinical features

- Acute loin pain +/− haematuria (due to haemorrhage, infection or stone formation)
- Loin discomfort (due to large kidneys)
- Subarachnoid haemorrhage (secondary to berry aneurysm rupture)
- Hypertension
- Liver cysts
- Chronic renal failure
- Large irregular palpable kidneys
- Hepatomegaly
- Ultrasound shows multiple renal cysts

Complications

- Progression to chronic renal failure ~ 70% by age 70
- Pain
- Cyst infection
- Renal stones
- Hypertension
- Liver cysts
- Berry aneurysms (10%)

Screening

- Children and siblings of patients should have renal ultrasound after age 20

TUMOURS OF THE UROGENITAL TRACT AND PROSTATE

Renal cell carcinoma (*K&C*, p. 683)

- Average age at presentation 55 years
- $\male > \female$ (2:1)

Clinical features

- Haematuria
- Loin pain
- Mass in flank
- Malaise
- Weight loss
- Polycythaemia (excess erythropoietin)

Investigations

- Excretion urography
- Ultrasound or CT
- MRI (for tumour staging)
- Raised ESR

Management

- Nephrectomy
- α-interferon/interleukin-2

Prognosis

- 60–70% 5-year survival for localised tumour
- 15–35% 5-year survival for lymph node involvement
- 5% 5-year survival for distant metastases

Urothelial tumours (*K&C*, p. 684)

- Transitional cell carcinoma, most common in the bladder

■ $\male > \female$ (4:1)
■ Present most commonly after 40 years

Risk factors

■ Cigarette smoking
■ Industrial carcinogen exposure (β-naphthylamine, benzidine)
■ Drugs (phenacetin, cyclophosphamide)
■ Chronic inflammation (schistosomiasis causes squamous cell carcinoma)

Clinical features

■ Painless haematuria
■ Clot retention

Investigations

■ Urine cytology
■ Excretion urography
■ Cystoscopy

Management

■ Local tumour ablation – endoscopic diathermy
■ Local tumour resection – endoscopic transurethral bladder tumour resection (TURBT)
■ Cystectomy
■ Radiotherapy
■ Local or systemic chemotherapy

Prognosis

■ 80% 5-year survival (T1 N0 M0)
■ 5% 5-year survival (distant metastases)

Prostate cancer (*K&C*, p. 685)

■ Fourth commonest cause of cancer death in men
■ Malignant change in prostate gland is very common in older men
■ About 80% >80 years
■ Usually dormant or asymptomatic

Clinical features

■ Bladder outflow obstruction
■ Distant metastases to bone, lung or brain

Investigations

■ Cystoscopy
■ Transrectal ultrasound
■ Prostatic biopsy

■ Prostate-specific antigen (PSA)
■ Bone scan

Management
  Local disease ■ Radical prostatectomy
  ■ Radiotherapy
Metastatic disease ■ Orchidectomy
  ■ LHRH analogues (buserelin, goserelin)

Prognosis

■ Variable

Testicular tumours (*K&C*, p. 522)

■ Commonest in young men aged 30–35
■ Seminomas 30%
■ Teratomas 70%
■ Higher risk in undescended testes and history of orchidopexy

Clinical features

■ Testicular swelling (painless or painful)
■ Distant metastases

Investigations

■ Testicular ultrasound
■ Surgical exploration and biopsy via the groin
Staging ■ Chest X-ray
■ α-fetoprotein
■ β-human chorionic gonadotrophin
■ Abdominal CT scan

Management
  Seminomas ■ Radiotherapy
■ Chemotherapy
  Teratomas ■ Orchidectomy
■ Chemotherapy

DISEASES OF THE PROSTATE

Benign prostatic enlargement (*K&C*, p. 685)

■ Common over 60 years

Clinical features

■ Bladder outflow obstruction
■ Urinary tract infection

BOX 14.3 ACUTE URINARY RETENTION	
Clinical features	**Management**
Anuria	Urethral catheterisation
Pain	Suprapubic catheterisation
Urgency	Look for a cause
Palpable bladder	

- Stones
- Acute urinary retention
- Chronic retention with overflow incontinence
- Bilateral hydronephrosis
- Smooth enlarged prostate on rectal exam

Investigations

- Urine culture
- Assessment of renal function
- PSA
- Cystoscopy

Management

- Observation
Medical
- α-receptor blockers
- Finasteride
Surgical
- Transurethral resection of prostate (TURP)
- Prostatic stents

SELF-ASSESSMENT QUESTIONS

Multiple choice questions

1. IgA nephropathy:
   A. May be associated with carcinoma of the bronchus
   B. Presents after streptococcal infections
   C. Presents with a purpuric rash
   D. Is caused by anti-GBM antibody
   E. Usually progresses to chronic renal failure

2. Goodpasture's syndrome:
   A. May present with haemoptysis
   B. Is caused by immune complex deposition
   C. Causes membranous glomerulonephritis
   D. Rarely progresses to chronic renal failure
   E. Is treated by nephrectomy

3. Acute nephritic syndrome:
   A. Occurs after *E. coli* infections
   B. Comprises oedema and low albumin
   C. Does not progress to acute renal failure
   D. Urine microscopy shows red cell casts
   E. Is commonly complicated by hypercholesterolaemia

4. In nephrotic syndrome:
   A. Urine protein excretion is >3 g/day
   B. The renal lesion is always proliferative glomerulonephritis
   C. The urine may be fatty
   D. The JVP is raised
   E. Renal biopsy is contraindicated

5. Urinary tract infection:
   A. Is commoner in males
   B. Is always symptomatic
   C. Usually indicates an abnormal renal tract in females
   D. May be treated with oral gentamicin
   E. Is most commonly caused by *E. coli* infection

6. Pyelonephritis:
   A. May present with rigors
   B. Is usually secondary to urinary tract obstruction
   C. Is associated with diabetes insipidus
   D. Causes infertility
   E. May be complicated by septicaemia

7. Renal calculi:
   A. Are most commonly composed of uric acid
   B. May be asymptomatic
   C. May be caused by hyperkalaemia
   D. Are usually radiolucent
   E. Over >2 cm pass spontaneously

8. Management of bladder outflow obstruction should include:
   A. Fluid restriction
   B. External beam shock wave lithotripsy
   C. Ventriculo-peritoneal shunt
   D. Urethral catheter
   E. Orchidectomy

9. Pre-renal uraemia:
   A. Is caused by hypertension
   B. May be due to gastrointestinal bleeding

C. Does not correct with fluid replacement

D. Usually requires emergency dialysis

E. Presents with pericarditis

10. Complications of acute renal failure include:
A. Subarachnoid haemorrhage
B. Encephalitis
C. Hypokalaemia
D. Pericarditis
E. Contrast nephropathy

11. Acute tubular necrosis:
A. Is the renal lesion of amyloidosis
B. May be part of multisystem failure
C. May be caused by a reaction to oral radiological contrast
D. Rarely requires dialysis
F. Has a good overall prognosis

12. Causes of chronic renal failure include:
A. Paracetamol toxicity
B. Sarcoidosis
C. Cirrhosis of the liver
D. Herbal therapies
E. Gilbert's syndrome

13. Management of chronic renal failure commonly includes:
A. Emergency urography
B. Bone marrow transplant
C. Abdominal paracentesis
D. Total dental extraction
E. AV fistula formation

14. Complications of chronic renal failure commonly include:
A. Anaemia
B. Pseudogout
C. Paget's disease
D. Haematuria
E. AV fistula formation

Extended matching questions

Question 1 *Theme: right-sided abdominal pain*

A. Pyelonephritis
B. Right ovarian cyst
C. Renal calculi
D. Appendicitis
E. Polycystic kidney disease
F. Crohn's disease
G. Gallstones
H. Right lower lobe pneumonia
I. Pancreatitis
J. Renal cell carcinoma
K. Hydronephrosis
L. Hepatitis
M. Irritable bowel syndrome

For each of the following questions, select the best answer from the list above:

I. A 39-year-old advertising executive, who suffers with gout, presents with sudden onset of excruciating colicky pain in the right loin. On examination he is distressed and tender in the right flank. He is apyrexial. Urinalysis shows blood^{+++} and no nitrite. What is the most likely diagnosis?

II. A 49-year-old woman with chronic multiple sclerosis, confined to a wheelchair, presents with fever, confusion and vomiting. She is incontinent of urine with a permanent indwelling catheter. She is pyrexial with a temperature of 39°C. There is reduced air entry to the right lung base. Her PO_2 is 7.6 and urinalysis shows protein^{++}, blood^{+}, nitrite^{+}. What is the most likely diagnosis?

III. A 39-year-old man presents with a 6-month history of a chronic dull ache in the right flank with a feeling of fullness on that side. Eighteen months ago he had emergency neurosurgical clipping of a berry aneurysm after suffering a subarachnoid haemorrhage. What is the most likely diagnosis?

Question 2 *Theme: acute renal failure*

A. Hepatorenal syndrome
B. Contrast nephropathy
C. Gentamicin toxicity
D. Acute GI haemorrhage
E. Hypertensive nephropathy
F. Haemolytic uraemic syndrome
G. Goodpasture's syndrome
H. Wegener's granulomatosis
I. Prostatic obstruction
J. Retroperitoneal fibrosis
K. Renal artery stenosis

For each of the following questions, select the best answer from the list above:

I. A 48-year-old alcoholic cirrhotic female was admitted 2 days ago with constipation and confusion. She has become pyrexial with low blood pressure and oliguria. Her blood tests show acute renal failure. What is the most likely diagnosis?

II. A 90-year-old man is admitted in a dehydrated, febrile and confused state. He was seen by his GP for a 'stomach upset' 2 days ago. His full blood count shows anaemia and thrombocytopenia with red-cell fragments on the blood film. His biochemistry shows acute renal failure. What is the most likely diagnosis?

III. A 74-year-old male is admitted with symptoms of a urinary tract infection. In the past 2 days he has developed increasing abdominal pain, fever and anuria. On examination he has a mass in the pelvis which is tender and dull to percussion. His blood tests show acute renal failure. What is the most likely diagnosis?

Haematology comprises the study of the components of the blood and the bone marrow, along with disorders of the lymphoreticular system. Common disorders include the anaemias and haematological malignancy.

BASIC SCIENCE IN HAEMATOLOGY

Components of blood
Cellular

- Erythrocytes (red cells)
- Reticulocytes (immature red cells)
- Leucocytes (white cells)
  - Lymphocytes
  - Monocytes
  - Eosinophils
  - Basophils
  - Neutrophils
- Platelets

Non-cellular

Plasma
- Liquid component of blood
- Includes
  - Fibrinogen
  - Clotting factors
  - Immunoglobulins
  - Albumin
  - Other plasma proteins
  - Electrolytes

Serum
- Fluid remaining after the formation of a fibrin clot (i.e. no fibrinogen)

Haemopoiesis (Fig. 15.1) (*K&C*, p. 420)

Sites of haemopoiesis

- Embryonic yolk sac – week 3
- Liver and spleen – week 6 – month 7
- Bone marrow – month 8 onwards
- All bones – at birth
- Central skeleton ⎫
- Proximal long bones ⎬ adulthood

Stem cells

- Progenitor cells for blood cells
- Proliferation and differentiation
- → Mature blood cells
- Self-renewal, so source cells not depleted

Growth factors

- Glycoproteins, e.g. granulocyte colony-stimulating factor (G-CSF)

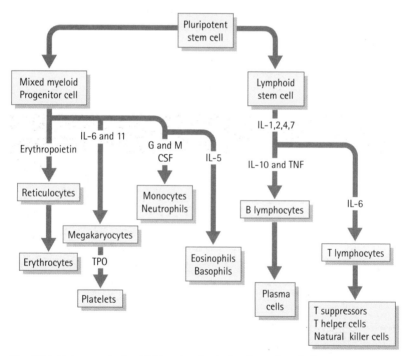

Fig. 15.1 Haemopoiesis. All blood cells derive from the pluripotent stem cell. Differentiation into cell lineages depends on a range of cytokines, hormones and growth factors. IL: Interleukin. G-CSF: Granulocyte colony stimulating factor. M-CSF: Monocyte colony stimulating factor. TNF: Tumour necrosis factor. TPO: Thrombopoietin.

I Stimulate proliferation and differentiation
I Used to increase number of white cells, e.g. after chemotherapy

Laboratory values (Table 15.1)
Red cell indices

I Size, number and haemoglobin content of erythrocytes
I Important in the classification of anaemia

Erythrocyte sedimentation rate (ESR)

I Rate of fall of red cells in a column of blood
I Measure of acute phase proteins and therefore of inflammation
I Increases with age
I Higher in ♀ than ♂

Plasma viscosity

I Measure of acute phase proteins
I No sex and little age variation

Reticulocyte count

I Immature red cells
I Measure of erythropoiesis
I Normally <2%

Table 15.1 Blood cell indices			
Measurement	Units	Male	Female
Haemoglobin (Hb) Hb concentration in blood	g dL^{-1}	13.5–17.7	11.5–16.5
Packed cell volume (PCV) Ratio of cell volume to plasma	L/L	0.42–0.53	0.35–0.45
Red cell count (RCC)	10^{12}/L	4.5–6.0	3.9–5.0
Mean corpuscular volume (MCV) Red cell size	fl	80–96	
Mean corpuscular Hb (MCH) Amount of Hb in each cell	pg	27–33	
Mean corpuscular Hb concentration (MCHC) Red cell Hb concentration	g dL^{-1}	32–36	
White cell count (WCC)	10^9/L	4.0–11.0	
Platelet count	10^9/L	150–400	
Reticulocyte count Proportion of immature red cell	%	0.5–2.5	

■ Increased by high marrow activity, e.g.
  – After bleeding
  – Anaemia
  – Haemolysis

Haemoglobin (*K&C*, p. 422)
Structure

■ Four globin (protein) chains
■ Four haem (iron-containing) molecules
■ Molecular weight 68 000

Function

■ Haem moiety can bind oxygen and CO_2
■ Acts as transporter for these gases

Genetics

■ Adult Hb (Hb A) consists of two α and two β globins
■ Hb A_2 consists of two α and two β globins (2% of adult Hb)
■ Fetal Hb consists of two α and two γ globins

ANAEMIA (*K&C*, P. 423)

■ A haemoglobin level below the reference range

Classification (Table 15.2)

■ By erythrocyte volume (MCV)

Macrocytic –
large red cells
■ B_{12} deficiency
■ Folate deficiency
■ Chronic alcohol misuse
■ Chronic liver disease
■ ↑ Reticulocytes
■ Hypothyroidism

Table 15.2 Iron indices in anaemia			
	Iron deficiency	Anaemia of chronic disease	Macrocytic anaemia
Hb	↓	↓	↓
MCV	↓	↓ or ↔	↑
Ferritin	↓	↑, ↓ or ↔	↑ or ↔
Serum iron	↓	↓	↔
Total iron binding capacity	↑	↓	↔
Transferrin saturation	↓	↓	↔

Microcytic – small red cells	▌ Iron deficiency
	▌ Thalassaemia
	▌ Sideroblastic anaemia
	▌ Anaemia of chronic disease
	▌ Myelodysplasia
Normocytic – normal red cells	▌ Acute blood loss
	▌ Anaemia of chronic disease
	▌ Haemolysis
	▌ Infection
	▌ Pregnancy
	▌ Hypopituitarism
	▌ Hypothyroidism (may be macrocytic)
	▌ Renal failure

Clinical features

Symptoms
▌ Fatigue
▌ Headache ⎫ Common in normal population
▌ Faintness ⎭
▌ Breathlessness
▌ Angina on effort
▌ Intermittent claudication
▌ Palpitations

Signs
▌ Pallor
▌ Tachycardia
▌ Systolic flow murmur
▌ Cardiac failure
▌ Koilonychia – spoon-shaped nails in iron deficiency
▌ Jaundice – haemolytic anaemia
▌ Bone deformity – thalassaemia major
▌ Leg ulcers – sickle cell disease
▌ Angular stomatitis
▌ Glossitis (Painful red tongue)

Investigations

▌ White cell count – if low may be dilutional or bone marrow failure
▌ Reticulocyte count – measures bone marrow activity
▌ Blood film for erythrocyte morphology – may show dimorphic picture (both large and small red cells); seen in combined iron and folate deficiency

Iron deficiency anaemia (*K&C*, p. 425)
Iron metabolism

▌ Iron requirements
 – ♂ 0.5–1 mg/day
 – ♀ 1.2–1.7 mg/day (2–3 mg/day in pregnancy)

■ Dietary iron 15–20 mg/day
■ 10% absorbed
■ Absorbed in duodenum and jejunum (Fig. 15.2)
■ Transported in blood bound to transferrin
■ Stored as ferritin and haemosiderin

Causes of iron deficiency

■ Blood loss (commonly menstrual)
■ Growth or pregnancy (↑ requirement)
■ Decreased absorption (e.g. gastrectomy)
■ Low dietary intake

Clinical features

■ Koilonychia and brittle nails/hair
■ Angular stomatitis
■ Dysphagia ⎫ Plummer–Vinson or
■ Glossitis ⎭ Paterson–Brown–Kelly syndrome

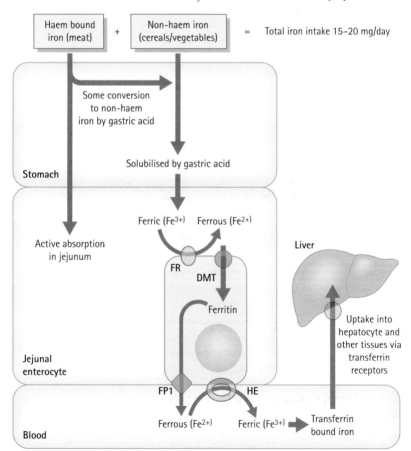

Fig. 15.2 Absorption of iron.

Investigations

- Blood count and film
- ↓ Serum ferritin
- ↓ Serum iron and ↑ iron-binding capacity
- ↓ transferin saturation

Management

- Treat cause
- Oral iron – ferrous sulphate or gluconate
- i.v. iron sucrose if unable to tolerate oral

Anaemia of chronic disease (*K&C*, p. 429)
Aetiology

- Reduced erythropoiesis
- Reduced red cell survival
- Chronic infection
  - Osteomyelitis
  - Infective endocarditis
  - TB
- Chronic inflammation
  - Rheumatoid arthritis
  - Systemic lupus erythematosus (SLE)
  - Polymyalgia rheumatica
- Malignancy

Investigations

- Low iron and iron-binding capacity
- Normal or high ferritin

Sideroblastic anaemia (*K&C*, p. 429)
Aetiology

- Abnormal haem metabolism
- Excess iron deposited in erythrocytes (ring sideroblasts)
- Inherited (X-linked) or acquired
  - Myelodysplastic syndrome
  - Drugs, e.g. isoniazid
  - Alcohol/lead

Megaloblastic anaemia (*K&C*, p. 430)
Aetiology

- B_{12} deficiency (Fig. 15.3 and Table 15.3)
- Folate deficiency (Table 15.4)
- Myelodysplasia

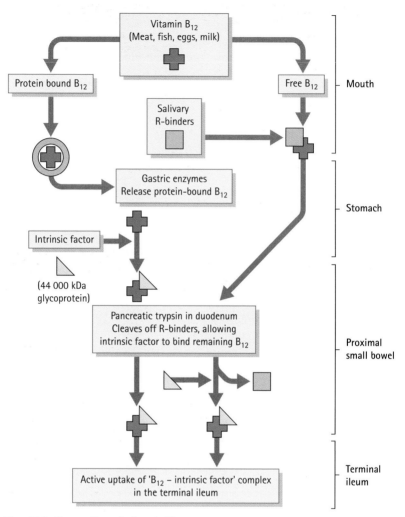

Fig. 15.3 Absorption of vitamin B$_{12}$.

Investigations

▮ ↑ MCV > 96 fl (macrocytosis)
▮ Blood film – hypersegmented neutrophils
▮ Serum B$_{12}$ and folate
▮ Red cell folate – better measure of tissue folate
▮ Look for underlying cause
▮ Schilling test (Fig. 15.4) (now rarely done)

Pernicious anaemia (*K&C*, p. 432)

▮ – → Megaloblastic anaemia

Table 15.3 Causes of B₁₂ deficiency anaemia

Low dietary intake
Vegan diet – B_{12} high in meat, fish, eggs and milk

Impaired absorption (stomach)
Pernicious anaemia
Gastrectomy ⎫ Lack of intrinsic factor
Congenital lack of intrinsic factor ⎭

Impaired absorption (small bowel)
Pancreatic insufficiency – failure to cleave off R-binders
Terminal ileal disease – loss of absorption site
Bacterial overgrowth – bacterial utilisation of B_{12}

Abnormal metabolism
Transcobalamin II deficiency – congenital lack of B_{12} transporter

Table 15.4 Causes of folate deficiency

Nutritional	↑ Utilisation
Poor intake	*Physiological*
Old age	Pregnancy
Poor diet	Lactation
Starvation	*Pathological*
Alcohol abuse	Increased red cell synthesis, e.g. haemolysis
Malabsorption	
Coeliac disease	**Inhibited metabolism**
Crohn's disease	Drugs
	Anticonvulsants, e.g. phenytoin
Anorexia	Methotrexate
Malignancy	Trimethoprim
GI disease	Increased cell turnover, e.g. malignancy
	Inflammatory disease
	Metabolic disease, e.g. homocystinuria
	Haemodialysis

Aetiology

▎ Autoimmune disease
▎ Common (esp. in elderly)
▎ Anti-intrinsic factor antibodies in 50%
▎ Anti-parietal cell antibodies in 90%
▎ → Intrinsic factor deficiency due to auto-immune gastritis
▎ → B_{12} malabsorption

Disease associations

▎ Autoimmune thyroid disease
▎ Addison's disease

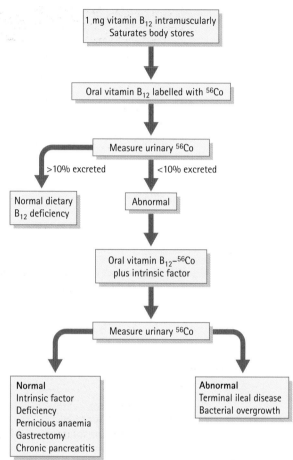

Fig. 15.4 Schilling tests. These are designed to diagnose the cause of vitamin B$_{12}$ deficiency (now rarely done).

▌ Vitiligo
▌ Blond hair and blue eyes, Blood group A
▌ Higher risk of gastric cancer in males

Pathology

▌ Gastric mucosal atrophy
▌ Achlorhydria (loss of gastric acid synthesis)

Clinical features

▌ Pallor and mild jaundice
▌ Glossitis (sore red tongue)
▌ Angular stomatitis
▌ Progressive polyneuropathy
▌ Subacute combined degeneration of the cord

Table 15.5 Causes of macrocytosis without anaemia

Physiological	Reticulocytosis
Pregnancy	Hypothyroidism
Newborn babies	Aplastic anaemia
	Drugs, e.g. azathioprine
Pathological	
Alcohol excess	
Liver disease	

- $\rightarrow$ Paraesthesia, weakness and ataxia
- $\rightarrow$ Paraplegia
- Rarely, optic atropy or dementia

Management

- 1 mg vitamin B_{12} per day for 7 days i.m.
- Then 1 mg every 3 months for life

Folate deficiency (*K&C*, p. 433)

- $\rightarrow$ Megaloblastic anaemia (Table 15.5)

Folate absorption

- Found in spinach, broccoli, liver and kidney
- Cooking destroys folate
- Daily requirement 100 mg
- B_{12} required for folate metabolism

Clinical features

- Anaemia
- Glossitis
- No neuropathy

Management

- Oral folate 5 mg per day

Prophylaxis

- Advised prior to and during pregnancy
- Reduces risk of neural tube defects

Sickle cell disease (*K&C*, p. 443)
Aetiology

- Mutation $\rightarrow$ abnormal β globin (Hb S)
- $\rightarrow$ Sickle cell trait (heterozygote Hb AS)
- Or sickle cell disease (homozygote Hb SS)

BOX 15.1 ACUTE SICKLE CRISIS

Give	**Investigations**
High-flow oxygen	Full blood count – extent of anaemia and
I.v. access and fluids	leucocytosis
	Chest X-ray if there are chest signs
History	Urea and electrolytes for renal dysfunction
Previous crises	
Chest or cardiac crises	**Analgesia**
Previous ITU admissions	i.v. or i.m. pethidine, diamorphine or fentanyl
Recent fever or evidence	Patient controlled analgesia
of infection	
Recent travel	
Check for	
Chest sickling	
Pleuritic pain, cough, crackles,	
pleural rub	
Hypoxia on blood gases	

- Hb S is insoluble when deoxygenated
- → Hb forms crystals and deforms red cells
- → Sickle shape
- → Reduced red cell survival and microvascular obstruction

Epidemiology

- 25% of Africans carry abnormal gene
- Also India, Middle East and southern Europe

Precipitation of crisis

- Infection
  - Notably chest → hypoxia
  - Parvovirus → marrow aplasia → pancytopenia
  - Haemolysis due to sepsis
- Sequestration of red cells in liver and spleen
- Dehydration → increased plasma viscosity

Clinical features

- Onset after 6 months (as Hb F level drops)
- Chronic haemolytic anaemia
- Recurrent painful crises
- Bone pain
- Chest – pleuritic pain, common cause of death
- Cerebral – fits, neurological signs

- Kidneys – papillary necrosis, inability to concentrate urine
- Spleen – splenic infarcts → hyposplenism
- Liver – pain and abnormal liver function
- Penis – priapism

Long-term
- Hyposplenism → risk of infection
- Chronic leg ulcers
- Gallstones
- Necrosis of femoral heads
- Chronic renal disease
- Stroke

Investigations

- Full blood count
  - Anaemia
  - Infection (leucocytosis)
- Blood film
  - Sickling
  - Hyposplenism
- Hb electrophoresis demonstrates Hb S

Management

Acute
- i.v. fluids
- Oxygen
- Antibiotics if evidence of infection
- Adequate analgesia
- Exchange transfusions if severe crisis

Long-term
- Pneumococcal vaccine
- *Haemophilus influenzae* vaccine
- Folic acid
- Transfusions if very anaemic
- Hydroxyurea increases Hb F production

Thalassaemia (*K&C*, p. 440)
Aetiology

- Inherited failure of synthesis of one globin type
- Accumulation of remaining globin type
- → Haemolysis and ineffective erythropoiesis

β-thalassaemia

Minor (trait)
- Carrier state (heterozygote)
- Asymptommatic
- Low MCV and MCH

Major
- Homozygote
- Severe anaemia requiring transfusions

- Onset 3–6 months old
- Anaemia and infections
- Extramedullary haemopoiesis
- → Skull expansion and bossing

Treatment
- Regular transfusions to suppress haemopoiesis and avoid deformity and anaemia
- Iron chelation to reduce overload
- Bone marrow transplantation

α-thalassaemia

- Deletion in one to four of the four a globin genes
- All four deleted → fetal death (hydrops fetalis)
- Three of four → moderate anaemia
- Two of four → carrier state, no anaemia

Haemolytic anaemia (*K&C*, p. 436)

- Anaemia due to the premature breakdown of erythrocytes, resulting in reduced red cell survival
- If haemolysis is acute, anaemia, jaundice and haemoglobinuria are seen

Aetiology

Inherited
- Sickle cell disease
- Thalassaemia
- Hereditary spherocytosis
- Hereditary elliptocytosis
- Glucose-6-phosphate dehydrogenase deficiency
  - X-linked recessive
  - → Haemolysis due to drugs, e.g. aspirin
  - Favism (fava beans → haemolysis)
  - Haemolysis due to infection
- Pyruvate kinase deficiency
  - Autosomal recessive
  - → Anaemia and splenomegaly

Acquired
- Autoimmune haemolytic anaemia (Table 15.6)
  - Autoantibodies against red cell membrane
  - Positive direct Coombs' test (Fig. 15.5)
- Drug-induced autoimmune haemolysis
  - Quinine
  - Penicillin
  - Methyldopa
- Haemolytic disease of the newborn
  - Maternal anti-red cell IgG crosses placenta
  - → Fetal red cell destruction (Rhesus disease)

Table 15.6 **Autoimmune haemolytic anaemia (AIHA)***

	Warm AIHA	Cold AIHA
Antibody type	IgG	IgM
Optimal antibody binding	37°C	< 37°C
Direct Coombs' test	Strong positive	Positive
Causes	Idiopathic (primary)	Idiopathic (primary)
	SLE	Lymphomas
	Lymphomas	Infectious mononucleosis
	Chronic lymphatic leukaemia	*Mycoplasma* infection
	Malignancy	
	Drugs, e.g. methyldopa	

*These anaemias are classified based on the temperature at which the autoantibody best binds to the red cell membrane.

❙ Paroxysmal nocturnal haemoglobinuria
  – Red cell destruction by complement
  – → Haemolysis due to infection or surgery
  – → Early morning haemoglobinuria
  – Increased risk of venous thrombosis
❙ Mechanical haemolysis
  – Cardiac prosthetic valves
  – Marching
  – Microangiopathic haemolytic anaemia
❙ Others
  – Extensive burns
  – Renal and liver disease
  – Malaria

BLOOD GROUPS AND BLOOD TRANSFUSION
(*K&C*, P. 458)

❙ The blood group of a particular patient is determined by red cell surface antigens
❙ The two common and most important groupings are ABO and Rhesus status
❙ The process of typing blood is based on a series of indirect Coomb' tests to analyse the blood for the presence of these antigens
❙ Cross-matching blood for transfusion is carried out by looking for agglutination when blood cells to be donated are mixed with the patient's serum (Fig. 15.5)

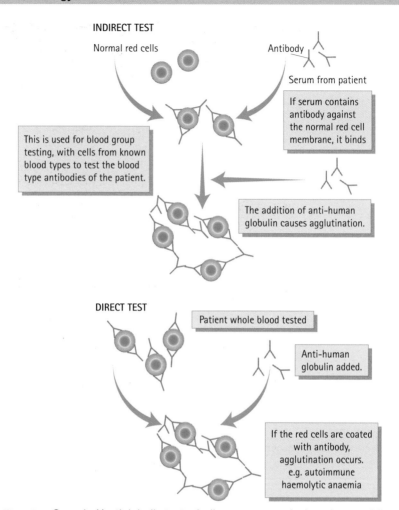

Fig. 15.5 Coombs'/antiglobulin tests. Indirect tests are designed to establish whether there is an anti-red cell antibody in the patient's serum. They are used for blood group testing, using cells from known blood types to test the blood type antibodies of the patient. Direct tests establish whether there is an autoantibody already attached to the patient's red cells.

ABO blood group (Table 15.7)

▮ Presence of A or B antigens on red cells
▮ Presence of anti-A or anti-B in serum
▮ Mixing incompatible blood → haemolysis

Rh blood group

▮ Presence or absence of D antigen
▮ Antibodies form if a D-negative patient is given D-positive blood

Table 15.7 The ABO and Rhesus blood groups

Group	Genotype	Red cell antigens	Antibodies	Frequency	Notes
O	OO	None	Anti-A and anti-B	44%	Universal donor
A	AO or AA	A	Anti-B	45%	
B	BO or BB	B	Anti-B	8%	
AB	AB	A and B	None	3%	Universal recipient
D +ve	C or D or E	D	None		Three genes determine genotype: C, D and E
D −ve	CDE	None	Anti-D*		* After exposure

Fetal Rhesus D syndrome

❙ RhD-negative mother with a D-positive child will be sensitised at the first delivery
❙ Subsequent D-positive fetuses will be subjected to anti-D antibodies → hydrops fetalis
❙ Prophylaxis with anti-D antibodies given to the mother at each delivery suppresses the mother's own antibody production, protecting future fetuses

Blood products

❙ Whole blood ~ 500 mL
❙ Packed cells – 250 mL of plasma removed
❙ Red cell concentrate – all plasma removed
❙ Platelet concentrate
❙ Fresh frozen plasma – replacement of clotting factors
❙ Cryoprecipitate – factor VIII, fibrinogen and von Willebrand factor
❙ Human albumin
❙ Normal immunoglobulin

Procedure for blood transfusion (*K&C*, p. 459)

❙ Type patient's blood
❙ Cross-match donor blood with patient serum
❙ Donor blood is coded and labelled with the patient's name; a record sheet with the unit number of the donor blood and the patient's name and identification number is produced

When administering blood

■ Two members of staff check the following

Between the patient and record sheet
■ Name of the patient
■ Date of birth of the patient
■ Identification number of the patient

Between the blood and record sheet
■ Blood unit number
■ Blood group
■ Name, age and date of birth of the patient

Complications of blood transfusion (*K&C*, p. 460)

■ Incompatibility → poor red cell survival

Transfusion reactions

■ Usually ABO incompatibility
■ Haemolysis and haemoglobinuria
■ Rigors
■ Dyspnoea
■ Hypotension
■ Renal failure
■ Disseminated intravascular coagulation

Febrile transfusion reactions

■ Mild fever and flushing
■ Rarely due to haemolysis

Transmission of infection

■ Previously HCV + HIV
■ All blood screened for known infections

BLOOD COAGULATION (FIG. 15.6) (*K&C*, P. 466)

Vessel wall injury leads to

■ Vasoconstriction → reduced blood flow
■ Platelet activation → serotonin and thromboxane
■ Coagulation → fibrin clot formation

Platelet adhesion

■ Adhesion to collagen exposed by vessel damage via glycoprotein Ia receptor on platelets and in combination with von Willebrand factor via glycoprotein Ib receptors
■ Fibrinogen then binds to platelets, is converted to fibrin and forms cross-links, producing a platelet plug

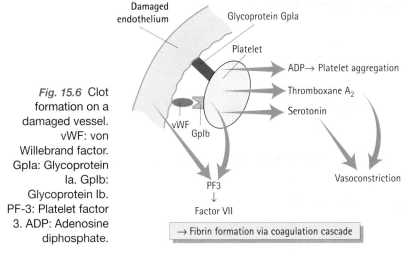

Fig. 15.6 Clot formation on a damaged vessel. vWF: von Willebrand factor. Gpla: Glycoprotein Ia. Gplb: Glycoprotein Ib. PF-3: Platelet factor 3. ADP: Adenosine diphosphate.

Platelet prostaglandin

▮ Prostaglandin metabolism → thromboxane production
▮ → Vasoconstriction and platelet activation
▮ Process is inhibited by aspirin

Coagulation cascade (Fig. 15.7) (K&C, p. 467)

▮ Enzymatic reactions
▮ → Activation of coagulation proteins
▮ → Conversion of fibrinogen to fibrin
▮ Old classification into extrinsic and intrinsic
▮ This is based on in vitro coagulation; in vivo cascade differs

Coagulation factors

▮ Synthesised in the liver
▮ Enzyme precursors (XII, XI, X, IX)
▮ Enzyme cofactors (V, VIII)

Coagulation inhibitors

▮ Anti-thrombin inactivates clotting factors
▮ Activated protein C destroys factors V and VIII and initiates fibrinolysis
▮ Protein S – cofactor for protein C

Fibrinolysis (Fig. 15.8)

▮ Plasminogen converted to plasmin by tissue plasminogen activator (t-PA)

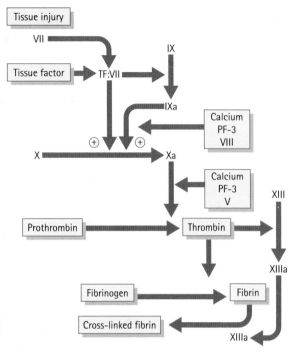

Fig. 15.7 The
coagulation cascade
in vivo.

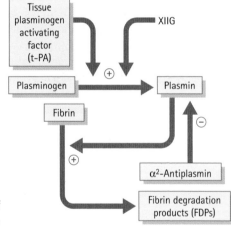

Fig. 15.8 The breakdown of
fibrin.

▌ Converts fibrin to fibrin degradation products and
D-dimer fragments

Measurements of coagulation
Prothrombin time (PT, normal 10–16 seconds)

▌ Lengthened by factor VII, X, V or II abnormality
▌ Also increased by warfarin

International normalised ratio (INR, normal = 1–1.3)

▋ Comparison of prothrombin time to a known
standard
▋ Used to monitor warfarin

*Activated partial thromboplastin time (APTT, normal 23–31
seconds)*

▋ Abnormalities of factors XI, IX, VIII, X, V, II or I
▋ Increased by heparin

Thrombin time (TT, normal 12 seconds)

▋ Prolonged by fibrinogen deficiencies and heparin

Bleeding time

▋ Standard cut made and time taken for bleeding to
stop is measured

Correction tests – addition of normal plasma

▋ If this corrects an abnormal test, then a factor
deficiency is the cause of the coagulopathy
▋ If no correction occurs, it suggests the presence of
an inhibitor in the patient's plasma

D-dimer assay

▋ Increased during fibrinolysis, e.g. after pulmonary
embolus
▋ If negative, PE is very unlikely

Fibrin degradation products (FDPs)

▋ Increased by fibrinolysis, e.g. pulmonary
embolus

Inherited coagulation defects (*K&C*, p. 472)

Haemophilia A

▋ X-linked inheritance found in 1:5000 men
▋ Factor VIII:C deficiency

*Factor VIII < 1%
of normal*
▋ Frequent spontaneous bleeding
▋ Joint bleeds → deformity

*Factor VIII < 5%
of normal*
▋ Severe bleeding after injury

*Factor VIII > 5%
of normal*
▋ Mild disease
▋ Prolonged bleeding after trauma

Investigations

▋ See Table 15.8

Table 15.8 Blood results in coagulopathy

	Prothrombin time (PT)	Activated partial thromboplastin time (APTT)	Bleeding time	Factor VIII:C level	Von Willebrand factor (vWF)
Platelet disorders	Normal	Normal	↑	Normal	Normal
Vitamin K deficiency	↑	↑	Normal	Normal	Normal
Haemophilia A and B	Normal	↑	Normal	↓	Normal
Von Willebrand's disease	Normal	↑	↑	↓	↓

Management

- Factor VIII:C i.v.
- DDAVP (vasopressin) intranasal spray (increases factor VIII:C levels)
- Minor bleeding – aim for 30% of normal
- Major bleeding – aim for 50% of normal
- Surgery – aim for 100% preoperatively

Complications of treatment

- Antibodies against factor VIII:C
- Complications of blood transfusion

Haemophilia B (Christmas disease) (*K&C*, p. 474)

- X-linked inheritance found in 1:30 000 men
- Factor IX deficiency
- Clinically identical to haemophilia A

Management

- i.v. factor IX

Von Willebrand's disease (*K&C*, p. 474)

- Three types (all chromosome 12)
  - Type 1: mild disease, autosomal dominant
  - Type 2: mild disease, autosomal dominant
  - Type 3: severe disease, autosomal recessive
- Bleeding follows trauma and surgery
- Spontaneous epistaxis
- Defect of platelet adhesion combined with factor VIII:C deficiency

Management

- Intranasal DDAVP (vasopressin)
- Factor VIII/von Willebrand factor if required

Acquired coagulation defects

Vitamin K deficiency (*K&C*, p. 475)

- Failure of synthesis of vitamin K-dependent factors
- Reduced factors II, VII, IX and X
- Reduced protein C and S

Aetiology

- Inadequate stores (newborn children)
- Malabsorption (fat-soluble vitamin)
- Oral anticoagulants, e.g. warfarin

Investigations

- Elevated prothrombin time and APTT

Management

- Intravenous vitamin K

Chronic liver disease (*K&C*, p. 475)

- Vitamin K deficiency
- Reduced clotting factor synthesis
- Thrombocytopenia
- Abnormal platelet function

Disseminated intravascular coagulation (DIC) (*K&C*, p. 475)

- Uncontrolled fibrin production in blood vessels
  - Malignancy
  - Septicaemia
  - Transfusion reactions
  - Placental abruption
  - Trauma
  - Burns
  - Snake bites

Investigations

- Elevated prothrombin time
- Low platelets
- Elevated FDPs and D-dimers

Clinical features

- Haemorrhage
- Shock
- Epistaxis, bleeding gums

Management
- Platelets
- Fresh frozen plasma (FFP)
- Cryoprecipitate
- Blood if required

Massive blood transfusion
- Lack of factors VIII and V in transfusion blood
- Few platelets
- Citrate in transfusions lowers serum calcium
- If giving > 10 units check clotting and platelets
- Consider platelets and fresh frozen plasma
- Calcium i.v.

Clotting factor autoantibodies
- 10% of haemophiliacs – antibodies against factor VIII
- SLE
- Post-childbirth

Antiphospholipid antibodies (see also Chapter 11)
- Found in 10% of those with SLE
- → Recurrent arterial and venous thrombosis
- Recurrent miscarriages
- Patients have elevated APTT
- Management
  - Anticoagulation
  - Aspirin

Anticoagulant drugs (*K&C*, p. 479)
Warfarin
- Oral Vitamin K antagonist
- Increases prothrombin time

BOX 15.2 UNCONTROLLED BLEEDING DUE TO ANTICOAGULATION WITH WARFARIN

Severe bleeding
Stop warfarin immediately
i.v. access
Give 5 mg of i.v. vitamin K by slow infusion
Fresh frozen plasma or clotting factors II, IX, X and VII
Blood transfusion if required

Less severe bleeding
e.g. Epistaxis or haematuria or INR > 8
Withhold warfarin
Consider vitamin K 0.5 mg i.v.

Heparin
- Parenteral administration (usually i.v.)
- Potentiates antithrombin III
- Elevates APTT

Low molecular weight heparin
- Can be given subcutaneously
- Predictable anticoagulant effect

Fibrinolytics
- Activate plasmin
- Recombinant t-Pa
- Streptokinase

Anti-platelet drugs
- Aspirin
- Clopidogrel
- Dipyridamole

Thromboembolic disease (*K&C*, p. 476)
- Thromboembolic disease is a very common cause of death; just under 50% of adult deaths result from its manifestation
  - Coronary artery thrombosis
  - Cerebral artery thrombosis
  - Pulmonary embolism (PE)

Thrombus
- Formation of solid clot in a vessel

Embolus
- Fragment of clot carried to a distant site
- → Obstruction of a vessel

Arterial thrombus
- Associated with atheroma
- → Platelet attachment
- → Propagation of thrombus

Venous thrombus
- Occurs in normal vessels
- Commonly deep leg veins
- Risk factors – Table 15.9

Table 15.9 Risk factors for deep vein thrombosis	
Patient	**Diseases**
Age	Previous DVT/PE
Obesity	Malignancy
Immobility	Thrombophilia
Smoking	Myocardial infarction
	Infection
	Inflammatory bowel disease
	Nephrotic syndrome
	Polycythaemia
	Surgery or trauma

Thrombophilia (*K&C*, p. 477)

- Recurrent venous thrombosis
- Venous thrombosis under the age of 40
- Often a family history

Aetiology

- Factor V Leiden syndrome
- Antithrombin deficiency
- Protein C and S deficiency
- Antiphospholipid syndrome (p. 318)

Deep vein thrombosis (DVT) (*K&C*, p. 870)

- Formation of thrombus in
  - Deep calf vein
  - Axillary vein

Clinical features

- Pain and tenderness
- Swelling of the limb
- Redness of overlying skin
- Pulmonary embolism

Investigations

- Doppler ultrasound of the vein
- Venography (intravenous contrast)

Management

- Low molecular weight heparin *or*
- Intravenous heparin
- Warfarin
- Bed rest
- Graduated pressure stockings

BOX 15.3 PULMONARY EMBOLUS

Patient is
In pain – pleuritic chest pain
Dyspnoeic
Shocked – hypotension
  and tachycardia

Give
High-flow oxygen
i.v. access

History
Risk factors for PE
Presence of a DVT
Thrombophilia
Oral contraceptive pill
Smoking
Concomitant illness/
  surgery/immobility

Investigations
Full blood count
Coagulation screen
D-dimer or FDPs (raised in PE)
Chest X-ray – oligaemic patch
ECG
Tachycardia
Right axis deviation and bundle
  branch block
S wave in lead I, Q wave and inverted
  T in lead III

Consider
Thrombolysis if shocked with no
  contraindications

Anticoagulate
Low molecular weight heparin or
Heparin bolus and i.v. infusion

Confirm diagnosis
$\dot{V}/\dot{Q}$ scan, CT pulmonary angiogram

Complications

- Phlebitis
- Venous eczema

Pulmonary embolism (*K&C*, p. 844)

- Obstruction of a branch of the pulmonary artery by clot from a DVT

Clinical features

Small or — Pleuritic chest pain
medium PE — Shortness of breath
- Haemoptysis in 30%
- Tachypnoea
- Pleural rub
- Coarse crackles
- Pleural effusion
Massive PE — Collapse
- Shock
- Cardiac arrest electromechanical dissociation
- Elevated JVP ('a' wave)
- Gallop rhythm

Recurrent PE
- Breathlessness
- Weakness
- Syncope
- Gradual deterioration

Investigations

- Chest X-ray – oligaemic area
- ECG
  - S wave in lead I, Q wave and inverted T in lead III
  - Right axis deviation
  - Right bundle branch block
- Fibrin degredation products (FDPs) and D-dimers in blood are elevated
- $\dot{V}/\dot{Q}$ scan (Fig. 5.51)
  - Radionucleotide scan
  - Demonstrates defects in perfusion of the lung in areas with normal ventilation
- Blood gases – hypoxia and low $PaCO_2$
- Echocardiogram – high PA pressure
- Pulmonary angiography/CT pulmonary angiogram

Management

- High-flow oxygen
- Analgesia
- Intravenous heparin *or*
- Low molecular weight heparin
- Consider thrombolysis (rtPa)

HAEMATOLOGICAL MALIGNANCY (*K&C*, P. 500)

These are malignant proliferations of:

- Lymphocytes
  - Hodgkin's disease
  - Non-Hodgkin's lymphoma
  - Chronic lymphocytic leukaemia
  - Myeloma (plasma cells)
- Immature lymphocytes
  - Acute lymphoblastic leukaemia
  - Hairy cell leukaemia
- Myeloid cells
  - Acute myelogenous leukaemia
  - Chronic myeloid leukaemia

Table 15.10 Staging of Hodgkin's Disease (modified Ann Arbor classification)

Stage*	Features
I	Single organ or single lymph node region
II	Two or more lymph node regions on the same side of the diaphragm
	One lymph node region and one other organ
III	Lymph nodes on both sides of the diaphragm
	Splenic involvement
IV	Extralymphatic involvement
	Lung
	Liver
	Bone
	Bone marrow

*Presence of B symptoms is denoted with a 'b' after the stage. Bulky disease is denoted with an 'x' after the stage. Lack of both is denoted with an 'a'.

Lymphomas

Hodgkin's disease (Table 15.10) (*K&C*, p. 508)

- B or T cell malignant clone

Clinical features

- Lymphadenopathy
- Fever
- Drenching sweats B symptoms
- Weight loss
- Alcohol-induced pain
- Hepatomegaly
- Splenomegaly

Investigations

- Blood count – anaemia
- ESR ↑
- Uric acid sometimes ↑
- Chest X-ray – mediastinal mass or hilar lymph nodes
- CT scan
  - Lymphadenopathy
  - Liver or spleen enlargement or infiltration
- Lymph node biopsy and histology
- Bone marrow biopsy (shows Sternberg–Reed cells)

Management

- Depends on
  - Stage and histology
  - Site of tumour
  - Presence of B symptoms

- Radiotherapy
- Chemotherapy
- Myeloablation and stem cell support

Prognosis

- 40–70% survival at 20 years
- Depends on stage of original tumour

Non-Hodgkin's lymphoma (*K&C*, p. 512)
Aetiology

- 70% B cell
- Associated with EBV and HIV infection

Clinical features

- Lymphadenopathy
- Symptoms due to site of tumour
- May involve GI tract, lungs, brain

Investigations

- Blood count
  - Anaemia
  - Thrombocytopenia
- Liver chemistry
- Chest X-ray
- CT scan of abdomen and thorax
- Bone marrow biopsy
- Lymph node biopsy

Management

- Depends on grade
- Radiotherapy
- Chemotherapy

Burkitt's lymphoma

- Associated with Epstein–Barr virus
- Endemic in West Africa
- Jaw, abdominal and ovarian tumours
- Curable

Acute leukaemias (*K&C*, p. 501)
Epidemiology

- Rare: 5 in 100 000

Aetiology

- Unknown in most cases
- T-cell leukaemia – retrovirus (HTLV-1)

- Specific genetic mutations
- Chromosome translocations, e.g. t(15; 17)
- Environmental factors
- Ionizing radiation

Clinical features

- Bone marrow failure
- → Weakness and tiredness due to anaemia
- → Bruising due to thrombocytopenia
- → Repeated infections

Investigations

- Blood count
- Blood film – leukaemic blast cells
- Bone marrow – blast cells

Management

- Correct anaemia and thrombocytopenia
- Treat any infection
- Chemotherapy to achieve remission
- Myeloablation with stem cell support to clear marrow of malignant cells

Acute myeloid leukaemia (AML)

- Classified by cell type (Table 15.11)
- 70% alive at 1 year → 30% alive at 5 years
- Treatment aims for complete remission
- Followed by bone marrow ablation

Acute lymphoblastic leukaemia (ALL)

- Predominantly a disease of children
- Cure rate 50–60% in children, 30% in adults

Table 15.11 Classification of acute myelogenous leukaemia (AML)

FAB (French, American, British) type	Description	Notes
M1	Myeloblastic	No maturation of blasts
M2	Myeloblastic	Maturation of blasts seen
M3	Promyelocytic	Associated with DIC
		All-trans-retinoic acid (ATRA) → remission
M4	Myelomonocytic	Skin and gum lesions, CNS involvement
M5	Monoblastic	
M6	Erythroblastic	Very rare
M7	Megakaryoblastic	

- Central nervous system involvement common
- $\rightarrow$ Prophylactic intrathecal chemotherapy

Chronic leukaemias (*K&C*, pp. 505–507)

- Chronic leukaemias occur in older patients, most of whom die within 5 years of diagnosis
- Clinical course consists of a chronic illness lasting 3–4 years, followed by transformation into an acute leukaemia or sometimes myelofibrosis in the case of chronic myeloid leukaemia

Chronic myeloid leukaemia (CML)
Clinical features

- Anaemia
- Night sweats and fever
- Weight loss
- Splenomegaly $\rightarrow$ pain

Investigations

- Blood count – raised white count
- Multiple myeloid precursors
- Bone marrow biopsy
- Genetic testing for the Philadelphia chromosome (9: 22 translocation) (positive in 90–95%)

Management

- Interferons $\rightarrow$ remission in 10%
- Hydroxyurea reduces white cell count
- Myeloablation with bone marrow transplant

Chronic lymphocytic leukaemia (CLL)
Clinical features

- Often an incidental finding
- Infections due to neutropenia
- Anaemia (may be due to haemolysis)
- Lymphadenopathy
- Hepatosplenomegaly

Investigations

- Haemoglobin low or normal
- White count $> 15 \times 10^9/L$
- 40% lymphocytes
- Platelets low or normal
- Serum immunoglobulins may be low

Management

■ Nothing if asymptomatic
■ Steroids for haemolysis
■ Fludarabine or chlorambucil

Hairy cell leukaemia

■ Rare
■ Usually a B cell tumour
■ Cells have filament-like projections

Myeloproliferative disorders (*K&C*, pp. 453–455)

■ Uncontrolled proliferation of a blood cell line
■ Can transform into acute leukaemias or from one myeloproliferation to another

Polycythaemia vera (Table 15.9)

■ Red cell proliferation
■ Patients usually > 60 years old

Clinical features

■ Tiredness
■ Depression
■ Tinnitus
■ Vertigo
■ Visual disturbance
■ Itching after a hot bath
■ Gout (due to increased cell turnover)
■ Thrombosis or haemorrhage
■ Plethora and cyanosis
■ Splenomegaly

Investigations

■ Haemoglobin raised
■ Packed cell volume (haematocrit) ↑
■ 50% have ↑ platelets
■ 75% have ↑ white cells
■ Uric acid ↑
■ Leucocyte alkaline phosphatase ↑

Management

■ Venesection
■ Chemotherapy
■ Allopurinol to avoid gout

Prognosis

▌ 30% → myelofibrosis
▌ 5% → AML

Essential thrombocythaemia

▌ Platelet count $> 1000 \times 10^9/\text{L}$
▌ → Bruising and bleeding (poor platelet function)
▌ Increased risk of thrombosis

Myelofibrosis

▌ Stem cell proliferation
▌ Bone marrow fibrosis

Clinical features

▌ Anaemia
▌ Weight loss
▌ Splenomegaly
▌ Bone pain
▌ Gout

Investigations

▌ Anaemia
▌ High platelets
▌ 'Dry' bone marrow aspirate
▌ High uric acid

Management

▌ Blood transfusion
▌ Folic acid
▌ Chemotherapy and radiotherapy
▌ Splenectomy may be required

Prognosis

▌ 10–20% → AML

Myelodysplasia

▌ Stem cell defects
▌ → Bone marrow failure
▌ Abnormal red cells, leucocytes and platelets

Management

▌ Supportive therapy
▌ Low-intensity chemotherapy

Multiple myeloma and hyperglobulinaemia (*K&C*, pp. 516–517)

▌ Clonal expansion of plasma cells resulting in
very high production of a single immunoglobulin
(paraprotein) or an immunoglobulin component

Table 15.12 Complications of hyperviscosity syndrome

Headaches
Visual disturbance – retinal artery and vein occlusion
Cerebrovascular accidents – indication for urgent plasmapheresis
Thrombophilia

Myeloma

▮ Elderly patients

Clinical features

▮ Bone lesions → pain and fractures
▮ Hypercalcaemia
▮ Bone marrow infiltration
▮ → Anaemia, neutropenia
▮ Renal impairment
▮ Hyperviscosity syndrome (Table 15.12)

Investigations

▮ Blood count (anaemia, low white cells)
▮ Elevated ESR and CRP
▮ Elevated calcium, urea and creatinine
▮ Protein electrophoresis – monoclonal band
▮ Skeletal X-ray survey – lytic lesions, e.g. skull (Fig. 5.17)
▮ 24-hour urine for light chain proteins
▮ Bone marrow aspirate – plasma cells

Management

▮ Supportive treatment
▮ Steroids and radiotherapy for bone lesions
▮ Chemotherapy

Waldenström's macroglobulinaemia

▮ Older males
▮ IgM paraprotein
▮ → Hyperviscosity syndrome (Table 15.12)
▮ Lymphadenopathy
▮ Malaise and weight loss

PLATELET DISORDERS (*K&C*, PP. 470–472)

▮ Platelets, derived from megakaryocytes, are involved in the formation of clots (see p. 429)

Table 15.13 Causes of eosinophilia

Parasites	Lung disease
Ascaris	Asthma
Hookworm	Allergic bronchopulmonary
Strongyloides	aspergillosis
	Churg–Strauss syndrome
Allergy	
Allergic rhinitis	**Skin disorders**
Drug reactions	Urticaria
	Pemphigus
Malignancy	Eczema
Hodgkin's disease	
Carcinoma	**Others**
	Sarcoidosis

Table 15.14 Causes of thrombocytopenia

Reduced production	Immune destruction
Leukaemia	Autoimmune idiopathic
Aplastic anaemia	thrombocytopenic purpura
Megaloblastic anaemia	SLE
Myeloma	
	Coagulation
Drugs	DIC
Co-trimoxazole	Haemolytic uraemic syndrome
Infections	**Other**
Viral infection	Hypersplenism

Thrombocytopenia

❚ Low platelet count
❚ Low production in bone marrow
❚ High destruction in circulation
❚ Causes – see Table 15.14

Autoimmune thrombocytopenic purpura

❚ Follows viral infection in children (acute)
❚ Idiopathic in adult women (chronic)
❚ 60% have anti-platelet antibodies
❚ → Purpuric rash
❚ Epistaxis and menorrhagia
❚ Treat with steroids/splenectomy

Thrombocytosis

❚ High platelet count
❚ Haemorrhage
❚ Inflammation (any site)
❚ Essential thrombocythaemia (see above)

SELF-ASSESSMENT QUESTIONS

Multiple choice questions

1. Which of the following statements about haemoglobin are correct:
   A. Adult haemoglobin comprises two α and two γ chains
   B. Each haemoglobin molecule comprises four globin chains and one haem group
   C. Deoxyhaemoglobin is insoluble in water
   D. β -thalassaemia is an inherited inability to synthesise β globin chains
   E. Each haemoglobin molecule can carry four oxygen molecules

2. The following are true of vitamin B_{12} absorption:
   A. It requires the presence of intrinsic factor
   B. Intrinsic factor is produced by gastric G cells
   C. Active absorption takes place in the jejunum
   D. Chronic pancreatic insufficiency is a cause of vitamin B_{12} deficiency
   E. Oral B_{12} is useful in the treatment of pernicious anaemia

3. In autoimmune haemolytic anaemia:
   A. The direct Coombs' (globulin) test will be positive
   B. The autoantibody is always IgG class
   C. Haemoglobinuria may occur
   D. *Mycoplasma* pneumonia is a recognised cause

E. Jaundice is a recognised symptom

4. Regarding pernicious anaemia:
   A. Anti-parietal cell or anti-intrinsic factor antibodies are detectable
   B. Chronic hyperplastic gastritis results
   C. There is an increased risk of gastric cancer
   D. Oral intrinsic factor will reverse the vitamin B_{12} deficiency
   E. Men are as commonly affected as women

5. The following are appropriate blood transfusion options:
   A. Group O donor to group A recipient
   B. Group A Rhesus-positive donor to group A Rhesus-negative recipient
   C. Group AB Rhesus-negative donor to group O Rhesus-negative recipient
   D. Group B Rhesus-positive donor to group A Rhesus-positive recipient
   E. Group A donor to group AB recipient

6. The following are recognised complications of blood transfusions:
   A. Urticarial rash
   B. Hepatitis C infection
   C. Fever
   D. Anaphylactic shock
   E. Disseminated intravascular coagulation

Best one of five questions

7. A 36-year-old woman has the following full blood count: Hb 10.1 g/dL, MCV 76 fl, MCH 24, WCC 9.4, Platelets 187. Which one of the following is the most likely diagnosis?:
- **A.** Megaloblastic anaemia
- **B.** Iron deficiency anaemia
- **C.** Aplastic anaemia
- **D.** Folate deficiency
- **E.** Polycythaemia rubra vera

8. A 25-year-old man presents with a fever, night sweats and abdominal pain. Which one of the following is the most likely diagnosis?
- **A.** Polycythaemia rubra vera
- **B.** Acute myeloid leukaemia
- **C.** Non-Hodgkins lymphoma
- **D.** Chronic lymphocytic leukaemia
- **E.** Acute lymphoblastic leukaemia

9. A 78-year-old man is found to have a white cell count of 32×10^9/ml, 95% lymphocytes. What is the most likely diagnosis?
- **A.** Chronic myeloid leukaemia
- **B.** Chronic lymphocytic leukaemia
- **C.** Acute lymphoblastic leukaemia
- **D.** Malignant myeloma
- **E.** Myelodysplasia

10. Which one of the following is the best test for measuring the anti-coagulant effect of warfarin?
- **A.** Activated partial thromboplastin time
- **B.** Bleeding time
- **C.** Prothrombin time
- **D.** Whole blood clotting time
- **E.** Thrombin time

Extended matching questions

Question 1
- **A.** Iron deficiency
- **B.** Vitamin B_{12} deficiency
- **C.** Folic acid deficiency
- **D.** Sickle cell disease
- **E.** Alpha-thalassaemia
- **F.** Hereditary spherocytosis
- **G.** Haemolytic anaemia
- **H.** Anaemia of chronic disease
- **I.** Acute haemorrhage
- **J.** Hypersplenism

For each of the following select the most appropriate diagnosis from the list:

- **I.** A 43-year-old woman with a microcytic, hypochromic blood film
- **II.** A 17-year-old man with severe joint pain and abnormal red blood cells
- **III.** An 87-year-old woman with a macrocytosis following a gastrectomy

Question 2
- **A.** Erythrocytes
- **B.** Platelets
- **C.** Monocytes
- **D.** Neutrophils
- **E.** Basophils
- **F.** Eosinophils
- **G.** Lymphocytes
- **H.** Reticulocytes
- **I.** Megakaryocytes
- **J.** Plasma cells

For each question choose the correct answer from the list above
I. The cell type from which platelets derive
II. Cell type responsible for antibody production
III. A nucleated cell that increases in numbers after acute blood loss

Question 3
A. Blood group O
B. Blood Group A
C. Blood Group B
D. Blood Group AD
E. D-Rhesus positive
F. D-Rhesus negative

For each question choose the correct answer from the list above
I. Blood group with a frequency of 8% in the population
II. Blood group characterised by the presence of anti-A and Anti-B antibodies in the blood
III. Blood group of a mother whose foetus suffers Rhesus D syndrome

Oncology and genetic disease 16

(K&C, p. 483)

Oncology studies the management of 'malignant disease', illness arising from the uncontrolled proliferation of a cell clone. The clone characteristically is able to invade adjacent tissues (local spread) and seed to distant sites via the vascular or lymphatic circulation (metastasis). Malignancy is an important cause of death worldwide, most notably in the developed

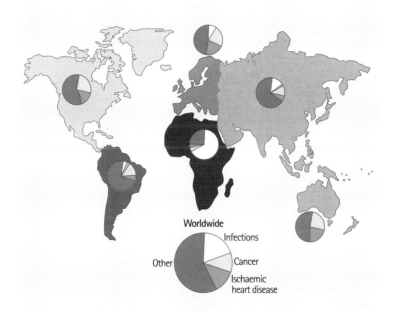

Fig. 16.1 Causes of mortality by continent demonstrating the relative importance of infection, malignancy and heart disease. Malignancy is responsible for roughly 13.5% of all male and 11.7% of all female deaths worldwide. (Data from the World Health Organisation, 1999).

Table 16.1 Age-standardised mortality for the ten highest causes of malignancy-related death in the UK in 2000 (Globocan 2000, International Agency for Research on Cancer)

Rank	Male		Female	
	Site	Mortality	Site	Mortality
1	Lung	48.6	Breast	26.8
2	Colon and rectum	18.7	Lung	21.1
3	Prostate	18.5	Colon and rectum	13.8
4	Stomach	10.1	Ovarian	8.3
5	Oesophagus	8.7	Pancreas	5.3
6	Bladder	7.0	Stomach	4.8
7	Pancreas	6.6	Oesophagus	4.0
8	Lymphoma	5.8	Lymphoma	3.9
9	Leukaemia	4.9	Leukaemia	3.3
10	Brain	4.5	Brain	3.0

world (Fig.16.1). Specific malignancies are discussed in the appropriate system chapter.

CANCER EPIDEMIOLOGY

Sex differences (Table 16.1)

- Sex-specific tumours (e.g. prostate)
- Risk factors (e.g. smoking, diet, alcohol intake)
- Genetic variation
- Hormonal variation (tumours dependent on hormones for growth)

Age differences
Childhood cancers (age 3–13 years)

- Hereditary, e.g. retinoblastoma
- Haematological, e.g. acute leukaemia

Adult cancers

- Frequency increases with age

Geographical differences (*K&C*, p. 484)

- Variation in population genotype distribution
- Variation in environmental factors, e.g.
  - Diet in gastric cancer
  - Hepatocellular carcinoma secondary to chronic viral hepatitis

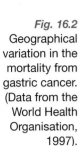

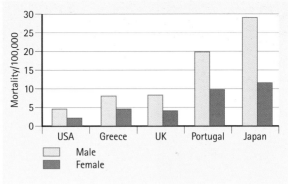

Fig. 16.2 Geographical variation in the mortality from gastric cancer. (Data from the World Health Organisation, 1997).

CANCER AETIOLOGY (*K&C*, P. 483)

Smoking

▎ Associated with 30% of cancer deaths in the UK
▎ Implicated in several cancers
  – Lung carcinoma
  – Oral cavity cancers
  – Oesophageal carcinoma
  – Bladder (transitional cell carcinoma)

Alcohol

▎ Oral cavity cancers
▎ Oesophageal carcinoma
▎ Colorectal carcinoma
▎ Hepatocellular carcinoma

Environmental risks
Asbestos

▎ Mesothelioma
▎ Lung carcinoma

Hydrocarbons

▎ Lung carcinoma
▎ Skin cancers

UV light

▎ Melanoma
▎ Basal cell carcinoma
▎ Squamous cell carcinoma

Drugs
Oestrogens

▎ Vaginal carcinoma
▎ Endometrial carcinoma

Alkylating agents

▎ Acute myeloid leukaemia

Infections

▎ Viral hepatitis – hepatocellular carcinoma
▎ *Schistosoma* – bladder cancer
▎ Helicobacter pylori – gastric cancer
▎ Epstein–Barr virus – Burkitt's lymphoma
▎ Papillomavirus – cervical cancer

CANCER GENETICS (*K&C*, P. 486)

▎ Malignancy results from genetic mutations that lead to uncontrolled proliferation of a cell clone
▎ These mutations and abnormalities can arise in several ways

Chromosome abnormalities

▎ Chronic myeloid leukaemia – 9:22 translocation (Philadelphia chromosome) positive in 95%
▎ Acute promyelocytic leukaemia – 15:17 translocation positive in >90%
▎ Burkitt's lymphoma 8:14 translocation → *myc* gene over-expressed

Failure of DNA repair

▎ Mutation of DNA repair systems → hereditary cancer syndromes, e.g.
  – Xeroderma pigmentosum
  – Ataxia telangiectasia
  – *BCRA1* and 2 in breast cancer
  – Mismatch repair mutations in colon cancer

Tumour suppressors

▎ Mutation of tumour suppressor genes → over-expression of mutated gene product
▎ Failure of control of cell cycle → uncontrolled proliferation
▎ e.g. *p53* mutations in GI cancers

Inherited cancers

▌ Specific mutations increase the risk of malignancy if inherited, e.g.
  - *apc* gene: familial adenomatous polyposis
  - *BCRA* genes: breast and ovarian cancer
  - *Rb* gene: hereditary retinoblastoma

Oncogenes

▌ Genes which, if activated inappropriately by a mutation, → malignancy, e.g.
  - *C-Myc*: cervical cancer, Burkitt's lymphoma, breast cancer
  - *K-Ras*: colorectal cancer

▌ The gene may have a cell cycle regulatory role
  - *bcl-2* expression → resistance of apoptosis → a proliferating clone that is open to further mutations → malignant transformation

CANCER BIOLOGY (*K&C*, PP. 485–486)

Cell proliferation

▌ Uncontrolled proliferation
▌ Often loss of cell differentiation
▌ → Exponential growth curve
▌ 'Doubling time' describes the growth rate
▌ → Very variable between tumour types
▌ As tumour enlarges, growth may slow due to:
  - Limitation of blood supply
  - Local production of growth inhibitors

Local invasion

▌ Penetration of malignant cells into other tissues
▌ Associated with loss of intercellular adhesion
▌ Increased production of proteolytic enzymes

Lymphatic spread

▌ Tumours seed to locally draining lymph nodes

Dissemination (Table 16.2)

▌ Invasion into blood vessels or lymphatics
▌ Allows seeding of cells to distant sites
▌ Metastases → organs with a dense vasculature, e.g.
  - Liver
  - Lungs
  - Bone marrow

Table 16.2 Common sites of metastasis

Site	Origin	Site	Origin
Bone	Breast	Liver	GI tract
	Bronchus		Breast
	Thyroid		Bronchus
	Prostate	Adrenal	Bronchus
	Kidney	Lung	Kidney
Intracerebral	Bronchus		Prostate
	Breast		Breast
	Stomach		Bone
	Prostate		GI tract
	Thyroid		Cervix
	Kidney		Ovary
			Testicular

▌ Tumour cells express ligands for endothelial receptors

▌ → Increased adhesion and invasion

▌ → Specific metastatic patterns, e.g. breast cancer → long bones

DIAGNOSIS OF CANCER (K&C, P. 488)

Clinical features

▌ Specific combinations of symptoms and signs can suggest particular malignancies

▌ E.g. painless jaundice and weight loss → pancreatic cancer, dysphagia → oesophageal carcinoma

▌ Personality change with complex focal neurology → intracerebral tumour

▌ Cough, haemoptysis and weight loss → bronchogenic carcinoma

▌ Characteristics of a palpable mass suggesting malignancy:
  – Fixed to deep tissues
  – Fixed to overlying skin
  – Hard/'craggy' texture
  – Overlying ulceration
  – Lymphadenopathy

▌ Family history of malignancy
  – Colorectal carcinoma

▌ Exposure to specific risks (see above)

Table 16.3 The TNM system		
T		Extent of primary tumour
N	N0	No involved lymph nodes
	N1–4	Lymph node groups involved
M	M0	No metastases
	M1	Metastases present

- Associated diseases that increase risk
  - Hepatitis B or C (hepatocellular carcinoma)
  - Pernicious anaemia (gastric cancer)
  - Barrett's oesophagus (oesophageal carcinoma)
  - asbestosis (bronchogenic carcinoma)

Imaging

- Can be highly suggestive of malignancy
- E.g. chest X-ray in lung cancer

Tissue diagnosis

- Vital for confirmation of diagnosis and guiding treatment
- Tumour type
- Degree of differentiation (tumour grade)

Methods

- CT- or ultrasound-guided biopsy
- Endoscopic biopsy
- Laparoscopic/open surgical biopsy
- Fine needle aspiration (FNA) of subcutaneous mass

Tumour staging (Table 16.3)

- Assessment of distribution of tumour
- Classification varies with tumour
- Staging investigations required, e.g.
  - CT scanning
  - Lymph node sampling
  - PET
  - Laparoscopy

Tumour markers

- Serum markers for the presence of malignancy
- Useful in following response to treatment

- Can help demonstrate relapse post-therapy
- Rarely useful in initial diagnosis
- E.g.
  - Ca-125 – pancreatic/ovarian/GI cancer
  - Ca-19–9 – GI and pancreatic cancers
  - α-foetoprotein – hepatocellular carcinoma
  - β-human chorionic gonadotrophin (HCG) – choriocarcinomas, testicular carcinoma
  - Chorioembryonic antigen (CEA) – colorectal carcinoma

Screening

- Investigations used to detect premalignant tissue or malignancy in those in whom cancer has not been diagnosed
- E.g.
  - Mammograms for breast cancer
  - Smears for cervical cancer
  - Faecal occult blood and colonoscopy for colorectal carcinoma

Surveillance

- Investigations to detect recurrence of malignancy following treatment for a previous cancer
- E.g.
  - Mammography after breast cancer
  - Prostate-specific antigen (PSA) for progression of prostatic cancer

TREATMENT OF MALIGNANCY (K&C, P. 490)

- Therapeutic efforts in oncology are aimed at:
  - Complete destruction of the tumour (curative therapy)
  - Reduction of the tumour mass in order to improve life expectancy
  - Reduction of symptoms of the cancer (palliative care)

Surgical resection

- May be curative (complete tumour removal)
- May be palliative (symptomatic relief but not curative)

Radiotherapy

- High-energy electromagnetic radiation
- Targeted at specific site
- Useful adjuvant therapy to reduce relapse rate as well as curative intent

Chemotherapy

- Drug therapy aimed at killing tumour cells
- Also kills normal cells
- Given in cycles to allow normal cells to recover

Antimetabolites

- Block cell metabolism
  - Folic acid antagonists: methotrexate
  - Nucleic acid analogues: 5-fluorouracil

Plant alkaloids

- Inhibit microtubule formation
- → Block cell replication
  - Vincristine

Taxanes

- Inhibit microtubule formation
- Useful in breast and ovarian cancers
  - Docetaxel

Cytotoxic antibiotics

- Block DNA replication
  - Doxorubicin

Platinum analogues

- Cross-link DNA strands
- → Block DNA replication
  - Cisplatin

Alkylating agents

- Block DNA synthesis
  - Cyclophosphamide

Endocrine therapy

- Hormonal manipulation of tumour cells that express hormone receptors on their surface
  - Tamoxifen – blocks oestrogen receptor

Biological therapy

- Use of immunologically active substances
  - E.g. α-interferon in melanoma/myeloma

Adjuvant therapy

❚ Specific therapy after a primary therapy modality
❚ Used to treat undetected metastases
– Breast and colon cancers

Neoadjuvent therapy

❚ Given before primary therapy to reduce the risk of metastasis

Myeloablation with stem cell support

❚ High-dose chemotherapy and radiotherapy
❚ Aims to kill all dividing cells
❚ Haemopoietic stem cells then given
❚ → Reverses resultant bone marrow failure
❚ Stem cells may be
– Allogenic: from a matched donor
– Autologous: taken from patient before therapy
❚ Collection of stem cells may be via
– Bone marrow sampling
– Peripheral blood sampling

COMPLICATIONS OF TREATMENT (K&C, P. 494)

Failure of therapy

❚ Incomplete surgical resection
❚ Tumour resistance to chemotherapy
❚ Failure of response to radiotherapy

Nausea and vomiting

❚ Common
❚ Treat with antiemetics (Fig. 16.3)
– Metoclopramide
– Domperidone
– $5HT_3$ antagonists (ondansetron)

Hair loss

❚ Difficult to avoid, but regrows after therapy

Bone marrow suppression

❚ Dose-dependent effect of therapy

Neutropenia

❚ ↑ Bacteria, viral and fungal infection
❚ Treat with antibiotics
❚ Stem cell stimulating factors, e.g. GM-CSF

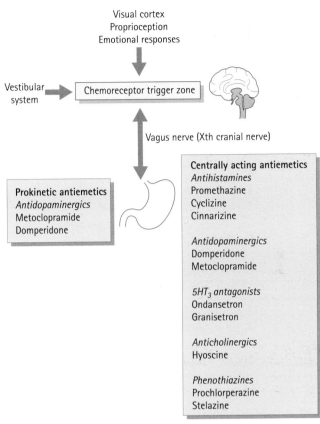

Fig. 16.3 Mechanisms of action of antiemetics.

Thrombocytopenia

    ▐ → Bleeding
    ▐ Treat with platelet transfusion

Anaemia

    ▐ Treat with blood transfusion

Cardiotoxicity

    ▐ Dose-dependent effect of doxorubicin

Neurotoxicity

    ▐ Occurs with vincristine
    ▐ Must never be given intrathecally

Sterility

    ▐ Common with alkylating agents
    ▐ ♂ Sperm storage prior to therapy
    ▐ ♀ Ovum storage (still experimental)

Mucositis

▮ Mucosal inflammation – notably of the mouth and GI tract after radiotherapy

PALLIATIVE CARE (K&C, PP. 524–527)

▮ Therapy aimed at reducing symptoms due to the malignancy

Pain

▮ Occurs in 70% of cancers
▮ → Step up analgesia until relief obtained (WHO analgesia ladder, Fig. 16.4)
  – Paracetamol and non-steroidal anti-inflammatory drugs (NSAIDs)
  – Weak opioids – codeine +/– paracetamol
  – Strong opioids – morphine or diamorphine

Specific analgesics

▮ Naproxen for bone pain
▮ Amitriptyline/gabapentin for pain due to nerve damage
▮ Carbamazepine/gabapentin for neuropathic pain

Continuous subcutaneous infusions

▮ Allow continuous delivery of analgesia, antiemetics and sometimes anxiolytics

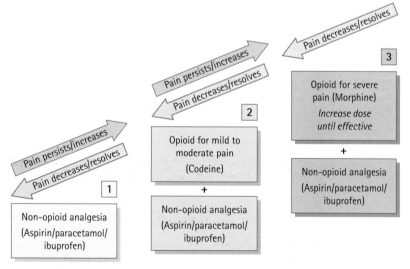

Fig. 16.4 The World Health Organisation Analgesia ladder.

Patient-controlled analgesia
    ❚ Continuous analgesia with the ability for the patient to give limited extra doses

Complications of analgesics
  Opioids ❚ Constipation, nausea vomiting
    ❚ Respiratory and CNS depression
    ❚ Drowsiness, hallucinations
  NSAIDs ❚ GI ulceration
    ❚ GI bleeding
    ❚ Renal failure

Non-drug approaches
    ❚ Surgery to reduce tumour mass
    ❚ Radiotherapy
    ❚ Nerve blocks
    ❚ Steroids to reduce local inflammation

Gastrointestinal symptoms
Anorexia
    ❚ → Nasogastric feeding if appropriate

Nausea and vomiting
    ❚ → Appropriate antiemetic therapy

Bowel obstruction
    ❚ → Surgical bypass
    ❚ Antispasmodics – hyoscine
    ❚ Antiemetics
    ❚ Nasogastric tube to reduce vomiting

Psychological support
    ❚ Effective communication with the patient
    ❚ Honesty about diagnosis and prognosis
    ❚ Support for emotional crisis
    ❚ Full explanations of symptoms
    ❚ Human genetics and inherited disease

HUMAN GENETICS (*K&C*, P. 171)

Chromosomal disorders
    ❚ Majority → spontaneous abortion

Abnormal chromosome numbers
    ❚ Down's syndrome: trisomy 21,1:650 live births
    ❚ Edward's syndrome: trisomy 18,1:3000

Table 16.4 Autosomal dominant, autosomal recessive and X-linked recessive disorders

Autosomal dominant	Autosomal recessive
Achondroplasia	Albinism
Adult polycystic kidney disease	Cystic fibrosis
Familial Alzheimer's disease	β-thalassaemia
Familial hypercholesterolaemia	Friedreich's ataxia
Huntington's chorea	Haemochromatosis
Marfan's syndrome	Phenylketonuria
Neurofibromatosis type I	Sickle cell disease
Von Willebrand's disease	Wilson's disease
	X-linked recessive
	Duchenne muscular dystrophy
	Haemophilia A
	Haemophilia B
	Red–green colour blindness
	Wiskott–Aldrich syndrome

- Pataú's syndrome: trisomy 13,1:5000
- Klinefelter's syndrome: XXY, 1:1000 males
- Turner's syndrome: XO, 1:2500 girls

Abnormal chromosome structure

- Deletion of chromosome segment
  - Prader–Willi syndrome
- Duplication of chromosome segment
  - Charcot–Marie–Tooth syndrome

Mitochondrial DNA abnormalities (*K&C*, p. 173)

- Inherited mitochondrial DNA mutations
- Passed via maternal line (sperm do not donate mitochondria)
- → Myopathies and neuropathies
- E.g. DIDMOAD syndrome (Diabetes insipidus, diabetes mellitus, optic atrophy and deafness)

Gene defects (Table 16.4) (*K&C*, p. 176)

- Result in abnormal protein being synthesised
- Homozygous: both gene copies abnormal
- Heterozygous: one gene copy abnormal

Autosomal dominant disorders (Fig. 16.5)

- One of the two gene copies is mutated
- Normal gene not sufficient to compensate
- Or mutated protein is toxic
- Effect may vary in each generation
- Varying penetrance

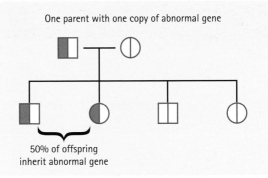

One parent with one copy of abnormal gene

Fig. 16.5
Autosomal
dominant
inheritance.

50% of offspring
inherit abnormal gene

▌ → Disease skipping generations
▌ New cases arise due to germ-line mutations

Autosomal recessive disorders (Fig. 16.6)

▌ Both gene copies have mutation (homozygous)
▌ No functioning protein synthesised
▌ Carrier state exists if only one copy affected
(usually no clinical significance)
▌ → Inborn errors of metabolism

Sex-linked inheritance

▌ Mutations of genes on the X chromosome
▌ Vast majority are recessive (Fig. 16.7), but
– Males only have one X chromosome, therefore
are affected by mutation
– Females act as carriers if heterozygotes

X-linked dominant

▌ Heterozygote ♀ has the disease
▌ Rare
▌ E.g. vitamin D-resistant rickets

Trinucleotide repeats

▌ Multiple repeats of three nucleotides
▌ Severity of the disease α number of repeats
▌ Number of repeats increases with each generation
▌ Therefore severity increases with each
generation = genetic anticipation
– Myotonic dystrophy (CTG triplets)
– Huntington's chorea (CAG triplets)

Genetic imprinting

▌ Disease phenotype varies
▌ Depends on origin of mutant gene

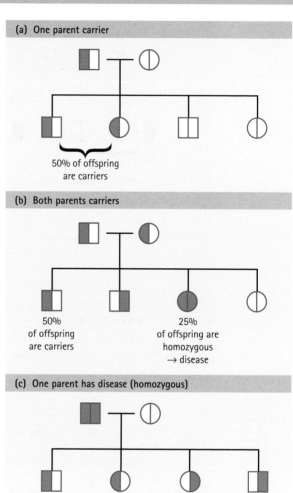

(a) One parent carrier

50% of offspring are carriers

(b) Both parents carriers

50% of offspring are carriers

25% of offspring are homozygous → disease

(c) One parent has disease (homozygous)

All offspring are carriers

Fig. 16.6 Autosomal recessive inheritance.

▌ E.g. deletion of long arm of chromosome 15
  – If inherited from mother → Prader–Willi syndrome
  – If inherited from father → Angelman syndrome

Multifactorial inheritance (K&C, p. 185)

▌ Encoded for by multiple genetic loci (polygenic)
  – Height
  – Hair colour
  – Hypertension

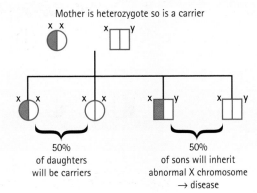

Mother is heterozygote so is a carrier

50%
of daughters
will be carriers

50%
of sons will inherit
abnormal X chromosome
→ disease

Fig. 16.7 X-linked
recessive
inheritance.

- Pyloric stenosis
- Ankylosing spondylitis

Genetic screening and counselling (*K&C*, p. 191)

Provision of information to prospective parents who are carriers of an inherited disease is vital for informed decisions to be made. Determination of these risks is important and requires screening.

Screening

❙ Detection of carrier of a mutation, e.g.
  - Thalassaemia
  - Sickle cell disease
  - Tay–Sachs disease
  - Haemophilia
  - Cystic fibrosis

Prenatal diagnosis
Maternal serum

❙ Maternal α-fetoprotein – neural tube defects
❙ Bart's triple test on maternal serum assesses risk of foetal trisomy 21
  - α-fetoprotein (low)
  - β-human chorionic gonadotrophin (high)
  - Unconjugated oestriol (low)

Imaging

❙ Ultrasound for anatomical abnormalities
❙ Nuchal fold translucency for Down's syndrome

Amniocentesis

■ Sampling amniotic fluid for fetal cells
■ α-fetoprotein and biochemical analysis
■ Risk to foetus <1%

Chorionic villus sampling

■ Chromosome/DNA analysis
■ Risk to foetus 1–2%

Cordocentesis

■ Fetal blood sampling
■ Chromosome and DNA analysis
■ Risk to foetus 1–2%

Counselling

■ Risk of passing on genetic abnormality to child depends on inheritance and parental genome

SELF-ASSESSMENT QUESTIONS

Multiple choice questions

1. Smoking has been associated with an increased risk of the following:
   A. Bronchial cancer
   B. Oesophageal cancer
   C. Transitional cell carcinoma
   D. Pharyngeal cancer
   E. Breast cancer

2. Regarding malignancy:
   A. A translocation between chromosomes 9 and 22 is seen in 10% of chronic myeloid leukaemia
   B. *p53* mutations are common in gastrointestinal malignancy
   C. *Helicobacter pylori* is associated with a decreased risk of gastric cancer
   D. Kaposi's sarcoma is only seen in immunocompromised patients
   E. Family history is important in determining the risk of breast cancer

3. The following are common sites of metastasis for the named primary cancer:
   A. Intracerebral: breast carcinoma
   B. Long bones: osteosarcoma
   C. Vertebral column: prostatic carcinoma
   D. Liver: bronchial carcinoma
   E. Liver: cutaneous basal cell carcinoma

4. The following are autosomal dominant:
   A. Haemophilia A
   B. Achondroplasia
   C. Haemochromatosis
   D. Red–green colour blindness
   E. Leprosy

5. The following genetic abnormalities result in the named condition:
   A. Trisomy 19 – Down's syndrome
   B. XO – Turner's syndrome
   C. XXY – Klinefelter's syndrome
   D. Trisomy 21 – Pataú's syndrome
   E. XXO – Smith's syndrome

6. The following are inherited in an X-linked recessive manner:
   A. Down's syndrome
   B. Polycystic kidney disease
   C. Wiskott–Aldrich syndrome
   D. Haemophilia A
   E. Acute intermittent porphyria

Best one of five questions

7. Which one of the following is an $5HT_3$ antagonist antiemetic:
   A. Metoclopramide
   B. Cyclizine
   C. Granisetron
   D. Prochlorperazine
   E. Diazepam

8. A 55-year-old man presents with abdominal distension. He has a long history of chronic hepatitis C infection. Which one of the following is he at an increased risk of suffering?
   A. Pancreatic adenocarcinoma
   B. Cholangiocarcinoma
   C. Gallbladder carcinoma

D. Hepatocellular carcinoma

E. Gastric adenocarcinoma

9. A 29-year-old man requests information about his risk of colonic carcinoma. His father has just died of the disease at the age of 54. What is the man's risk of developing a colonic carcinoma?

A. 1 in 250

B. 1 in 100

C. 1 in 50

D. 1 in 20

E. 1 in 3

10. A 45-year-old woman was seen with a palpable mass in her left breast. What is the most appropriate way of confirming the diagnosis?

A. Bilateral mammography

B. Ultrasound guided fine needle aspiration

C. Breast lumpectomy

D. Whole body PET scan

E. Local lymph node excision

11. A 66-year-old man with a previous history of a bronchogenic carcinoma is admitted with confusion, nausea and diplopia. Which one of the following may provide most effective symptom control?

A. Diazepam

B. metaclopramide

C. Dexamethasone

D. Odansetron

E. Domperidone

12. In the treatment of malignancy

A. Surgery is always carried out with the aim of a cure

B. Nausea is a rare side-effect of chemotherapy

C. Combination chemotherapy is rarely more efficacious than single therapy

D. Methotrexate is a folate metabolism antagonist

E. Vincristine can be given intrathecally

EXAMINING THE NERVOUS SYSTEM
(*K&C*, P. 1176)

This is explained in some detail here as it is often dreaded but need not be if an organised and thoughtful approach is taken.

General rules

- Explain carefully to patients what you want them to do for each part of the examination and why
- Ask the patient to copy your actions, rather than trying to explain a complicated manoeuvre
- Always compare one side with the other
- Organise your examination into categories
  - Mental state
  - Cranial nerves
  - Motor function
  - Reflexes
  - Coordination and gait
  - Sensation

Equipment

- Pen torch
- Snellen eye chart or pocket vision card
- Ophthalmoscope
- Tendon hammer
- 128 and 512 Hz tuning forks
- Cotton wool
- 'Neuropins' or paper clips
- Orange stick

Mini-mental status examination (see p. 37)

Ten questions give an indication of cerebral function, including orientation in time, place, long- and short-term memory; mark correct responses out of 10.

- Name?
- Age?
- Address?
- Where are you now?
- Name of the monarch?
- Name of the prime minister?
- Dates of the Second World War?
- Remember the following address and repeat it when asked: 42 West Street, Edinburgh (ask the patient to recall this after asking of the rest of the questions)
- What time is it now?
- Count backwards from 20 to 10

Cranial nerves

General observation (*K&C*, p. 1179)

- Ptosis (III)
- Facial droop or asymmetry (VII)
- Hoarse voice (X)
- Articulation of words, dysarthria (V, VII, X, XII)
- Abnormal eye position (III, IV, VI)
- Abnormal or asymmetrical pupils (II, III)

I Olfactory

- Ask the patient about changes in or absence of sense of smell

II Optic

- Examine the optic fundi for
  - Papilloedema
  - Optic atrophy
  - Maculopathy
  - Hypertensive or diabetic retinopathy

Test visual acuity

- Allow the patient to use glasses
- Ask the patient to read a Snellen eye chart with each eye
- Record the smallest line the patient can read for each eye
- Visual acuity is reported as a pair of numbers (20/20) where the first number represents how far

the patient is from the chart and the second number is the distance from which the 'normal' eye can read a line of letters. For example, 20/40 means that at 20 feet the patient can only read letters a 'normal' person can read from twice that distance

Test visual fields

▌ Position yourself at eye level a metre or so in front of the patient and ask him/her to look into your eyes

▌ Hold your hands out to the sides halfway between you and the patient and wiggle a finger on both hands asking the patient to indicate which side he/she sees the finger move; if the patient only sees one side this indicates a lateral field defect or sensory neglect on that side

▌ Test the four quadrants of each eye while asking the patient to cover the opposite eye comparing with your own fields of vision for the appropriate eye

Test pupillary reactions

▌ Ask the patient to look into the distance

▌ Shine a bright light obliquely into each pupil in turn

▌ Look for both the direct (same eye) and consensual (other eye) reactions

▌ Test accommodation
  – Hold your finger about 10 cm from the patient's nose
  – Ask him/her to look into the distance and then at your finger
  – Look for constriction of the pupil and convergence of the eyes to near vision

III Oculomotor (*K&C*, p. 1183)

▌ Look for ptosis

▌ Test extraocular movements (superior, medial and inferior rectus and inferior oblique muscles)
  – Holding your finger about 1 metre in front of the patient, ask him/her to follow your finger with the eyes without moving the head
  – Check horizontal, vertical and oblique gaze using a cross or 'H' pattern, ask about diplopia
  – Pause during upward and lateral gaze to check for nystagmus

▌ Test pupillary reactions to light

IV Trochlear (superior oblique muscle)

I Inward and downward movement of eyes (see above)

VI Abducens (lateral rectus muscle)

I Lateral eye movement (see above)

V Trigeminal (*K&C*, p. 1185)
Motor

I Ask the patient to first open the mouth and then clench the teeth
I Palpate the temporal and masseter muscles as this is done

Sensory

I On both sides, use cotton wool to test
- The forehead (olfactory division)
- The cheeks (maxillary division)
- The jaw (mandibular division)

Corneal reflex

I Ask the patient to look up and away
I From the other side, touch the cornea (not sclera) lightly with a fine wisp of cotton wool
I Look for the normal blink reaction of both eyes
I Repeat on the other side

VII Facial (*K&C*, p. 1186)

I Observe for any facial droop or asymmetry
I Ask the patient to do the following, noting any weakness or asymmetry
- Raise eyebrows
- Close both eyes tightly
- Smile or show the teeth
- Puff out the cheeks
I Central vs peripheral
- With an upper motor neurone lesion (stroke), crossover of innervation means function is preserved over the upper part of the face (forehead, eyebrows, eyelids)
- With a lower motor neurone lesion (Bell's palsy), the entire side of the face droops

VIII Vestibulocochlear (*K&C*, p. 1188)

- Rub your fingers together next to one ear while whispering a number in the other and ask the patient to tell you the number
- Repeat for the other side

Weber's test

- Use a 512 Hz tuning fork
- Place the base of the vibrating tuning fork firmly on top of the patient's head
- Ask the patient where the sound appears to be coming from (normally in the midline)
  - In sensorineural deafness there will be deafness in the affected ear
  - In conductive deafness, the sound will be heard better in the deaf ear

Rinne's test (to compare air and bone conduction)

- Use a 512 Hz tuning fork
- Place the base of the vibrating tuning fork against the mastoid bone behind the ear
- When the patient no longer hears the sound, hold the end of the fork near the patient's ear and ask if he or she can hear it now (air conduction is normally greater than bone conduction)
  - In conductive deafness bone conduction is better than air conduction

IX and X Glossopharyngeal and vagus (tested together) (*K&C*, p. 1190)

- Ask the patient to swallow a sip of water, look for choking or dribbling
- Ask patient to say 'Agh', watching the movements of the soft palate and the pharynx. The uvula deviates away from the affected side
- Test the gag reflex (unconscious patient)
  - Touch the back of the throat on the soft palate with an orange stick on each side
  - It is normal to gag after each stimulus

XI Accessory

- From behind, look for wasting of the trapezius muscles
- Ask the patient to shrug the shoulders against resistance

■ Ask the patient to turn the head against resistance. Watch and palpate the sternomastoid muscle on the opposite side

XII Hypoglossal

■ Look at the tongue for wasting or fasciculation (lower motor neurone lesion)
■ Ask the patient to
  – Protrude the tongue
  – Move the tongue from side to side
■ The tongue moves towards the side of any lesion

Motor function (corticospinal or pyramidal tracts)
(*K&C*, p. 1191)

Observation

■ Involuntary movements (e.g. tremor, tics, fasciculation)
■ Wasting and asymmetry (pay particular attention to the hands, and shoulder and thigh girdles)

Muscle tone

■ Ask the patient to relax
■ Holding the patient's hand, flex and extend his/her wrist and elbow
■ Place both your hands on the thigh and gently roll the leg from side to side watching for corresponding movement of the foot
■ There is normally a small, continuous resistance to passive movement
■ Observe for decreased (flaccid) or increased (rigid/cogwheeling/spastic) tone

Power
Pronator drift

■ This is a short screening test for muscle strength
■ Ask the patient to hold both arms straight out in front, palms up and eyes closed
■ With an upper motor neurone lesion, the patient will not be able to maintain extension and supination (and 'drifts' into pronation and flexion)

Muscle strength

■ Test strength by asking the patient move against your resistance
■ Always compare one side to the other

Other tests of power

- Flexion (C5, C6, biceps) and extension (C6, C7, C8, triceps) at the elbow
- Extension at the wrist (C6, C7, C8, radial nerve)
- Squeeze two of your fingers as hard as possible ('grip', C7, C8, T1)
- Finger abduction (C8, T1, ulnar nerve)
- Opposition of the thumb (C8, T1, median nerve)
- Flexion (L2, L3, L4, iliopsoas) and extension at the hip (S1, gluteus maximus)
- Adduction (L2, L3, L4, adductors) and abduction at the hips (L4, L5, S1, gluteus medius and minimus)
- Extension (L2, L3, L4, quadriceps) and flexion (L4, L5, S1, S2, hamstrings) at the knee
- Dorsiflexion (L4, L5) and plantar flexion (S1) at the ankle
- Grade strength on a scale from 0 to 5 (Table 17.1)

Tendon reflexes

- Use a tendon hammer with as little force as needed to provoke a response
- Reinforcement
  - If the reflexes are not elicited as above then ask the patient to clench the teeth or grasp the hands together and then pull apart
  - Retest reflexes as this task is performed
- Reflexes should be graded on a 0 to 4 'plus' scale (Table 17.2)

Biceps (C5, C6)

- Position the patient with the arms relaxed across the lap and partially flexed at the elbow with the palm down
- Place your thumb or finger on the biceps tendon

Table 17.1 Muscle strength grading scale	
Grade	**Description**
0/5	No muscle movement
1/5	Visible muscle movement, but no movement at the joint
2/5	Movement at the joint, but not against gravity
3/5	Movement against gravity, but not against added resistance
4/5	Movement against resistance, but less than normal
5/5	Normal strength

Table 17.2 Tendon reflex grading scale

Grade	Description
0	Absent
1+or +	Hypoactive
2+or ++	'Normal'
3+or +++	Hyperactive without clonus
4+or ++++	Hyperactive with clonus

▌ Tap your finger with the reflex hammer
▌ Watch for flexion of the elbow

Triceps (C6, C7)

▌ Hold the patient's hand across the chest
▌ Tap the triceps tendon above the elbow with the reflex hammer
▌ Watch for extension of the elbow

Brachioradialis (C5, C6)

▌ Rest the forearm on the abdomen or lap
▌ Tap the radius about 3–5 cm above the wrist
▌ Watch for flexion and supination of the forearm

Knee (L2, L3, L4)

▌ Hold your arm under the patient's flexed knees, taking the weight of the legs on your forearm
▌ Tap the patellar tendon just below the patella
▌ Note contraction of the quadriceps and extension of the knee

Ankle (S1, S2)

▌ Dorsiflex the foot at the ankle with your hand, with the knee slightly bent and the leg rotated laterally
▌ Tap the Achilles tendon
▌ Watch and feel for plantar flexion at the ankle

Clonus

▌ Support the knee in a partly flexed position
▌ With the patient relaxed, quickly pull the foot into dorsiflexion
▌ Observe for sustained rhythmic beats of dorsiflexion

Plantar response (Babinski)

▌ Run a key or orange stick firmly along the lateral aspect of the sole of each foot

- Flexion of the big toe is normal
- Extension of the big toe with fanning of the other toes is abnormal and indicates an upper motor neurone lesion

Coordination and gait (cerebellospinal connections)
(*K&C*, p. 1194)

Rapid alternating movements (dys-diadochokinesis)

- Ask the patient to tap the back of one hand with, alternately, the palmar and dorsal aspects of the other hand as accurately and quickly as possible

Point-to-point movements (finger–nose and heel–shin)

- Ask the patient to touch your index finger and his/her nose alternately several times. Move your finger about slowly as the patient performs this task. Holding your finger still, ask the patient to touch his/her nose and then your finger with the eyes closed. Repeat for the other side
- Ask the patient to place one heel on the opposite knee and run it down the shin to the big toe and back again. Repeat with the patient's eyes closed
- Look for past-pointing, intention tremor and clumsiness

Romberg's test (cerebellar connections and dorsal columns)

- Ask the patient to stand with the feet together and eyes closed for 5–10 seconds without support (be prepared to catch the patient if unstable)
- The test is positive if the patient becomes unstable (indicating a vestibular or proprioceptive problem)

Gait

- Ask the patient to walk across the room, turn and come back and then walk heel-to-toe in a straight line

Sensation (*K&C*, p. 1197)

General

- Compare symmetrical areas on the two sides of the body and distal and proximal areas of the extremities
- When you detect an area of sensory loss map out its boundaries in detail
- Test the following areas

– Shoulders (C4)
– Inner and outer aspects of the forearms (C6 and T1)
– Thumbs and little fingers (C6 and C8)
– Front of both thighs (L2)
– Medial and lateral aspect of both calves (L4 and L5)
– Little toes (S1)

Light touch (dorsal columns)

▮ Use a piece of cotton wool to touch the skin lightly
▮ Ask the patient to respond whenever a touch is felt

Pain (spinothalamic tracts)

▮ Use a suitable sharp object (e.g. Neuropin or paperclip) to test 'sharp' or 'dull' sensation

Temperature (spinothalamic tracts)

▮ This can be left out if pain sensation is normal
▮ Use a tuning fork heated or cooled by water and ask the patient to identify 'hot' or 'cold'

Vibration (dorsal columns)

▮ Use a low-pitched tuning fork (128 Hz)
▮ Place the stem of the fork over the radial head or medial malleolus, and ask the patient to tell you if he/she feels the vibration

Position sense (dorsal columns)

▮ Hold the patient's big toe away from the other toes with your fingers on each side of the toe
▮ Show the patient 'up' and 'down.'
▮ Ask the patient to close the eyes and to identify the direction in which you move the toe
▮ Test the fingers in a similar fashion

Dermatomes

▮ See Fig. 17.1

NEUROLOGICAL INVESTIGATIONS

Routine

▮ See Table 17.3

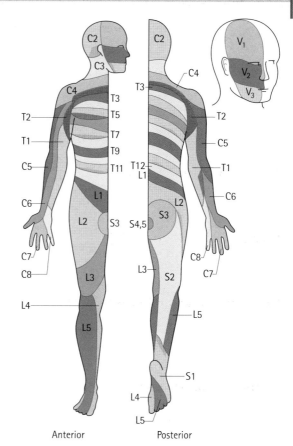

Fig. 17.1
Dermatomes of spinal roots and ophthalmic (V_1), maxillary (V_2) and mandibular (V_3) divisions of the trigeminal nerve.

Anterior   Posterior

Neuroradiology

Skull X-ray

❚ Skull fracture
❚ Paget's disease
❚ Myeloma
❚ Intracranial calcification
❚ Intrasellar tumour

Pituitary fossa X-ray

❚ Enlargement with pituitary tumours

Spinal X-rays

❚ Fractures/vertebral collapse
❚ Metastases
❚ Spondylosis
❚ Tuberculosis

Table 17.3 Abnormalities in routine investigations and possible causes

Test	Result	Potential cause/effect
Urinalysis	Glycosuria	Polyneuropathy
	Bence Jones protein	Cord compression
Blood film	Raised MCV	Vitamin B_{12} deficiency
ESR	Prolonged	Vasculitis
Serum electrolytes	Low potassium	Weakness
	Low sodium	Confusion/coma
Serum calcium	Low	Tetany/spasms
Serum creatine phosphokinase (CPK)	Raised	Muscle disease
Chest X-ray	Tumour	Metastases
		Paraneoplastic syndrome
Thyroid function	Hypothyroidism	Confusion/dementia
Vitamin B_{12}	Low	Polyneuropathy
		Confusion/dementia
		Subacute combined degeneration of the cord

Computed tomography (CT)

Brain

- Cerebral tumours
- Intracranial haemorrhage
- Infarction
- Subarachnoid haemorrhage
- Midline shift
- Hydrocephalus
- Cerebral atrophy
- Pituitary lesions

Spine

- Cord/bone lesions

Magnetic resonance imaging (MRI)

- Greater resolution than CT for small lesions and does not require contrast injection
- No radiation
- Contraindicated in patients with metal implants, e.g. aneurysm clips
- Plaques (multiple sclerosis, MS)
- Nerve root compression
- Spinal cord lesions
- Blood vessel imaging

Cerebral angiography

- Intra-arterial or intravenous contrast is injected to demonstrate arterial or venous systems, e.g. berry aneurysms, arteriovenous malformations

Myelography

- Contrast is injected into lumbar subarachnoid space and imaged with CT scanning or X-ray to demonstrate spinal cord compression and lesions

Positron electron tomography (PET)

- Maps function of specific areas of brain

Electrical studies (*K&C*, p. 1203)

Electroencephalography (EEG)

- Records electrical brain activity from scalp electrodes on 16 channels
- Used in
  - Epilepsy (spikes or spike and wave abnormalities)
  - Diffuse brain disorders (slow waves, e.g. hepatic encephalopathy)

Electromyelography (EMG)

- Demonstrates abnormal muscle innervation and myopathies

Nerve conduction studies

- Nerve entrapment
- Neuropathies

Visual evoked potentials (VEP)

- Record time for visual stimulus to reach the visual cortex
- Document previous retrobulbar neuritis

Lumbar puncture (LP) and cerebrospinal fluid (CSF) examination (*K&C*, p. 1204)

Indications for lumbar puncture

- Diagnosis of meningitis or encephalitis
- Intrathecal injection of contrast or drugs
- Diagnosis of subarachnoid haemorrhage
- Measurement of CSF pressure (Table 17.4)
- Therapeutic removal of CSF
- Detection of miscellaneous CSF abnormalities, e.g. oligoclonal bands in MS

Table 17.4 Normal CSF

Appearance	**Protein**
Crystal clear, colourless	0.2–0.4 g/L
Pressure	**Glucose**
60–150 mmH$_2$O	{2/3}–{1/2} blood glucose level
Cell count	**Microbiology**
5/mm^3	Sterile
No polymorphs	
No red blood cells	

Contraindications for lumbar puncture

▌ Raised intracranial pressure
▌ Suspected intracranial or spinal cord mass lesion
▌ (Unconscious patients and those with papilloedema must have CT scan to exclude raised intracranial pressure or mass lesion before LP)
▌ Platelet count <40 × 10^9/L
▌ Abnormal coagulation

Brain biopsy

▌ Inflammatory and degenerative brain diseases
▌ CT-guided sampling of mass lesions

UNCONSCIOUSNESS AND COMA (K&C, P. 1205)

▌ Coma is a state of unrousable unresponsiveness
▌ Consciousness is graded using the Glasgow Coma Scale (GCS – Table 17.5)

Aetiology of coma

▌ Diffuse brain dysfunction (see Table 17.6)
▌ Brainstem lesion
▌ Brainstem compression (coning)

EPILEPSY (K&C, P. 1219)

▌ A continuing tendency to suffer epileptic seizures, a seizure being a convulsion or transient abnormal event resulting from paroxysmal discharge of cerebral neurones

Prevalence

▌ 2% of the population has two or more seizures

BOX 17.1 COMA

Check A B C (airways, breathing, circulation)
Immobilise cervical spine if head or spinal injury suspected
Look for warning cards/bracelets etc, e.g. diabetics, epileptics

Examination
Glasgow Coma Score
Rectal temperature
Smell breath for alcohol/ketones
Blood pressure
Pupils
    Bilateral fixed dilated – brainstem death, barbiturates, hypothermia
    Single fixed dilated – coning
    Pinpoint – pontine lesions, opiates
Fundi for papilloedema
Eye movements
    Doll's head reflex
    Fixed lateral gaze
Lateralizing signs
    Facial drooping
    Muscle tone
    Plantar responses
    Tendon reflexes

Investigations
Drug screen
Serum biochemistry
Serum glucose
Thyroid function tests
Blood cultures
ECG
CT scan or MRI of brain
LP and CSF examination (only after raised intracranial pressure excluded)
EEG
Serum cortisol

Immediate management
Careful observation to detect changes in vital functions or depth of coma
Protect airway
Ventilate if necessary

Longer-term management
Skin care
Pressure area care
Oral hygiene
Nutrition (nasogastric feeding or percutaneous endoscopic gastrostomy tube)
Eye care
Urinary catheter only if essential

Classification

    ❚ By clinical pattern of seizures
      (Table 17.7)
Generalised ❚ Absence (petit mal)

Table 17.5 Glasgow Coma Scale

Eye opening (E)		Verbal function (V)	
Spontaneous	4	Orientated	5
To speech	3	Confused conversation	4
To pain	2	Inappropriate words	3
None	1	Incomprehensible sounds	2
		None	1
Motor function (M)			
Obeys commands	6		
Localises to pain	5		
Withdraws	4		
Flexion	3		
Extension	2		
None	1		

Table 17.6 Causes of diffuse brain dysfunction

Drug overdose, alcohol	Adrenal failure
Hypoglycaemia	Hyponatraemia
Hyperglycaemia	Hypernatraemia
Hypoxia	Metabolic acidosis
Hypertensive encephalopathy	Hypothermia, hyperpyrexia
Uraemia	Epilepsy
Hepatic encephalopathy	Encephalitis
CO_2 retention	Head injury
Hypothyroidism	Subarachnoid haemorrhage

BOX 17.2 STATUS EPILEPTICUS

Definition
Seizures which follow each other without recovery of consciousness

Management
Nurse the patient in an area with full ventilatory support available if required and with cardiac monitoring facilities
Give oxygen and monitor pulse, O_2 saturation and BP
Exclude hypoglycaemia
Diazepam 10–20 mg i.v. at a rate of 2.5 mg/30 seconds until fitting stops (up to a maximum of 40 mg); beware of respiratory depression
Loading dose of i.v. phenytoin, 15 mg/kg at a rate <50 mg/minute
Maintenance phenytoin i.v. or oral depending on patient's ability to take it
If status continues unresponsive to treatment for more than 90 minutes, the patient needs to be anaesthetised with thiopental or propofol and ventilated

❚ Myoclonic
❚ Tonic-clonic (grand mal)
❚ Tonic
❚ Akinetic

Table 17.7 Clinical pattern of epileptic seizures

Generalised tonic-clonic seizures
Warning – vague
Tonic phase – body becomes rigid before patient falls (often with a cry), biting the tongue and with urinary incontinence
Clonic phase – a generalised convulsion with rhythmic jerking of muscles and frothing at the mouth
Recovery – patient is drowsy or confused, or in a coma for several hours (post-ictal)

Absence seizures
Patient becomes still and staring and looks pale
Eyelids may twitch
Attack lasts a few seconds usually, during which the patient is unresponsive
No recollection of the event

Partial (focal) seizures
Aura, e.g. strange smell, tingling in a limb
Motor (Jacksonian)
Jerking movements begin at the angle of the mouth or in the hand, spreading to involve the limbs on the side opposite from the epileptic focus
Patient remains conscious
Paralysis of the affected limbs may follow for several hours (Todd's paralysis)
Temporal lobe epilepsy
May be simple or complex
Feeling of unreality, often déjà-vu, associated with absence attacks, vertigo or visual hallucinations

Partial
- Simple (e.g. Jacksonian, no impairment of consciousness)
- Complex (impairment of consciousness)

Aetiology
- Genetic
- Developmental abnormalities
- Trauma
- Surgery
- Pyrexia (in children, febrile convulsions)
- Intracranial mass
- Infarction
- Alcohol/drug withdrawal
- Encephalitis
- Metabolic abnormalities, e.g. hyponatraemia, hypoglycaemia

Investigations

- EEG (abnormal during seizures, often normal in between)
- CT scan/MRI scan
- Serum biochemistry
- Chest X-ray

Management

During seizure
- Maintain airway and physical safety
- Rectal or i.v. diazepam 5–10 mg if seizure does not stop spontaneously

Prophylactic
- For recurrent seizures
- First-line drugs
  - Sodium valproate
  - Carbamezepine
  - Phenytoin
  - Ethosuximide (petit mal)
- Newer drugs
  - Lamotrigine
  - Vigabatrin
  - Gabapentin
  - Clobazam
  - Phenobarbital

Toxic drug effects

All drugs
- Ataxia
- Nystagmus
- Dysarthria

Phenytoin
- Gum hypertrophy
- Hypertrichosis
- Osteomalacia
- Folate deficiency
- Polyneuropathy

Driving

- It is illegal to drive if any form of seizure or unexplained loss of consciousness has occurred during the past year
- In the UK it is essential that a doctor inform patients of the driving regulations; it is then the patient's responsibility to inform the licensing authority

Other causes of drop attacks, blackouts and episodes of disturbed consciousness (*K&C*, p. 1226)

- Diagnosis can usually be determined from the history

- A witness account of an attack is especially valuable

Aetiology

- Syncope, e.g. simple, micturition
- Transient ischaemic attack (see p. 502)
- Panic attack
- Cardiac arrhythmia, e.g. Stokes–Adams attack
- Aortic stenosis
- Hypoglycaemia
- Vertigo

MOVEMENT DISORDERS (*K&C*, P. 1227)

Parkinson's disease

- Combination of tremor, rigidity and akinesia

Prevalence

- Increases with age
- 1:200 over 70 years of age
- Less prevalent in smokers

Aetiology

- Idiopathic
- Drug-induced, e.g. phenothiazines
- MPTP (methylphenyltetrapyridine, impurity in illegally synthesised opiates)
- Encephalitis lethargica

Pathology

- Cell degeneration in the substantia nigra
- Loss of dopamine in the extrapyramidal nuclei

Clinical features

- Tremor – 4–7 Hz resting tremor (pill-rolling)
- Micrographia
- Rigidity – increased tone throughout the range of movement
- Cogwheel rigidity (stuttering rigid tone combined with tremor)
- Bradykinesia – poverty of movement
- Falls
- Mask-like facies
- Reduced blinking
- Stooping, shuffling gait (festinant)
- Poor arm swinging

- Monotonous speech, slurring dysarthria
- Normal power
- Brisk reflexes
- Downgoing plantars
- Cognitive function initially preserved; late dementia sometimes occurs

Investigations

- No diagnostic test; diagnosis made on clinical grounds

Management

- Levodopa plus dopa decarboxylase inhibitor e.g. Sinemet or Madopar; start gradually increasing the dose until adequate response or limiting side-effects (see below)
- Dopaminergic agonists, e.g. bromocriptine
- Selegeline – monoamine oxidase B inhibitor
- Neurosurgery (occasionally for intractable tremor)
- Physiotherapy
- Physical aids

Side-effects of levodopa

Short-term
- Nausea and vomiting
- Confusion
- Visual hallucinations
- Chorea

Long-term
- End-of-dose dyskinesia
- On–off syndrome
- Chorea
- Dystonic movements

Prognosis

- Variable
- Usually worsens over 10–15 years with death from bronchopneumonia

Huntington's disease (*K&C*, p. 1231)

- Inherited progressive chorea and dementia in middle life

Prevalence

- 5:100 000

Aetiology

- Autosomal dominance with full penetrance
- Children of an affected parent have a 50% chance of inheriting the mutation on chromosome 4

Pathology

- Cerebral atrophy
- Loss of neurones in caudate nucleus and putamen
- Depletion of γ-aminobutyric (GABA), angiotensin-converting enzyme (ACE) and met-enkephalin in substantia nigra

Clinical features

- Chorea (sudden involuntary jerky semi-purposeful movements, flitting from one part of the body to another)
- Progressive dementia

Investigations

- MRI or CT shows atrophy of caudate nucleus

Management

- Phenothiazines may reduce chorea

Prognosis

- Death 10–20 years after onset

Screening

- Mutation analysis is available for presymptomatic screening in families but no effective treatment is known to alter disease progression

Other causes of chorea

- Sydenham's chorea (rheumatic fever)
- Drugs, e.g. phenytoin
- Thyrotoxicosis
- Stroke
- Systemic lupus erythematosus (SLE)

MULTIPLE SCLEROSIS (*K&C*, P. 1233)

- Multiple plaques of demyelination in the brain and spinal cord disseminated in time and place
- Clinical diagnosis: two neurological events separated in time and neurological location

Prevalence

- Increases moving north from the Equator
- 60–100/100 000 in the UK

Aetiology

- Increased concordance among monozygotic twins
- HLA haplotype A3, B7, D2 and DR2 is more common

Environmental	❚ ?Viral infection
	❚ ?Dietary antigens

Pathology

❚ Plaques of demyelination particularly in
- Optic nerves
- Periventricular region
- Brainstem and cerebellar connections
- Cervical spinal cord
- Corticospinal tracts
- Posterior columns

Clinical patterns

❚ Relapsing/remitting
❚ Chronic progressive
❚ See below

Investigations

Imaging	❚ MRI brain and spinal cord (visualises multiple plaques)
CSF	❚ Oligoclonal bands in 80%
	❚ Raised mononuclear cell count 5–60 cells/mm^3
Visual evoked responses	❚ Delayed following optic neuropathy

Management

❚ No treatment has been shown to alter long-term outcome
❚ Corticosteroids – i.v. methylprednisolone or ACTH may speed recovery in acute relapses
❚ β-interferon – reduces relapse rate but not long-term outcome
❚ Physiotherapy
❚ Occupational therapy
- Walking aids
- Wheelchairs
- Car/house conversions
❚ Speech therapy
❚ Counselling

Prognosis

❚ Unpredictable course ranging from grave disability to mild and benign

Optic neuropathy
Clinical features

❚ Blurred vision in one eye
❚ Mild ocular pain

- Recovery within 1–2 months
- Optic disc swelling (optic neuritis)
- Normal disc (retrobulbar neuritis)
- Optic atrophy
- Relative afferent pupillary defect (dilatation of the affected eye when light is transferred from the good eye to the affected eye)

Brainstem demyelination
Clinical features

- Double vision
- Vertigo
- Facial numbness
- Weakness
- Dysphagia
- Pyramidal tract signs
- Nystagmus
- Ataxia
- Cranial nerve defects
- Internuclear ophthalmoplegia

Spinal cord lesion
Clinical features

- Difficulty walking
- Sensory abnormalities
- Electric shock-like pains radiating down trunk and limbs caused by neck flexion (Lhermitte's sign)
- Urinary symptoms (incontinence, retention)
- Spastic paraparesis
- Increased tone
- Weakness
- Brisk reflexes
- Up-going plantars
- Sensory level

Other presentations of MS

- Epilepsy
- Trigeminal neuralgia
- Tonic spasms of a hand
- Organic psychosis
- Dementia

INFECTIONS AND INFLAMMATORY CONDITIONS OF THE NERVOUS SYSTEM (*K&C*, P. 1236)

Meningitis

Aetiology

- See Table 17.8

Clinical features

- Headache
- Neck stiffness
- Fever
- Photophobia
- Vomiting
- Rigors
- Positive Kernig's sign
- Petechial/purpuric rash (meningococcal septicaemia)
- Drowsiness/focal signs (suggest complication, e.g. raised intracranial pressure/abscess)

Investigations

- CT of brain to exclude raised intracranial pressure
- Lumbar puncture (Table 17.9)
- Blood cultures
- Blood glucose
- Chest X-ray

Table 17.8 Causes of meningitis

Bacteria	**Chronic inflammatory conditions**
Neisseria meningitides	Sarcoidosis
Streptococcus pneumoniae	Behçet's disease
Staphylococcus aureus	Syphilis
Listeria monocytogenes	
Gram-negative bacilli	**Malignancy**
Haemophilus influenzae	
Mycobacterium tuberculosis	**Blood**
Treponema pallidum	Following subarachnoid haemorrhage
Viruses	
Enterovirus	
Echovirus	
Coxsackie virus	
Herpes simplex	
HIV	
Epstein–Barr virus (EBV)	
Fungi	
Cryptococcus neoformans	
Candida	

Table 17.9 CSF findings in meningitis

	Appearance	Mononuclear cells (per mm^3)	Polymorphs (per mm^3)	Protein (g/L)	Glucose (% blood glucose)
Normal	Crystal clear	<5	Nil	0.2–0.4	>50
Viral	Clear/turbid	10–100	Nil	0.4–0.8	>50
Pyogenic	Turbid/purulent	<50	200–300	0.5–2	<50
TB	Turbid/viscous	100–300	0–200	0.5–3	<30

Table 17.10 Antibiotics in meningitis

Suspected organism	Antibiotic
Unknown	Cefotaxime
Meningococcus	Benzylpenicillin
	Cefotaxime
Pneumococcus	Cefotaxime
TB	Rifampicin

▌ Skull X-ray (if trauma)
▌ Throat swab for *Neisseria*

Management

▌ Immediate parenteral antibiotics (Table 17.10); do not wait for LP/CT
▌ Further treatment depends on results of blood or CSF culture and sensitivities
▌ Viral meningitis requires no specific treatment
▌ I.v. steroids with first dose of antibiotics

Prophylaxis

▌ Meningococcus is notifiable
▌ Family and very close contacts should be treated with ciprofloxacin or rifampicin to eradicate carriage
▌ Meningococcal vaccine to close contacts

Acute viral encephalitis
Aetiology

▌ Herpes simplex
▌ Echovirus
▌ Coxsackie virus
▌ Mumps
▌ EBV
▌ Adenovirus
▌ Varicella zoster

- Influenza
- Measles
- Rabies

Clinical features

- Often mild and self-limiting
- HSV-1 infection may be more serious
- Headache
- Fever
- Mood change
- Drowsiness
- Seizures
- Focal signs
- Coma

Investigations

- CT scan (may show diffuse oedema)
- EEG (characteristic slow wave changes in HSV)
- CSF (increased mononuclear cells, slightly raised protein)

Management

- I.v. aciclovir for suspected HSV-1

Prognosis

- 20% mortality in serious cases, with many others suffering long-term severe brain damage

Herpes zoster (shingles) (*K&C*, p. 1240)

- Recrudescence of varicella zoster virus infection within a dorsal root ganglion

Clinical features

- Typical blistering rash affecting dermatome supplied by the affected nerve root

Trigeminal nerve (ophthalmic division)
- Rash affects the eye and may cause corneal scarring

Facial nerve (Ramsay Hunt syndrome)
- Facial palsy
- Vesicles on ear lobe, external auditory meatus and fauces

Treatment

- Aciclovir

Complications
- Post-herpetic neuralgia

Neurosyphilis (*K&C*, p. 1240)

Meningovascular syphilis
- Subacute meningitis with cranial nerve palsies or paraparesis

Tabes dorsalis
- Demyelination of dorsal roots
- Charcot's joints (neuropathic)
- Ataxia
- Stamping gait
- Widespread sensory loss
- Argyll Robertson pupils (small irregular pupil, fixed to light, constricts to accommodation)
- Ptosis
- Optic atrophy

Generalised paralysis of the insane (GPI)
- Dementia
- Weakness
- Tremor
- Brisk reflexes
- Extensor plantars
- Argyll Robertson pupils

Taboparesis
- Congenital neurosyphilis
- Features of tabes dorsalis and GPI in childhood

Management
- Parenteral penicillin for 2–3 weeks

Sporadic Creutzfeldt–Jakob disease (CJD) (*K&C*, p. 1242)
Aetiology
- Prion disease
- Can be passed on from surgical specimens, autopsy material (e.g. corneal grafts) and human pituitary hormones

Pathology
- Spongiform changes in brain

Clinical features
- Slowly progressive dementia develops after age 50

Variant CJD
- First noted in Britain in 1995

Aetiology

- Prion disease
- Linked to ingestion of meat from cattle infected with bovine spongiform encephalopathy (BSE)

Clinical features

- Younger patients
- Early neuropsychiatric symptoms
- Ataxia
- Dementia
- Myoclonus
- Chorea
- Death

Brain abscess (*K&C*, p. 1243)

- A focal area of bacterial infection causing an expanding mass lesion in the cerebrum or cerebellum

Aetiology

- *Streptococcus milleri*
- *Bacteroides* spp
- *Staphylococcus* spp
- Fungi
- Parameningeal infection, e.g. ear, nose, paranasal sinuses
- Skull fracture
- Distant infection, e.g. pneumonia, infective endocarditis
- Immunosuppression, e.g. HIV infection

Clinical features

- Headache
- Fever
- Focal signs
- Seizures
- Vomiting
- Drowsiness
- Papilloedema

Investigations

- Imaging (mass lesion on CT or MRI +/− hydrocephalus)
- Blood cultures
- Raised ESR
- Raised white cell count

■ Look for a local/distant focus of infection
■ Lumbar puncture is contraindicated

Management

■ Parenteral antibiotics
■ Surgical decompression

Prognosis

■ Mortality 25%
■ Persistent epilepsy common in survivors

INTRACRANIAL TUMOURS (TABLE 17.11) (*K&C*, P. 1243)

■ Primary intracranial tumours account for about 10% of all neoplasms

Clinical features

■ Direct mass effect on function, e.g. hemiparesis
■ Raised intracranial pressure (Table 17.12)
■ Seizures

Table 17.11 Intracranial tumours

Type	Prevalence		
Metastases	50%	**Primary malignant**	35%
Bronchus		Astrocytoma	
Breast		Oligodendroglioma	
Stomach		Lymphoma	
Prostate		Medulloblastoma	
Thyroid		**Benign**	15%
Kidney		Meningioma	
Lymphoma (associated with AIDS)		Neurofibroma	

Table 17.12 Symptoms and signs of raised intracranial pressure

Headache	Bradycardia
Vomiting	Decerebrate posturing (coning)
Papilloedema	False localizing signs
Impaired consciousness	VI nerve lesion
Respiratory depression	III nerve lesion

Investigations

- CT or MRI scanning
- Brain biopsy

Management

- Reduce cerebral oedema using corticosteroids and/or i.v. mannitol
- Anticonvulsants
- Surgery
- Radiotherapy

Prognosis

- 50% survival at 2 years for high grade malignant tumours

HEADACHE AND MIGRAINE (*K&C*, P. 1247)

Tension headache

- The vast majority of chronic and recurrent headaches

Clinical features

- Throbbing headache
- Tight band sensation
- Pressure behind eyes

Management

- Avoid precipitating causes
- Simple analgesia

Migraine

- Recurrent headaches associated with visual and gastrointestinal disturbance

Pathology

- Vasodilatation and oedema of blood vessels
- Release of vasoactive substances

Classical migraine
Clinical features

- Prodrome
  - Teichopsia (flashes)
  - Jagged lines
  - Unilateral patchy scotoma
  - Lasts 15 minutes to 1 hour
- Headache hemicranial or generalised

- Nausea and vomiting
- Generally irritable
- Preference for the dark
- Sleeping

Other patterns

- Migraine without aura
- Hemiplegic migraine

Differential diagnosis

- Subarachnoid haemorrhage
- Transient ischaemic attack
- Partial seizures

Management

- Avoid precipitating features

During attack
- Paracetamol
- Antiemetics
- Sumatriptan (5HT agonist)
- Ergotamine

Prophylaxis
- Pizotifen, methysergide (5HT antagonists)
- Propranolol
- Amitriptyline (low-dose)

Cluster headaches

- Affect adults in third and fourth decades
- ♂ > ♀

Clinical features

- Recurrent bouts of excruciating pain centred around one eye
- Wakes patient at night
- Vomiting
- Watering and congestion of affected eye
- Transient ipsilateral Horner's syndrome

Management

- Usually unhelpful
- No analgesia effective for headache
- Lithium carbonate for prophylaxis
- Oxygen during attack

Other causes of headache

- Subarachnoid haemorrhage
- Meningitis
- Sinusitis

- Brain tumours
- Temporal arteritis
- Benign intracranial hypertension
- Head injury

CEREBROVASCULAR DISEASE AND STROKE
(TABLE 17.13) (*K&C*, P. 1209)

- Stroke is the third commonest cause of death in the UK
- A stroke is a focal neurological deficit due to a vascular lesion lasting >than 24 hours (if the patient survives)
- A transient ischaemic attack (TIA) is a focal neurological deficit lasting <24 hours

Risk factors

- Hypertension
- Smoking
- Family history
- Hyperlipidaemia
- Afro-Caribbean race
- High-dose oral contraceptive pill

Transient ischaemic attacks (*K&C*, p. 1211)
Clinical features

- Focal deficit depends on part of brain affected

Carotid system
- Amaurosis fugax
  – visual loss
- Aphasia (dominant side)
- Hemiparesis
- Hemianopic visual loss

Vertebrobasilar
- Diplopia

Table 17.13 Types of cerebrovascular disease

Thromboembolic infarction
Cerebral and cerebellar haemorrhages
Dissection of carotid or vertebral arteries
Subarachnoid haemorrhage
Subdural and extradural haemorrhage
Cortical venous and dural sinus thrombosis

system
- Vertigo
- Vomiting
- Dysarthria, choking
- Ataxia
- Transient global amnesia

Evidence of source of embolus
- Atrial fibrillation
- Carotid bruit
- Valvular heart disease
- Subclavian artery stenosis

Cerebral infarction (*K&C*, p. 1212)
Clinical features
- Focal deficit depends on part of brain affected (see below)
- Initially flaccid areflexic weakness followed by spastic tone, brisk reflexes and extensor plantars
- See Fig. 17.2 for arterial supply to the cerebral cortex

Dysphasia
- Dominance
  - Almost all right-handed and 50% of left-handed people have language function in the left hemisphere
- Expressive dysphasia
  - Lesion in Broca's area in frontal lobe
  - Reduced fluency of speech
  - Failure to construct sentences
  - Comprehension preserved
- Receptive dysphasia
  - Lesion in Wernicke's area in temporo-parietal region
  - Fluent speech with incorrect words
  - Use of jargon
  - Sounds like nonsense
  - Failure of comprehension

Middle cerebral/ internal carotid artery (internal capsule stroke)
- Hemiparesis (limbs and face)
- Aphasia (dominant side)
- Hemianopic visual loss
- Dysarthria

Posterior inferior cerebellar artery (brainstem stroke)
- Coma, altered consciousness
- Vertigo
- Vomiting
- Dysphagia, choking
- Ataxia
- Contralateral loss of pain on face

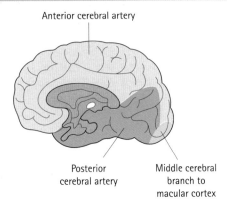

Medial view of right hemisphere

Anterior cerebral artery

Posterior cerebral artery

Middle cerebral branch to macular cortex

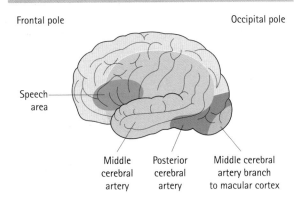

Lateral view of left hemisphere

Frontal pole

Occipital pole

Speech area

Middle cerebral artery

Posterior cerebral artery

Middle cerebral artery branch to macular cortex

Fig. 17.2 Arterial supply to the cerebral cortex.

Important parts of examination of patients with cerebrovascular disease

- Neurological signs
- Source of embolus (e.g. carotid bruit, atrial fibrillation)
- Blood pressure (in both arms)
- Optic fundi (hypertensive retinopathy, papilloedema)

Investigations

- Acute (*K&C*, Box 21.1)
- Long term risk management (*K&C*, Box 21.2)
- CT/MRI imaging of brain (Chapter 5)
  - Demonstrates site
  - Distinguishes between infarct or haemorrhage

- Carotid Doppler scanning
- Magnetic resonance angiography (for possible surgery)
- Blood count
- ESR
- Blood glucose, lipids
- Syphilis serology
- Chest X-ray
- ECG
- Echocardiogram

Management

- Identify and treat risk factors where possible
- Antihypertensive therapy
- Aspirin 300 mg initially then 75 mg per day or other antiplatelet therapy
- Anticoagulation (for atrial fibrillation)
- Surgery (internal carotid endarterectomy)
- Thrombolysis in acute stroke (effective if given within 3 hrs of onset)

Rehabilitation

- Physiotherapy
- Speech therapy
- Occupational therapy

Prognosis

- 30–40% survival at 3 years (among initial survivors)
- 10% chance of further stroke within a year

Intracerebral haemorrhage (*K&C*, p. 1216)

- Accounts for 10% of strokes

Aetiology

- Rupture of microaneurysms

Risk factors

- Hypertension

Clinical features

- Difficult to distinguish between haemorrhage and infarction
- Haemorrhage may be accompanied by headache and coma

Investigations

- CT head (Fig. 5.40)

Management

▌ As for infarction except avoid antiplatelet and anticoagulant drugs

Prognosis

▌ 70% death within 2 years

Subarachnoid haemorrhage (*K&C*, p. 1217)

▌ Spontaneous arterial bleeding into subarachnoid space

Prevalence

▌ 6:100 000/year
▌ Accounts for 5% of strokes

Aetiology

▌ Saccular 'berry' aneurysms (70%)
▌ Arteriovenous malformation (AVM) (10%)
▌ No lesion (20%)

Clinical features

▌ Sudden onset of severe occipital headache
▌ Vomiting
▌ Loss of consciousness
▌ Neck stiffness
▌ Positive Kernig's sign
▌ Papilloedema and retinal haemorrhages

Investigations

▌ CT scan
▌ Lumbar puncture (if CT undiagnostic) – red cells and/or xanthochromia in CSF
▌ Carotid and vertebral angiography

Management

Immediate ▌ Bed rest
▌ Treat hypertension
▌ Dexamethasone
▌ Nimodipine
Later ▌ Neurosurgical aneurysm clipping or coil insertion

Prognosis

▌ 50% mortality at presentation
▌ 10–20% more die in early weeks

Chronic subdural haematoma (*K&C*, p. 1218)

▌ Accumulation of blood in subdural space following rupture of a vein after head injury (sometimes trivial)

Clinical features

▊ May be delayed
▊ Headache
▊ Drowsiness
▊ Confusion
▊ Focal deficits

Management

▊ Often conservative
▊ Usually resolve spontaneously without surgical drainage

DEGENERATIVE DISORDERS

Motor neurone disease (*K&C*, p. 1253)

▊ Progressive degeneration of lower motor neurones and upper motor neurones of the cortex, cranial nerve nuclei and spinal cord

Incidence

▊ 2:100 000: year
▊ Slight male predominance

Clinical patterns

▊ Progressive muscular atrophy – progressive weakness and wasting of arm and hand muscles
▊ Amyotrophic lateral sclerosis – progressive spastic tetraparesis or paraparesis with wasting and fasciculation
▊ Progressive bulbar palsy – degeneration of lower cranial nerve nuclei

Clinical features

▊ Muscle wasting
▊ Fasciculation
▊ Reflexes absent or exaggerated
▊ Dysarthria
▊ Dysphagia
▊ Nasal regurgitation of fluids
▊ Choking
▊ Bulbar and pseudobulbar palsy (see p. 516)
▊ Ocular movements are not affected
▊ Cerebellar or extrapyramidal signs do not occur
▊ Dementia is unusual
▊ Sphincter function is usually preserved
▊ No sensory signs

Investigations

- Diagnosis made on clinical grounds
- EMG – denervation of muscles with preserved motor conduction velocity

Prognosis

- Relentlessly progressive course
- Death within 3 years

Management

- Riluzole (sodium channel blocker, inhibits glutamate release) slows progress
- No treatment affects outcome

Friedreich's ataxia (*K&C*, p. 1258)

- Progressive degeneration of dorsal root ganglia, spinocerebellar tracts and corticospinal tracts

Aetiology

- Abnormal gene for fraxitin (unknown function)
- Autosomal recessive

Clinical features

- Difficulty walking from about 12 years of age
- Ataxia of gait and trunk
- Nystagmus
- Dysarthria
- Absent reflexes in legs
- Optic atrophy
- Pes cavus
- Cardiomyopathy

NEUROPATHY

- A pathological process affecting peripheral nerves

Pathology

- Demyelination
- Axonal degeneration
- Wallerian degeneration (after nerve section)
- Compression
- Infarction
- Infiltration

Mononeuropathies

- Caused by peripheral nerve compression

Carpal tunnel syndrome (*K&C*, pp. 539 and 1260)

▌ Median nerve compression in carpal tunnel (at wrist)

Aetiology

▌ Idiopathic
▌ Hypothyroidism
▌ Diabetes mellitus
▌ Pregnancy
▌ Rheumatoid arthritis
▌ Obesity
▌ Acromegaly

Clinical features

▌ Tingling in fingers (especially at night)
▌ Weakness of thenar muscles
▌ Wasting of thenar eminence
▌ Weakness of abductor pollicis brevis (raising thumb away from palm)
▌ Weakness of opposition of thumb and little finger
▌ Tinel's sign (reproduction of tingling by tapping over carpal tunnel)
▌ Sensory loss of palm and radial three and a half fingers

Management

▌ Splint wrist
▌ Surgical decompression

Ulnar nerve compression

▌ Usually occurs after trauma at elbow

Clinical features

▌ Wasting and weakness of interossei and hypothenar muscles
▌ Sensory loss in the ulnar one and a half fingers

Radial nerve compression ('Saturday night palsy')

▌ Occurs after nerve is compressed against humerus when arm is draped over a hard chair for several hours

Clinical features

▌ Wrist drop
▌ Weakness of finger extension

Mononeuritis multiplex

▌ Multiple mononeuropathies

Aetiology

▌ Diabetes mellitus
▌ Leprosy
▌ Vasculitis
▌ Sarcoidosis
▌ Amyloidosis
▌ Malignancy
▌ Neurofibromatosis
▌ HIV infection

Polyneuropathies

Guillain–Barré syndrome (*K&C*, p. 1260)

▌ Acute inflammatory post-infective polyneuropathy
▌ Follows 1–3 weeks after infection (often trivial, or Campylobacter infection)

Incidence

▌ 3/100 000/year

Clinical features

▌ Weakness of distal limb muscles $+/-$ numbness
▌ Weakness ascends over days for up to 3 weeks
▌ Can affect respiratory and facial muscles in 30%

Variants ▌ Autonomic neuropathy
▌ Miller–Fisher syndrome (affecting ocular muscles, and with ataxia)

Investigations

▌ Diagnosis is made on clinical grounds
▌ Nerve conduction studies (demyelinating neuropathy)
▌ CSF (cell count normal, protein raised 1–3 g/L)

Management

▌ Measurement of respiratory function (arterial blood gases, vital capacity, FEV_1)
▌ Assisted ventilation if necessary
▌ High-dose i.v. γ-globulin
▌ Plasmapheresis
▌ Subcutaneous heparin for prevention of thromboembolism

Prognosis

▌ Spontaneous gradual recovery
▌ 15% disability or death

Table 17.14 Other polyneuropathies	
Metabolic	**Vitamin deficiencies**
Diabetes mellitus	Thiamin (B$_1$)
Uraemia	Pyridoxine (B$_6$)
Porphyria	Vitamin B$_{12}$
Amyloidosis	Nicotinic acid
Toxic	**Non-metastatic manifestation of malignancy**
Alcohol	
Drugs	
Phenytoin	
Isoniazid	
Metronidazole	
Thalidomide	
Vincristine	
Cisplatin	

Other polyneuropathies (table 17.14) (K&C, pp. 1262–1263)

Thiamin deficiency (Wernicke–Korsakoff syndrome)
Clinical features

- Ocular signs
  - Nystagmus
  - Bilateral rectal palsies
  - Fixed pupils
- Ataxia
- Confusion (amnestic syndrome, with loss of short-term memory)

Investigations

- Reduced red cell transketolase

Management

- Parenteral thiamine

Vitamin B$_{12}$ deficiency (subacute combined degeneration of the cord)
Aetiology

- See p. 417

Clinical features

- Distal sensory loss
  - Light touch
  - Vibration sense
  - Joint position sense
- Absent ankle jerks
- Extensor plantars
- Optic atrophy
- Dementia

Investigations

- Reduced serum B_{12}
- Macrocytosis
- Megaloblastic bone marrow

Management

- Parenteral B_{12}

Peroneal muscular atrophy (Charcot–Marie–Tooth disease)

- Inherited sensorimotor neuropathy
- Several types: autosomal dominant and recessive

Clinical features

- Distal limb wasting and weakness
- Inverted 'champagne bottle' legs
- Pes cavus
- Clawing of toes
- Loss of sensation
- Loss of reflexes

Autonomic neuropathy
Aetiology

- Diabetes mellitus
- Guillain–Barré syndrome
- Amyloidosis

Clinical features

- Postural hypotension
- Retention of urine
- Erectile dysfunction
- Diarrhoea
- Diminished sweating
- Cardiac arrhythmias

MUSCLE DISEASE (*K&C*, PP. 1266–1271)

Aetiology

- See Table 17.15

Myasthenia gravis

- Disorder of the neuromuscular junction

Prevalence

- 4:100 000
- ♀ > ♂ (2:1)
- Age of onset about 30 years

Table 17.15 Causes of myopathies	
Type	Example
Inflammatory	Polymyositis
Metabolic	Cushing's syndrome
Myasthenic	Myasthenia gravis
Hereditary	Duchenne muscular dystrophy
Myotonias	Myotonic dystrophy
Channelopathies	Periodic paralysis

Aetiopathogenesis

- Unknown aetiology
- IgG antibodies to acetylcholine receptor
- Immune complex deposits on postsynaptic membrane
- Destruction of acetylcholine receptor
- Thymic hyperplasia in 70%
- Associated with
  - Thyroid disease
  - Rheumatoid arthritis
  - Pernicious anaemia
  - SLE

Clinical features

- Weakness and fatigability of muscles
  - Proximal limb
  - Extraocular
  - Speech
  - Facial expression
  - Mastication
- Ptosis
- Reflexes preserved but fatigable

Investigations

- Tensilon test
- Serum acetylcholine receptor antibodies (positive in 90%)
- Mediastinal imaging for thymoma (chest X-ray, CT, MRI)

Management

- Oral anticholinesterases, e.g. pyridostigmine
- Thymectomy (improves prognosis)
- Corticosteroids
- Azathioprine
- Plasmapheresis

Lambert–Eaton myasthenic-myopathic syndrome

▮ Non-metastatic manifestation of small cell carcinoma of the bronchus due to defective acetylcholine release at the neuromuscular junction

Clinical features

▮ Muscle weakness and absent reflexes which improve with contraction

Dystrophia myotonica

▮ Autosomal dominant inheritance

Clinical features

▮ Cataracts
▮ Frontal baldness
▮ Ptosis
▮ Facial weakness
▮ Progressive distal muscle weakness
▮ Mild intellectual impairment
▮ Cardiomyopathy
▮ Hypogonadism
▮ Glucose intolerance

CRANIAL NERVE DEFECTS

▮ See Table 17.16

Specific cranial nerve and brainstem defects

Optic pathway (*K&C*, p. 1179)

▮ See Figure 17.3

Bell's palsy (*K&C*, p. 1187)

▮ Common acute, isolated facial nerve palsy

Aetiology

▮ Viral infection (often herpes simplex) causes swelling of nerve within petrous temporal bone

Clinical features

▮ Unilateral lower motor neurone facial weakness and droop
▮ Loss of taste on anterior two-thirds of tongue

Investigations

▮ Diagnosis made on clinical grounds

Table 17.16 Cranial nerve defects

Nerve	Causes	Features
I	Head injury	Loss of smell (anosmia)
II	Optic neuritis	See MS
	Optic nerve compression	Tunnel vision (if at chiasma)
	Visual pathway lesion	See Figure 17.3
III	Coning	Ptosis
	Aneurysm of posterior inferior carotid artery	Eye points down and out
	Diabetes	Fixed dilated pupil
IV	Rare	Diplopia looking away and down
V	Brainstem lesion	Sensory loss (face and tongue)
	Acoustic neuroma	Loss of corneal reflex
	Cavernous sinus thrombosis	Deviation of jaw towards lesion
VI	MS	Convergent squint
	Glioma	Diplopia looking towards lesion
	Raised intracranial pressure	
VII	Upper motor neurone lesion (infarction)	Facial muscle weakness
	Lower motor neurone lesion (Bell's palsy, Ramsay Hunt syndrome, parotid gland disease)	Loss of taste on anterior two-thirds of tongue
VIII	Acoustic neuroma	Sensorineural deafness
	Meningitis	Vertigo
	Head injury	Nystagmus
	Drugs – gentamicin	
IX and X	Brainstem infarct	Weakness of elevation of pharynx
	Motor neurone disease	Loss of gag reflex
	Carcinoma of nasopharynx	Hoarseness
		Dysphagia
		Bulbar or pseudobulbar palsy
XI	Syringobulbia	Weakness of sternomastoid and trapezius
	Motor neurone disease	
	Carcinoma of nasopharynx	
XII	Brainstem infarct	LMN lesion; unilateral wasting, weakness and fasciculation of tongue
	Motor neurone disease	UMN lesion; stiff, spastic tongue
	Carcinoma of nasopharynx	

Management

- Prednisolone 60 mg reducing to zero over 10 days plus aciclovir
- Closure of eyelid to protect cornea

Prognosis

- Spontaneous improvement begins during second week

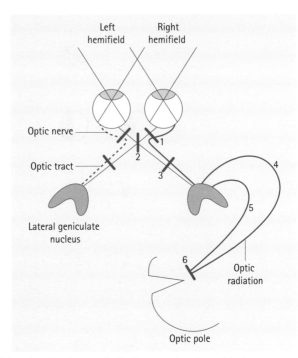

Fig. 17.3 Lesions of the visual pathway. A. Optic nerve tracts and lesions.

▌ Recovery takes up to 12 months
▌ Less than 10% have residual severe weakness

Bulbar palsy (*K&C*, p. 1191)
▌ LMN weakness of cranial nerve nuclei within medulla (IX, X, XI, XII)

Aetiology

▌ Motor neurone disease
▌ Syringobulbia
▌ Poliomyelitis
▌ Myasthenia gravis

Clinical features

▌ Weakness of elevation of palate
▌ Loss of gag reflex
▌ Paralysed vocal cords
▌ Dysphagia
▌ Nasal regurgitation of fluids
▌ Choking

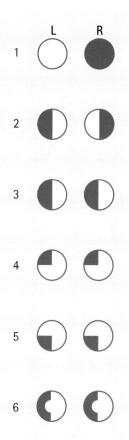

Fig. 17.3 (Continued) B. Visual field defects caused by lesions in the optic pathway. **Lesion 1:** This is analogous to losing an eye. One eye is completely blacked out. **Lesion 2:** Here only inputs from the nasal retinas are cut, so peripheral vision is lost on both sides. This can be caused by a pituitary tumour. (The pituitary lies just under the optic chiasm.) **Lesion 3:** Homonymous hemianopia: loss of the left hemifield. Both eyes are blind to anything on the left side of the world (assuming the eyes are pointed straight ahead). **Lesion 4:** The lower optic radiations are carrying information from the upper visual world so vision is lost in the upper quadrants of the left hemifield. **Lesion 5:** Here the parietal portion of the optic radiations are cut, so the lower visual world is affected on one side. **Lesion 6:** When the cortex itself is lesioned, vision at the fovea is spared, perhaps because there is such a large representation of the fovea in the cortex, or perhaps due to overlapping blood supply. The loss of vision is not a complete hemifield, then, but a notched hemifield. This is called macular sparing.

Pseudobulbar palsy (*K&C*, p. 1191)

▌ Bilateral upper motor neurone lesion of lower cranial nerve nuclei

Aetiology

▌ Motor neurone disease
▌ Multiple sclerosis
▌ Multi-infarct dementia
▌ Severe head injury

Clinical features

▌ Stiff, slow, spastic tongue (not wasted)
▌ Dysarthria
▌ Dry gravelly voice
▌ Preserved gag reflex
▌ Exaggerated jaw jerk
▌ Emotional lability

Horner's syndrome (*K&C*, p. 1183)

▌ Lesion of the cervical sympathetic pathway

Aetiology

▌ Brainstem stroke
▌ Coning
▌ Syringomyelia
▌ Apical lung cancer (Pancoast's tumour)
▌ Cervical rib
▌ Brachial plexus trauma

Clinical features

▌ Ptosis
▌ Myosis (constricted pupil)
▌ Enophthalmus
▌ Loss of sweating on side of face

SPINAL CORD DISEASE

Spinal cord compression (*K&C*, p. 1250)
Aetiology

▌ See Table 17.17

Clinical features

▌ Radicular pain
▌ Spastic paraparesis or tetraparesis
▌ Sensory loss to level of compression
▌ Sphincter disturbance (retention of urine and incontinence)

Table 17.17 Causes of spinal cord compression	
Within the cord Spinal cord neoplasms Transverse myelitis **In the meninges** Epidural abscess Epidural haemorrhage Ependymoma Meningioma	**Outside the cord** Vertebral neoplasms (metastases, myeloma) Disc lesions Vertebral collapse

Investigations

- Plain spinal X-rays
- Chest X-ray
- MRI
- Myelography

Management

- Surgical decompression if possible

Syringomyelia and syringobulbia (*K&C*, p. 1251)

- A fluid-filled cavity (syrinx) within the cervical spinal cord (syringomyelia) or extending up into the brainstem (syringobulbia)

Aetiology

- Arnold–Chiari malformation
- Spina bifida
- Hydrocephalus
- Intrinsic cord tumours

Pathology

- The expanding cavity within the cord destroys spinothalamic neurones, anterior horn cells, lateral corticospinal tracts, sympathetic trunk, trigeminal, IX, X XI and XII nuclei

Clinical features

- Loss of pain and temperature sensation in upper limbs
- Painless burns
- Trophic changes

- Normal light touch sensation
- Loss of upper limb reflexes
- Wasting of small muscles of hands
- Spastic paraparesis
- Neuropathic joints
- Brainstem signs, e.g. bulbar palsy, Horner's syndrome

Investigations

- MRI

Management

- No effective treatment or surgery

SELF-ASSESSMENT QUESTIONS

Best one of five questions

1. In epilepsy:
   - **A.** Generalised convulsions are characterised by maintenance of consciousness
   - **B.** Absence seizures are generalised
   - **C.** Absence seizures are commonest in adults
   - **D.** Temporal lobe seizures may affect the myocardium
   - **E.** Todd's paralysis follows temporal lobe seizure

2. In epilepsy:
   - **A.** The EEG is usually diagnostic between fits
   - **B.** All generalised seizures should be treated immediately with intravenous diazepam
   - **C.** It is the doctor's responsibility to inform the driving authorities when a patient is diagnosed with epilepsy
   - **D.** Ataxia usually signifies drug toxicity
   - **E.** Phenytoin causes alopecia

3. Which of the following statements is true in Parkinson's disease:
   - **A.** Smoking predisposes to Parkinson's disease
   - **B.** Males are more commonly affected
   - **C.** There is dopamine loss in the pyramidal nuclei
   - **D.** Incidence is 1:200 over 70 years of age
   - **E.** It may be caused by alcohol abuse

4. Common features of Parkinson's disease:
   - **A.** Intention tremor
   - **B.** Cogwheel rigidity
   - **C.** Dementia
   - **D.** Characteristic findings on CT brain scan
   - **E.** Extensor plantar reflexes

5. Which of the following is true about Huntington's disease?
   - **A.** It is inherited in an X-linked recessive manner
   - **B.** It is caused by a mutation on chromosome 5
   - **C.** It is associated with rheumatic fever
   - **D.** It is characterised by involuntary movements
   - **E.** It is associated with a higher than average IQ

6. The following are features of multiple sclerosis:
   - **A.** It may cause afferent pupillary defect
   - **B.** There is no concordance between monozygotic twins
   - **C.** The pathology is characterised by neurofibrillary tangles
   - **D.** Invariably leads to severe disability
   - **E.** Is associated with recent *Campylobacter* infection

7. The following are features of motor neurone disease:
   - **A.** Muscle hypertrophy
   - **B.** Ophthalmoplegia
   - **C.** Frontal balding
   - **D.** Cerebellar ataxia
   - **E.** Bulbar palsy

8. Causes of mononeuritis multiplex include:
   A. Diabetes mellitus
   B. Sarcoidosis
   C. Vitamin B_{12} deficiency
   D. HIV infection
   E. All of the above

9. Causes of polyneuropathy include:
   A. Porphyria
   B. Thalidomide
   C. Thyrotoxicosis
   D. A and B only
   E. A B and C

10. The clinical features of autonomic neuropathy are:
    A. Hypertension
    B. Erectile dysfunction
    C. Polydipsia
    D. Diarrhoea
    E. Infertility

11. The following statements about cerebrospinal fluid (CSF) are correct:
    A. It normally contains 5–10 red cells
    B. In bacterial meningitis the lymphocyte count is raised
    C. In viral meningitis glucose is lower than one-third of blood glucose
    D. In subarachnoid haemorrhage, xanthochromia occurs after 18 hours
    E. In Guillain–Barré syndrome protein is normal with a raised cell count

12. Which of the following statements about CNS infections is true:
    A. Herpes zoster causes a symmetrical rash
    B. Prion diseases are transferred by droplet spread
    C. Acute viral encephalitis is commonly caused by rotavirus
    D. Meningococcal septicaemia causes a vesicular rash
    E. Tuberculous meningitis is associated with high CSF protein

13. The following statements about Creutzfeldt–Jakob disease (CJD) are true:
    A. It is caused by a herpes virus infection
    B. It can be acquired during prosthetic heart valve replacement
    C. New variant CJD is more common in vegetarians
    D. It causes spongiform changes in the brain
    E. It is treatable with antiretroviral drugs

14. The following are aetiologically linked with brain abscess:
    A. Middle ear infection
    B. Lumbar puncture
    C. Skull fracture
    D. A B and C
    E. A and C

15. The following are symptoms and signs of raised intracranial pressure:
    A. Headache
    B. Tachycardia
    C. Papilloedema
    D. A and C
    E. All of the above

16. Which is the most important risk factor for cerebrovascular disease:
    A. Diabetes mellitus
    B. Hypertension

C. Asian race
D. Family history
E. Hypothyroidism

17. Aetiological factors in transient ischaemic attacks include:
    A. Atrial fibrillation
    B. Deep venous thrombosis
    C. Aortic sclerosis
    D. Warfarin therapy
    E. Polycystic kidney disease

18. Chronic subdural haematoma:
    A. Is due to arteriovenous malformation in 10% of cases
    B. Is usually precipitated by severe head injury
    C. Is characterised by a classical 'lucid period'
    D. Most often requires surgical drainage
    E. None of the above

Extended matching questions

Question 1 *Theme: difficulty walking/limb weakness*

A. Embolic stroke
B. Spinal cord compression
C. Guillain–Barré syndrome
D. Foot drop
E. Phenytoin toxicity
F. Motor neurone disease
G. Multiple sclerosis
H. Parkinson's disease
I. Huntington's disease
J. Friedreich's ataxia
K. Hysteria

For each of the following questions, select the best answer from the list above:

I. A 34-year-old housewife presents with difficulty walking due to weakness in her legs, 2 weeks after recovering from a bout of food poisoning. Examination shows absent tendon reflexes and {4/5} power in both legs. What is the most likely diagnosis?

II. A 70-year-old right-handed hypertensive smoker presents with sudden onset of weakness in the left leg and difficulty speaking. What is the most likely diagnosis?

III. A 61-year-old solicitor presents with a 1-year history of increasing difficulty walking. His wife has noticed his hands shaking and his secretary finds his handwriting has become too small to read. What is the most likely diagnosis?

Question 2 *Theme: headache*

A. Migraine
B. Temporal arteritis
C. Primary brain tumour
D. Hypertension
E. Subarachnoid haemorrhage
F. Meningitis
G. Encephalitis
H. Tension headache
I. Trigeminal neuralgia

For each of the following questions select the best answer from the list above:

I. A 24-year-old student presents with recent onset of flu-like symptoms, headache, vomiting, photophobia and neck stiffness. He is pyrexial (38.7°C), with a purpuric rash on the trunk. What is the most likely diagnosis?

II. A 32-year-old female legal secretary has a 6-month history of episodic throbbing right-sided headaches associated with nausea, often on Saturday mornings. What is the most likely diagnosis?

III. A 51-year-old Afro-Caribbean female with chronic renal failure and diabetes presents with a 3-week history of headache and blurred vision. Fundoscopy reveals retinal haemorrhages and papilloedema. What is the most likely diagnosis?

Question 3 *Theme: loss of consciousness/coma*

A. Grand mal epilepsy
B. Vasovagal faint
C. Hyperglycaemia
D. Hysteria
E. Hypothermia
F. Head injury
G. Drug overdose
H. Meningoencephalitis
I. Septicaemia
J. Stroke
K. Alcohol excess
L. Hypoglycaemia

For each of the following questions select the best answer from the list above:

I. A 48-year-old female diabetic is found unconscious in bed. Her husband died recently and she was last seen arguing with her son the previous day. She visited her GP complaining of insomnia a week ago. What is the most likely diagnosis?

II. A 75-year-old female is found unconscious in bed and smells of urine. She is pyrexial (38.5°C) and a urine dipstick shows positive nitrites. What is the most likely diagnosis?

III. An 88-year-old female not seen for several days is found unrousable in her front room on New Year's Day. On examination her pulse is 58 and regular, her BP is 90/60, there are no focal neurological signs but tendon reflexes are depressed. The ECG shows J waves. What is the most likely diagnosis?

Psychological medicine 18

- Patients with psychiatric problems can present with physical manifestations such as depression manifesting as irritable bowel syndrome
- Chronic/severe physical ill health can result in psychological disease such as depression after a stroke
- Psychiatric symptoms can be part of a physical disease such as depression in hypothyroidism
- Patients with psychiatric disease can develop physical problems which may or may not be as a result of their psychiatric disease (e.g. drug overdose) or its treatment (e.g. lithium toxicity)

THE PSYCHIATRIC HISTORY (*K&C*, P. 1274)

The psychiatric history is different in some ways from standard history taking. Corroboration and additional details should be sought from a relative or friend. The history should include the following:

Reason for referral

- Why and how the patient came to the attention of the doctor

Complaints

- As reported by the patient

Present illness

- Detailed account of the illness from its beginning to the present day
- Include the degree of insight on the patient's part

Family history

- Family atmosphere in childhood
- Early stresses (death or separation)
- Mental illness in family members

Personal history

- Short biography of childhood, school, jobs, marriage/divorce and children
- Present housing, social and financial situation

Personality

- Attitudes, beliefs, moral values and standards
- Leisure activities and interests
- Usual reaction to stress and setback

Medical history

- Health in childhood
- Menstrual and sexual history
- Previous mental health
- Use of alcohol, drugs and tobacco

Forensic history

- Legal problems or contact with the police or courts
- Note any violent or sexual offences (risk assessment)

EXAMINING THE MENTAL STATE (*K&C*, P. 1274)

Appearance/general behaviour

- Can give information about mood
- Facial appearance, eye contact, colour of clothes
- Posture
- Movement

Speech

- Disorders of thinking are recognised from speech

Disorders of stream (amount and speed) of thought
Pressure of thought

- Varied ideas arise in abundance
- Characteristic of mania
- Occurs in schizophrenia

Poverty of thought

- Patient reports lack/absence of thoughts

- Characteristic of depression
- Occurs in schizophrenia

Thought blocking

- Abrupt and complete interruption of stream
- Strongly suggests schizophrenia

Disorders of form of thought
Flight of ideas

- Quickly moving from topic to topic
- Distracted by clues in the immediate environment
- Clang associations (using words with similar sounds)
- Punning
- Rhyming

Perseveration

- Persistent and inappropriate repetition
- Occurs in dementia and other conditions

Loosening of associations

- Lack of clarity
- 'Knight's move' thinking
- 'Word salad'

Mood

- Affect/feeling/emotion

Changes in nature of mood

- Depression
- Anxiety
- Elation
- Phobia

Changes in fluctuation of mood

- Loss of emotion (apathy)
- Reduced variation in mood (blunted)
- Rapidly and excessively changeable mood (labile)

Inappropriate mood

- Incongruous mood such as laughing when describing death of close relative

Thought content (worries and preoccupations)
Obsession

- Recurrent persistent thoughts

Compulsion

- Repetitive, seemingly purposeful action
- Must be carried out
- Urge to resist

Insight

- Degree to which patient recognises own illness

Abnormal beliefs and interpretation of events (delusions)

- Delusions are abnormal beliefs arising from distorted judgements
- They are
  - False
  - Held with absolute conviction
  - Not modifiable by reason/experience
- Persecutory delusions – paranoid thoughts
- Delusions of worthlessness/grandeur
- Nihilism
- Thought insertion – the belief that thoughts are implanted from outside
- Thought withdrawal
- Thought broadcasting – the belief that unspoken thoughts are known to others

Abnormal experience referred to the environment, body or self

- Illusions
- Hallucinations
- Depersonalisation – the patient feels 'unreal'/detached/remote
- Derealisation – the external environment feels unreal/remote

Cognitive state/memory

- Assessed using mental test score ('Folstein score') (see Chapter 3)

ORGANIC MENTAL DISORDERS (K&C, P. 1309)

Delirium/toxic confusional state

- Impairment of consciousness associated with abnormalities of perception and mood

Table 18.1 Causes of delirium

Infection Any infection, particularly if high fever	**Drug intoxication** Anticonvulsants Anxiolytics/hypnotics/antidepressants Opiates/dopamine agonists
Metabolic disturbance Electrolyte upset Hepatic/renal failure Hypoxia	Digoxin **Drug/alcohol withdrawal** **Postoperative states**
Endocrine Hypoglycaemia Cushing's syndrome	**Vitamin deficiency** Thiamine (Wernicke–Korsakoff syndrome) Nicotinic acid (pellagra) Vitamin B_{12}
Intracranial Trauma Tumour Abscess Subarachnoid haemorrhage Epilepsy	

Aetiology

- See Table 18.1

Clinical features

- Acute – clears within days
- Fluctuant with lucid periods
- Worse at night
- Visual hallucinations may occur
- Patient is frightened, suspicious, restless and uncooperative
- More common in elderly patients

Investigations

- To determine underlying cause
- Bloods
  - Full blood count (FBC)
  - Urea and electrolytes (U&E), glucose, liver function tests (LFTs), calcium
  - Vitamin B_{12}
  - Thyroid function tests
- Blood & urine cultures
- ECG
- Chest X-ray
- CT of brain

Management

- Treat underlying cause
- Nurse carefully in a well-lit area

- Communicate clearly and concisely
- Give repeated information to orientate (family/carers can be useful for this)
- Ensure adequate hydration
- Sedate only if necessary, e.g. haloperidol i.m.
- Paracetamol if febrile
- Review all drugs and stop all but essential ones

Management of the agitated patient
Suggested by

- Agitated patient who is likely to harm him/herself or others

Emergency treatment

- Talk calmly to patient: if this fails, get help to restrain him/her
- Check blood sugar, oximetry, coma scale and for focal neurological deficit
- If not hypoglycaemic or hypoxic and has good coma scale with no focal neurology, then consider sedation with 5 mg i.m. haloperidol (repeat up to 20 mg if needed)
- If alcohol or benzodiazepine withdrawal likely, then use lorazepam 2 mg

Initial investigations

- Bloods – FBC, U&E, glucose, calcium, LFTs
- Blood and urine cultures if sepsis suggested
- Measure arterial blood gases
- ECG
- Chest X-ray

Dementia

- Progressive decline of cognitive function in the absence of clouded consciousness

Aetiology

- See Table 18.2

Differential diagnosis

- Depression

Investigations

- Blood
  - FBC
  - U&E, glucose, LFTs, calcium

Table 18.2 Causes of dementia

Degenerative	**Toxic**
Alzheimer's disease (65%)	Alcohol
Dementia with Lewy bodies (25%)	Occupational
Frontotemporal dementia	Lead or mercury poisoning
Huntington's disease	
Parkinson's disease	**Traumatic**
Normal pressure hydrocephalus	Boxing (punch drunk syndrome)
Primary progressive aphasia	
	Vitamin deficiency
Vascular	Thiamine
Cerebrovascular disease	Vitamin B_{12}
Cerebral vasculitis/cranial arteritis	
	Infections
Metabolic	Creutzfeldt–Jakob disease
Uraemia	HIV
Hepatic failure	Syphilis
Remote effects of carcinoma	Whipple's disease
Endocrine	**Psychiatric**
Hypothyroidism	Pseudodementia
Hypocalcaemia	
Intracranial	
Subdural haematoma	
Tumour	

- ESR, C-reactive protein
- Red cell folate, vitamin B_{12}
- Thyroid function tests
- Syphilis serology
- HIV antibodies if indicated and patient counselled
❙ Chest X-ray
❙ CT/MRI

Alzheimer's disease
Neuropathology

❙ Neuronal loss
❙ Neurofibrillary tangles
❙ Senile plaques
❙ Amyloid deposition

Aetiology

❙ Early onset – may be familial linkage to chromosomes 1, 14 and 21
❙ Late onset – ?apolipoprotein E gene

Clinical features

- Inability to learn new information or recall previously learnt information
- Decline in language, particularly names
- Apraxia – unable to carry out motor functions
- Agnosia – unable to identify/recognise objects
- Impairment of organizing/sequencing
- Behavioural change – wandering, agitation, aggression
- Paranoia and loss of insight

Management

- Cholinesterase inhibitors and drugs blocking glutamate transmission slow the rate of decline slightly but their use is clouded by complex cost–benefit arguments

Dementia with Lewy bodies
Clinical features

- Second commonest cause of dementia
- Fluctuating cognition with pronounced variation in attention/alertness
- Memory loss uncommon in early stages
- Sleep disorders, visual hallucinations, delusions and transient loss of consciousness

Management

- Avoid neuroleptic drugs

Vascular dementia/multi-infarct dementia
Clinical features

- History of transient ischaemic attacks or stroke
- Features depend on the site of ischaemic damage

Management

- Stroke prevention measures including anti-platelet drugs

SCHIZOPHRENIA (*K&C*, P. 1307)

- Abnormal integration of emotional and cognitive functions

Epidemiology

- 2–4/1000 annual incidence
- 1% lifetime risk

Aetiology

- Genetic – lifetime risk in patients with a parent affected is 12%
- Altered neurotransmitters
  - ↑ Dopamine activity
  - Altered serotonin metabolism
- Environmental triggers
  - High expressed emotion
  - More common in patients born in winter/ spring
  - Cannabis use is a possible risk factor

Clinical features

- Peak onset early twenties
- ♀ = ♂

Diagnosis

- Based on presence of first-rank symptoms:
- Auditory hallucinations
- Thought withdrawal
- Thought insertion
- Thought broadcasting
- Delusions
- External controlled emotions
- Somatic passivity and feelings (feeling that thoughts and acts are due to the influence of others)

Subtypes

Positive schizophrenia
- Acute onset
- Prominent delusions and hallucinations
- Good response to neuroleptics
- Better prognosis

Negative schizophrenia
- Insidious deterioration in personality
- Relative absence of acute symptoms
- Delusions and hallucinations absent
- Increasing apathy and eccentricity
- Slow withdrawal from society
- Poor response to neuroleptics

Management

- Combination of drug and social treatment delivered by multidisciplinary team

Table 18.3 Unwanted effects of neuroleptic drugs

Common effects

Extrapyramidal
Acute dystonia
Parkinsonism
Akathisia (restless, repetitive and irresistible need to move)
Tardive dyskinesia (mouthing and smacking of the lips, grimaces and contortions of the face/neck)

Autonomic
Hypotension
Failure of ejaculation

Anticholinergic
Dry mouth
Urinary retention
Constipation
Blurred vision

Metabolic
Weight gain

Rare effects

Hypersensitivity
Cholestatic jaundice
Leucopenia
Skin reactions

Others
Precipitation of glaucoma
Galactorrhoea
Amenorrhoea
Cardiac arrhythmias
Seizures
Retinal degeneration (high-dose thioridazine)

Neuroleptic malignant syndrome
Hyperthermia
Muscle rigidity
Tachycardia
Labile BP
Pallor
Elevated white cell count, creatine kinase, liver function tests
Treatment: lower temperature, bromocriptine, dantrolene

Drugs ▮ Antipsychotics/neuroleptics
  – Dopamine antagonists (chlorpromazine, haloperidol); unwanted side-effects are shown in Table 18.3
  – Atypical anti-psychotics (clozapine, risperidone, olanzapine) have less extrapyramidal side effects

Psychological treatment ▮ Reassurance and support

Social treatment ▮ Structured work and social programme

MOOD (AFFECTIVE) DISORDERS (K&C, P. 1288)

▮ Spectrum of disorders ranging from depression through to mania
▮ Patients who suffer attacks of both have bipolar disorder (Fig. 18.1)

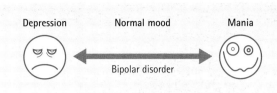

Fig. 18.1 Bipolar disorder.

Aetiology

Physical
- Genetic – monozygotic twin concordance 30–60%
- Neurotransmitter imbalance – downregulation of 5 HT receptors in depression
- Hormonal
  - cortisol (Cushing's syndrome induces depression and corticosteroids alter mood, moreover hypercortisolaemia occurs in patients with depression
  - Oral contraceptives/pregnancy/premenstrual
- CNS abnormalities – brain MRI/PET studies show:
  - increased ventricular volume, frontal lobe atrophy and altered blood flow
  - volume reduction in the hippocampus

Psychological
- Maternal deprivation
- Learned helplessness

Social
- Stressful life events e.g. divorce, unemployment
- Sexual abuse in childhood

Clinical features

- See Table 18.4
- Range of severity (Fig. 18.2)
  - Severe life-threatening disease
  - Minor forms

Differential diagnosis

Mania

- Drug-induced psychosis
  - Amphetamines/ecstasy/cocaine
  - Long term cannabis use
  - Steroids
- Acute schizophrenia
- Hyperthyroidism/Cushing's syndrome

Table 18.4 Clinical features of depression and mania

Characteristic	Depression	Mania
Mood	Depressed Miserable Unhappy	Elevated Labile Irritable
Talk	Slow Impoverished Monotonous	Fast Pressurised Flight of ideas
Energy	Reduced Apathetic/lethargic	Excessive

Ideation	Feelings of
	  Futility
	  Guilt
	  Self-reproach
	  Unworthiness
	Hypochondriasis
	Worrying
	Suicidal thoughts
	Delusions of guilt
	Nihilism
	Persecution
		Grandiose
		Self-confident
		Delusions of
		  Wealth
		  Power
		  Influence
		  Religious significance
		Persecutory delusions

Cognition	Impaired learning Pseudodementia if elderly	Disturbance of registration of memories
Physical	Early waking Poor appetite Weight loss Constipation Loss of libido Erectile dysfunction Fatigue Bodily aches and pains	Insomnia Weight loss
Behaviour	Poverty of movement/ expression Retardation/agitation	Disinhibition Increased sexual interest
Hallucinations	Auditory Hostile Critical	Excessive drinking/spending Fleeting auditory Occasionally visual

Depression

▌ Malignancy
▌ Hypothyroidism/hyperparathyroidism
▌ Cushing's syndrome
▌ Neurological diseases (multiple sclerosis, Parkinson's)
▌ Cerebral ischaemia or tumour
▌ Heart failure

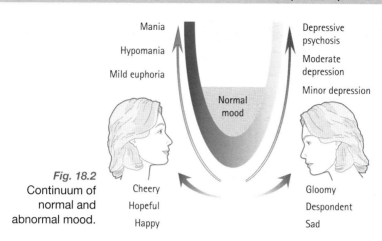

Fig. 18.2
Continuum of
normal and
abnormal mood.

Mania
Hypomania
Mild euphoria

Depressive
psychosis
Moderate
depression
Minor depression

Normal
mood

Cheery
Hopeful
Happy

Gloomy
Despondent
Sad

Table 18.5 Clinical features of normal grief reaction and depressive illness after bereavement (morbid grief reaction)

Characteristic	Normal bereavement	Morbid grief reaction
Onset	Immediately after loss	Delayed for weeks/months
Duration	Weeks	Months/years
Pattern	Slow acceptance and adjustment	Denial of loss and refusal to accept implications
Grief	Expressed openly	Expressed with difficulty
Guilt	Mild regret in early stage	Marked guilt often present

❚ Porphyria
❚ Drugs
  – Steroids
❚ Psychiatric disorders
  – Schizophrenia
  – Alcohol/drug (e.g. amphetamines) misuse or
    withdrawal
  – Borderline personality disorder
  – Dementia
❚ Normal bereavement reaction (Table 18.5)

Management (*K&C*, P. 1291)
Physical

❚ Stop depressing drugs including alcohol
❚ Regular exercise (good for mild/mod
  depression)

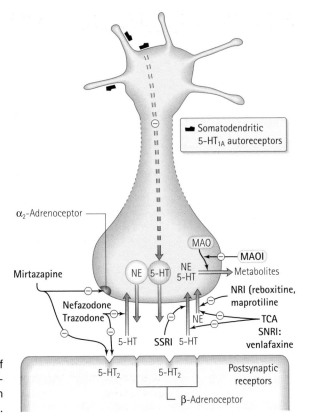

Fig. 18.3 Sites of action of anti-depressants with examples.

Depression (see Fig. 18.3)

▌ Drugs – choice depends on side-effects and safety
  – Serotonin reuptake inhibitors, e.g. fluoxetine
  – Tricyclic antidepressants (TCAs), e.g. amytriptyline; see Table 18.6 for unwanted effects
  – New generation antidepressants e.g. venlafaxine – serotonin and noradrenaline receptor blocker, mirtazapine increases both noradrenaline and selective serotonin transmission noradrenaline reuptake inhibitors, e.g. reboxetine
  – Monoamine oxidase inhibitors, e.g. phenelzine – used 2nd line

▌ Electroconvulsive therapy (ECT)
  – Used in life-threatening depression

Table 18.6 Unwanted effects of drugs used in affective disorders

Tricyclic antidepressants	Lithium
Anticholinergic effects	GI symptoms
Dry mouth	Hypothyroidism
Constipation	Fine tremor
Tremor	Weight gain (increased appetite)
Blurred vision	Polyuria/polydipsia
Urinary retention	Toxic symptoms
Postural hypotension	Drowsiness
Cardiac effects	Blurred vision
ECG changes	Tremor
Arrhythmias	Ataxia
Lowered seizure threshold	Dysarthria
Weight gain	Convulsions
Sedation	Coma and death
Mania	

Mania

▌ Acute attacks
- Lithium – Table 18.6 lists unwanted effects
- Neuroleptic drugs for severe hyperactivity, e.g. haloperidol

▌ Prophylaxis
- Lithium
- Regular check on drug levels (narrow therapeutic window)
- Regular check on renal function (renal excretion)
- Regular check on thyroid function
- Carbamazepine
- Valproate

Psychological

▌ Psychotherapy
▌ Cognitive/behavioural therapy

Social

▌ Assistance with social problems
▌ Group support
▌ Stress management
▌ Family/carer support

PUERPERAL AFFECTIVE DISORDERS
(*K&C*, P. 1291)

- Childbirth has a higher relative risk of depression than life events or physical illness
- Treatment of these disorders is as for any other affective disorder

Maternity blues
Clinical features

- Brief episodes of emotional lability, irritability and tearfulness
- Occurs in 50% of women 2–3 days post-partum
- Resolves spontaneously

Postpartum psychosis
Clinical features

- 1 in 500–1000 births
- Onset usually within 2 weeks of birth
- Classical features of affective psychosis plus confusion and disorientation
- If severe, patient may have delusions that child is deformed, evil or affected in another way which can lead to suicide or infanticide
- Responds well to treatment
- 20–30% recur in next puerperium

Postnatal depression
Clinical features

- Depression occurs in 10% of mothers in first post-partum year
- Clinically similar to other depressive illness
- Recovery after a few months

SUICIDE AND DELIBERATE SELF-HARM
(*K&C*, P. 1296)

Suicide
Risk factors

- Living alone
- Immigrant status
- Recent bereavement/separation/divorce
- Unemployment/retirement

Table 18.7 For deliberate self-harm-patients – indications for referral to psychiatrist

Absolute indications
Clinical depression
Psychosis
Clearly pre-planned suicide attempts
Persistent suicidal intent
Violent method used

Relative indications
Alcohol/drug abuse
Patients with risk factors for suicide (see above)
Patients with family history of suicide
Patients with serious (particularly incurable) physical illnesses
Those in whom there is a major unresolved crisis
Persistent suicide attempts
Any patient giving concern

- Male sex
- Older age
- Family or previous history of
  - Affective disorder
  - Suicide
  - Alcohol abuse
- Previous suicide attempt
- Drug/alcohol addiction
- Severe depression/early dementia
- Incapacitating, painful physical illness

Deliberate self-harm (DSH)
- ♀ > ♂
- Most patients < 35 years
- 90% involve self-poisoning
- Formal psychiatric disorder is unusual
- 1–2% kill themselves in the following year
- Assessment procedure – see Chapter 3
- Indications for referral to psychiatric team – see Table 18.7

NEUROSES AND STRESS-RELATED/SOMATOFORM DISORDERS (*K&C*, P. 1297)

Anxiety disorder
Clinical features
- See Table 18.8

Table 18.8 Clinical features of anxiety

Physical	*Nervous system*
Gastrointestinal	Fatigue
Dry mouth	Blurred vision
Dysphagia	Dizziness
Epigastric pain	Headache
Flatulence/aerophagy	Sleep disturbance
Diarrhoea	
	Psychological
Respiratory	Apprehension and fear
Sensation of chest constriction	Irritability
Difficulty inhaling	Difficulty concentrating
Over-breathing	Distractibility
	Restlessness
Cardiovascular	Sensitivity to noise
Palpitations, awareness of missed beat	Depression
Chest pain	Depersonalisation
	Derealisation
Genitourinary	
Frequency	
Failure of erection	
Lack of libido	

Differential diagnosis

Psychiatric disorders
- Depression
- Obsessive compulsive disorder
- Schizophrenia
- Dementia
- Drug/alcohol dependence
- Benzodiazepine withdrawal

Physical disorders
- Hyperthyroidism
- Hypoglycaemia
- Phaeochromocytoma

Management

Psychological
- Reassurance about physical symptoms
- Relaxation techniques
- Anxiety management training
- Biofeedback
- Behaviour therapies
- Cognitive behavioural therapy

Drugs
- Selective serotonin reuptake inhibitors (SSRIs)
- β-blockers for physical symptoms
- Short courses of benzodiazepines

Obsessive compulsive disorder

- Characterised by obsessional thinking and compulsive behaviour with varying degrees of anxiety/depression and depersonalisation

Clinical features

- Persistent and intrusive obsessions/compulsions
- Functioning impeded
- Constant need to check
- Repetitive/superstitious actions

Management

- Behaviour therapy
  - Response prevention
  - Modelling
- Serotonin reuptake inhibitors (may need higher doses than those used in depression)

Dissociative (conversion) disorder (previously known as hysteria)

- Characterised by
  - Absence of physical pathology
  - Unconscious production
  - Triggered by an unresolved conflict or life event
  - Absence of sympathetic overactivity

Table 18.9 Common dissociative/conversion symptoms

Dissociative (mental)	Conversion (physical)
Amnesia	Paralysis
Fugue	Gait disorder
Pseudodementia	Tremor
Dissociative identity disorder	Aphonia
Psychosis	Mutism
	Sensory symptoms
	Globus hystericus
	Hysterical fits
	Blindness

Clinical features

- ♀ > ♂
- Rarely occurs in those > 40 years
- See Table 18.9
- May confer advantage (secondary gain)
- Patients' emotional distress is less than expected

Management

- Psychotherapy

Somatoform disorders

▌ Patients
- Repeatedly present with physical problems
- Have repeatedly negative findings on clinical investigation
- Have no demonstrable physical cause

Clinical features

Hypochondriasis
▌ Preoccupation with ill health
▌ Disproportionate and unjustified concern

Somatisation disorder
▌ Repeatedly present with a variety of medical symptoms
▌ Undergo repeated investigations/operations
▌ May have medical connections

Management

▌ Explain and reassure
▌ Explore psychological/social problems
▌ Avoid repeated investigations
▌ Graded exercise programmes
▌ Trial of an antidepressant

Acute stress reaction and post-traumatic stress disorder

▌ Occur in individuals in response to exceptional physical or psychological stress

Acute stress reaction

▌ Lasts a few hours/days
▌ Initial state of 'daze'
▌ Then a phase of either
- Withdrawal/stupor *or*
- Agitation/over-activity
▌ Commonly associated with autonomic signs of anxiety

Post-traumatic stress disorder

▌ Delayed/protracted response to a stressful event
▌ 'Flashbacks'
▌ Intense distress in/avoidance of situations resembling the event (including anniversaries)
▌ Emotional blunting/numbness
▌ Detachment from others
▌ Hypervigilance
▌ Insomnia
▌ Anxiety and depression
▌ Occasionally suicide

Management

▋ Counselling

DRUG AND ALCOHOL ABUSE AND DEPENDENCE
(*K&C*, P. 1302)

▋ Current evidence suggests that drinking up to 21 units a week (for men) or 14 units a week for women carries no long-term health risk

Alcohol dependence syndrome
Clinical features

▋ Compulsive need to drink
▋ Altered alcohol tolerance
▋ Stereotyped pattern of drinking
▋ Drinking takes primacy over other activities
▋ Repeated withdrawal symptoms
▋ Relief drinking to avoid withdrawal, e.g. early morning drinking
▋ Rapid relapse if patient drinks again following a period of abstinence

Management

Psychosocial support and group therapy
▋ E.g. Alcoholics Anonymous

Drugs (effects are enhanced by combining them with counselling)
▋ Naltrexone reduces the risk of relapse into heavy drinking and the frequency of drinking
▋ Acamprosate alters neurotransmitters and reduces drinking frequency
▋ Disulfiram (Antabuse) reacts with alcohol to form acetaldehyde which produces unpleasant symptoms to discourage drinking

Drug abuse

▋ For commonly used illicit drugs the desired and adverse effects are shown in Table 18.10

Management

▋ Withdrawal programmes, e.g. using methadone
▋ Psychosocial support to help the addict live without drugs

Table 18.10 Desired and adverse effects of commonly used 'illicit' drugs

Drug	Desired effects	Adverse effects
Solvents ('glue sniffing')	Euphoria Floating sensation	Amnesia Visual hallucinations Inhalation of vomit Bone marrow/brain/liver/kidney toxicity Tolerance
Amphetamines	Stimulant Euphoria	Psychological dependence Restlessness Over-activity Paranoid psychosis
Cocaine	Stimulant Hyperarousal	Dependence Paranoid ideation Fits Coronary artery spasm/disease Perforation of nasal septum if inhaled
Cannabis	Exaggeration of pre-existing mood	No definite withdrawal syndrome or tolerance Psychosis
MDMA ('Ecstasy')	Psychedelic effects	Hyperpyrexia Acute hepatic/renal failure Possible chronic brain damage
Hypnotics (e.g. benzodiazepines)	Relaxation Sleep induction	Dependence Withdrawal syndrome Respiratory depression

Narcotics (morphine, heroin, codeine, methadone, pethidine)	Calm
	Slight euphoria
	Analgesia
	Flattening of emotions
		Marked and rapid tolerance
		Withdrawal syndrome
		Respiratory depression
		Complications of injecting
		  Infection (e.g. HIV/hepatitis B and C/endocarditis)
		  Vein thrombosis

EATING DISORDERS (K&C, P. 1310)

Anorexia nervosa
Aetiology

▌ Genetic
▌ Childhood sexual abuse
▌ Dietary problems in early life
▌ Social factors
 – Higher social class
 – Occupation – ballet dancers/nurses

Clinical features

- BMI (body mass index) <17.5
- Intense wish to be thin
- Morbid fear of fatness
- Amenorrhoea in women
- ♀ ≫ ♂
- Onset in adolescence, rare > 30 years
- Previous history of chubbiness/fatness
- Relentless pursuit of low body weight
- Distorted image of own body
- Eats little
- Avoids carbohydrates
- Vomiting/excess exercise/purging
- Loss of sexual interest
- Lanugo hair

Management

- Behaviour therapy – goal setting/reward for weight/dietary intake
- Psychotherapy
- Family therapy

Bulimia nervosa
Clinical features

- Binge eating
- Self-induced vomiting
- Laxative abuse
- Misuse of drugs, e.g. diuretics, thyroxine, anorectics
- ♀ ≫ ♂
- Often associated with anorexia nervosa
- Premorbid personality – neurotic traits
- May be associated with
  - Depression
  - Alcohol dependence
- Fluctuation in body weight
- Periods irregular

Consequences of vomiting

- Cardiac arrhythmias
- Renal impairment secondary to low K^+
- Muscular paralysis
- Tetany – hypokalaemic alkalosis
- Swollen salivary glands
- Eroded dental enamel

Table 18.11 Important sections of the Mental Health Act 1983

Section	Duration	Signatures required	Purpose
2	28 days	2 doctors (1 approved) plus nearest relative or social worker	Assessment and treatment
3	6 months	2 doctors (1 approved) plus nearest relative or social worker	Treatment
4	72 hours	1 doctor plus relative or social worker	Emergency admission
5(2)	72 hours	Doctor in charge of patient's care	Emergency detention of a patient already in hospital
5(4)	6 hours	Nurse (RMN)	Emergency detention of a patient already in hospital
136	72 hours	Police officer	Psychiatric assessment of patients in public places

Management

▋ Cognitive behaviour therapy
▋ SSRIs

PSYCHIATRY AND THE LAW (*K&C*, P. 1313)

Compulsory section under the Mental Health Act
Conditions

▋ For a patient to be held against his/her will under the Mental Health Act he/she must be
  – Suffering from a defined mental disorder
  – A risk to his/her and/or other people's health or safety
  – Unwilling to accept hospitalisation voluntarily

Sections

▋ See Table 18.11 for details

SELF-ASSESSMENT QUESTIONS

Best one of five questions

1. Of these first-rank symptoms of schizophrenia which also occurs in mania:
   A. Thought broadcasting
   B. Thought withdrawal
   C. Thought insertion
   D. Auditory hallucinations
   E. Persecutory delusions

2. In dementia the following are correct:
   A. Consciousness is clouded
   B. Multi-infarct dementia is the commonest cause
   C. Depression is a differential diagnosis
   D. Dementia with Lewy bodies accounts for 40%
   E. A CT scan is not indicated

3. The following management strategies in toxic confusional state may exacerbate the problem:
   A. Establish a corroborative history from a witness
   B. Nurse the patient in a darkened room
   C. Prescription of appropriate intravenous fluids if not drinking
   D. Minimise polypharmacy
   E. Prescription of antibiotics

4. In depression:
   A. Patients sleep well
   B. Patients usually have increased sexual interest
   C. Patients may have auditory hallucinations if disease is severe
   D. Monozygotic twin concordance is only 10% for unipolar depression
   E. Most patients are treated with psychotherapy alone

5. The following features of mania may also be seen in thyrotoxicosis:
   A. Delusions of wealth
   B. Weight loss
   C. Excessive drinking
   D. Flight of ideas
   E. Critical hallucinations

6. Lithium:
   A. Is used to prevent depression
   B. 50% undergoes renal excretion
   C. Causes hyperthyroidism
   D. Needs therapeutic drug level monitoring
   E. Is used to treat acute attacks of depression

7. The following are factors that increase the risk of suicide:
   A. Female sex
   B. Young age
   C. No previous history of depression
   D. Living with a large extended family
   E. A family history of suicide

8. In deliberate self-harm:
   A. 75% is by self-poisoning
   B. There is often an associated psychiatric disorder
   C. Patients with depression should be referred to a psychiatrist

D. A violent method makes suicide less likely

E. Patients who planned to be discovered are at higher risk of suicide

9. The following are physical symptoms of anxiety disorder except:
   A. Chest pain
   B. Diarrhoea
   C. Erectile dysfunction
   D. Urinary frequency
   E. Jaundice

10. Anorexia nervosa:
    A. Patients often have a BMI of over 30
    B. Patients have usually been thin since childhood
    C. Is more common in higher social classes
    D. Amenorrhoea occurs late in the disease
    E. Patients think they are thin

11. Regarding the sections of the Mental Health Act:
    A. Section 2 allows patients to be held for 6 months
    B. Section 3 is for psychiatric assessment only
    C. Section 5(2) relates to patients already in hospital
    D. Section 5(2) allows the patient to be detained for 6 hours
    E. Section 2 requires the signatures of one doctor and a social worker/relative

12. The following statements are correct:
    A. Obsessive compulsive disorder responds to low-dose serotonin reuptake inhibitors

B. Paralysis is a common symptom of a conversion disorder

C. Conversion disorder is produced consciously

D. Post-traumatic stress disorder occurs immediately after a stressful event

E. In acute stress reaction bradycardia is usual

13. The following are effects of illicit drugs:
    A. Cocaine causes hyperarousal
    B. Amphetamines induce sleep
    C. Cannabis use is associated with a withdrawal syndrome
    D. The development of tolerance to heroin is slow
    E. MDMA has no long term side effects

14. The following statements are correct about alcohol withdrawal:
    A. Delirium tremens occurs within hours of alcohol cessation
    B. Delirium tremens can be treated as an outpatient
    C. Acamprosate will help maintain abstinence
    D. Prevention with Disulfiram is usually effective
    E. Drugs to prevent alcohol dependence are enhanced by combining them with counselling

15. Antidepressant drugs:
    A. Are safe in overdose
    B. SSRIs are used in all patients
    C. Choice of drug depends on the side-effect profile

D. Tricyclic antidepressants are effective within a few days of starting treatment

E. Venlafaxine has no effect on serotonin

Extended matching questions

Question 1 *Theme: agitation*

A. Acute confusional state
B. Acute mania
C. Puerperal psychosis
D. Schizophrenia
E. Obsessive compulsive disorder
F. Alzheimer's disease
G. Anxiety disorder
H. Alcohol withdrawal syndrome
I. Cocaine abuse
J. Somatisation disorder

For each of the following questions, select the best answer from the list above:

I. A 59-year-old female smoker who lives with her husband presents with agitation. On direct questioning she cannot remember details of the distant past although her short-term memory seems intact. She has lost weight but there are no other physical signs or symptoms. What is the most likely diagnosis?

II. A 23-year-old female who was born in Jamaica but has lived in the UK since the age of 8 attends the accident and emergency department alone; she is agitated. She appears to have threatening auditory hallucinations. She also says that she is having difficulty sleeping. The casualty records show a previous attendance at a psychiatric outpatient clinic 2 years ago. The limited physical examination she allows is normal. What is the most likely diagnosis?

III. A 48-year-old male presents with agitation. On direct questioning he admits to visual hallucinations. He has a previous history of gastrointestinal bleeding. On examination he is sweaty and the pulse rate is 110/min. Blood tests reveal the following: Hb 14.4, MCV 101. What is the most likely diagnosis?

Question 2 *Theme: hallucinations*

A. Acute confusional state
B. Acute mania
C. Puerperal psychosis
D. Schizophrenia
E. Obsessive compulsive disorder
F. Alzheimer's disease
G. Anxiety disorder
H. Alcohol withdrawal syndrome
I. Amphetamine abuse
J. Somatisation disorder

For each of the following questions, select the best answer from the list above:

I. A 26-year-old man who lives with his mother presents with auditory hallucinations. He has recently been made redundant after he was said to be acting strangely at work. There are no physical signs or symptoms. He reports that he thinks people can hear his thoughts. On direct questioning his hallucinations are persecutory in nature. What is the most likely diagnosis?

II. A 33-year-old male attends the accident and emergency department alone and agitated. He appears to have paranoid auditory hallucinations. He also says that he is having difficulty sleeping. The A&E records show a previous attendance 2 years ago with an overdose of benzodiazepines. He denies problems with alcohol use now or in the past. The physical examination he allows is normal. What is the most likely diagnosis?

III. A 45-year-old male presents with agitation and complaining that he cannot sleep. He has recently been dismissed from his job. His wife is very upset and is accusing him of spending huge amounts of money and of having an affair. On direct questioning he admits to fleeting auditory hallucinations. He has lost weight and reports increased libido. What is the most likely diagnosis?

Question 3 *Theme: psychiatric treatments*

A. A tricyclic antidepressant
B. A selective serotonin reuptake inhibitor
C. ECT
D. Lithium
E. A monoamine oxidase inhibitor
F. Venlafaxine
G. Cognitive Behavioural Therapy
H. Carbamazepine
I. Chlorpromazine
J. Clozapine

For each of the following questions, select the best answer from the list above:

I. A 59-year-old female who lives with her husband presents with symptoms of depression. Her husband has just been diagnosed with lung cancer. She is overweight but there are no other physical signs or symptoms. What would be the most appropriate choice of treatment?

II. A 22-year-old female presents with an episode of hyperventilation. She describes panic attacks when trying to leave the house. The limited physical examination she allows is normal. You diagnose an anxiety disorder. She is unkeen to take any drug treatment. What would be the most appropriate choice of treatment?

III. A 48-year-old man is known to have bipolar disorder. He had been on lithium but was recently found to be hypothyroid so the lithium had been stopped. He requires another drug for his returning symptoms of mania. What would be the most appropriate choice of treatment?

Statistics and evidence-based medicine 19

The epidemiology of a disease is a description of the demographics of the affected population and the environment from which they originate. Statistical analysis is the manipulation of data about a patient group designed to reveal similarities or differences between groups of differing patients or between treatment types. Statistical analysis is also used to describe details about a population.

TYPES OF DATA

Nominal

- Mutually exclusive groups
  - Male or female

Ordinal

- Ranked exclusive groups
  - Mild/moderate/severe

Continuous

- Numerical values that may be anywhere along a continuum
  - Age

Descriptional statistics

- A method of describing a population or a sample from that population

Mean

- The mathematical average of a set of numerical data

Mode

- The most commonly occurring value

Median

▮ The middle number when the data set is arranged in numerical order
▮ If there is an even number of values it is the mean of the middle two

Sample mean

▮ The mathematical average of a variable measured in a sample

Population mean

▮ The mean calculated if the entire population under study were measured
▮ Note: this is rarely achievable

Distribution

▮ The pattern of spread of values
▮ Many biological values fit a 'normal' or Gaussian distribution, a bell-shaped curve

Normal distribution

▮ A symmetrical 'bell-shaped' curve distribution where the mean, mode and median are the same (Fig. 19.1)

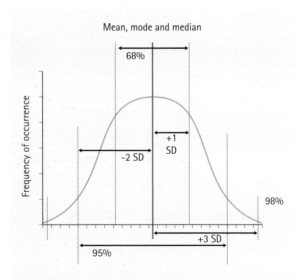

Fig. 19.1 Gaussian or normal distribution. This is symmetrical about the mean. Sixty-eight per cent of all values in the data set fall within ±1 standard deviation (SD), 95% between ±2 SD and 99% between ±3 SD. This is often described as the bell-shaped curve.

Skewed distribution

▌ Very high or low values may result in an asymmetrical distribution leading to a positive (high value) or negative (low value) skew (Fig. 19.2)

Variance

▌ Describes the spread of values either side of a mean

Standard deviation

▌ Gives the range of values within which a certain proportion of the sample will lie
▌ 68% will lie ±1 SD from the mean
▌ 95% will lie ±2 SD from the mean
▌ 99% will lie ±3 SD from the mean

Standard error

▌ The range within which the population mean will lie based on the sample mean
▌ It allows an estimation of the range in which the true population mean will lie when a

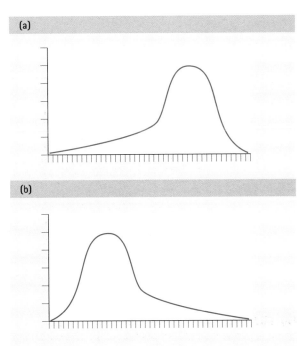

Fig. 19.2 Distributions. A. Negative skew. B. Positive skew.

representative sample from that population is analysed

Comparative statistics

❚ Allows data from two groups to be compared, with the aim of determining whether they originated from the same population or not, or, in the context of a trial, whether the differences between them are due to luck or really exist

Hypothesis

❚ The concept being tested

Null hypothesis

❚ That no difference exists between the two samples being analysed

Bias

❚ Inequalities between the groups being compared that lead to incorrect conclusions being reached

Errors in experimental design that cause incorrect results
Type 1 error

❚ A false positive result
❚ A difference is found between two groups where one does not exist

Type 2 error

❚ A false negative result
❚ No difference is detected although one does exist

Parametric data

❚ Data values fit a normal distribution

Statistical tests

❚ Tests that provide a probability value
❚ This value (the 'p' value) is the probability that the two sets of data being compared are from the same population or that no difference exists between them
❚ Statistical significance is stated to be a probability of 1 in 20 or lower that the two groups are the same ($p = 0.05$)

	Disease present	Disease absent	*Totals*
Treatment given	9	41	*50*
Placebo given	39	11	*50*
Totals	*50*	*50*	**100**

Fig. 19.3 The 2 × 2 table and Chi squared tests. If you consider a disease for which a treatment is given, 100 patients enter a study and are randomised to receive the treatment or a placebo. The groups are mutually exclusive. An individual cannot be in more than one group. A 2 × 2 table can then be drawn up of the outcomes. In this example, 50 patients received the treatment and 41 were cured, as were 11 of those who received the placebo. Analysis of this data can be carried out using a Chi squared test in order to determine whether the treatment is statistically better than the placebo.

Parametric tests

- Used on data following a normal distribution, e.g.
  - Student t test
  - Paired t test

Non-parametric tests

- Used on non-normally distributed data
  - Unpaired: Mann–Whitney
  - Paired: Wilcoxon

Nominal tests

- If data can be placed in a 2 × 2 square, for example, the response to a treatment or placebo (see Fig. 19.3) – then a Chi squared test can be used

95% confidence intervals

- The 95% confidence interval is the range of values around the mean within which the true population mean will lie in 95% of cases
- It is calculated from the standard error. We can state that in 95% of cases, the population mean will lie ±2 standard errors from our sample mean
- Data can therefore be expressed as a mean and 95% confidence interval, the values being the range provided by the mean ±2 standard errors

Correlation and regression (Fig. 19.4)
Correlation coefficient

- Reports on the relationship between two variables

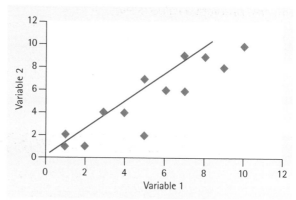

Fig. 19.4 Correlation and regression. When two variables are plotted against each other, a scatter plot results. A line of best fit can then be drawn through these points and the accuracy of the relationship between the two variables can be calculated based on the variance between each data point and the best fit line. This is the correlation coefficient.

- A value of 1 suggests a completely linear relationship
- 0 suggests that no relationship exists between them

Regression

- Allows calculation of the equation of a line drawn when two variables are plotted against each other
- Once this equation is defined, the value of one variable can be calculated when the other is known

Accuracy of test values
Normal range

- For any variable there is usually a range of normal values, usually defined as the mean value ± 2 or 3 standard deviations

Sensitivity

- The ability of a test to report an abnormal result when the disease is present
- It reports on what proportion of patients with a disease will have a positive test

Specificity

- The ability of a test to return a normal result when the disease is absent
- It reports on what proportion of patients without the disease will have a negative test

Positive predictive value (PPV)

▌ The proportion of positive tests where the disease is actually present

▌ A high PPV suggests that if the test is positive, then the disease is present, i.e. there are few false positives

CLINICAL TRIALS

▌ Designed to compare the effect of a therapy with either a placebo (i.e. an inactive substance) or another therapy

Randomisation

▌ Each patient entered into the trial has an equal chance of being in each of the therapy groups in the trial

Controlled trial

▌ Comparison of one therapy against another or a placebo

Blinded

▌ Patients do not know which therapy they are receiving

Double blind

▌ Neither the doctor nor the patient knows which therapy is being received

Bias

▌ Inequalities between the two groups other than the difference in therapy that they are receiving

Publication bias

▌ Failure of negative trials to be published, so only positive data about a therapy reaches the public domain

Intention to treat

▌ The analysis of the trial data includes all patients entered, irrespective of whether they completed the treatment course

Crossover trials

- Each subject undergoes both types of therapy, one after the other
- A comparison can then be made for each individual patient

EVIDENCE-BASED MEDICINE

Definition

- The conscientious, explicit and judicious use of current best evidence in making decisions about the care of individual patients

Role

- EBM leads to patient care guided by the best available data on therapies available, but it is specific to the patient; in other words it aims to take into account differences between individual patients
  - If a trial on hypertension were carried out in male Caucasians, its results may not be true of African women.

Resources
Cochrane Collaboration

- A collection of critical appraisals of trials on specific therapies

Medline/Pubmed/Index Medicus

- Databases of biomedical studies published worldwide

Critical appraisal

- The analysis of all the trials that have studied the same therapy in the same disease with a conclusion about the overall role of that therapy
- In general, only randomised controlled, preferably blinded trials are included and an intention to treat analysis is carried out

Relative risk

- The percentage change in the probability of an event occurring due to the therapy given
- If the chance of a stroke on aspirin is 2% and the chance off aspirin is 4%, the relative risk of a stroke

on aspirin is 50% (the proportion of strokes that would have been avoided)

▮ A relative risk of 100% (≡1) suggests that the risk in each group is identical

Absolute risk

▮ The proportion of all patients who would benefit from the therapy

▮ In the above example, the chance of a stroke off aspirin is 4% while on aspirin it is 2%; therefore the absolute reduction in risk from taking aspirin is 4%–2% = 2%

Number needed to treat

▮ An estimation of the number of patients who would need to receive a therapy in order for a defined event to be avoided.

▮ In the example, 2 in every 100 patients taking aspirin will be prevented from having a stroke; to avoid 1 stroke, therefore, 50 patients have to be given aspirin

SCREENING AND SURVEILLANCE

Screening

▮ The investigation of a population in order to identify those who have a specific disease

Surveillance

▮ The investigation of an individual in order to detect recurrence of a disease

Ransom's criteria

▮ Criteria for an appropriate screening test

▮ That there is a safe and sensitive test for the disease with a high positive predictive value; the test should not have a high complication rate

▮ The yield of the test needs to be high enough to merit the cost of the test and the inconvenience and discomfort for both those in whom the disease is detected and those in whom it is not

▮ Earlier treatment of the disease has to have a benefit to the patient compared with late treatment; in other words, an effective therapy has to be available

Number needed to screen

▌ The number of individuals who have to be screened in order to prevent one death due to the disease

Lead time

▌ The time difference between detection of a disease by screening and the point at which it would have presented by causing symptoms

EPIDEMIOLOGY

▌ The study of disease and the way it is distributed within the population
▌ The risk of developing a specific disease can depend on a wide variety of factors

Genetic predisposition

▌ Genetic variation between individuals alters their susceptibility to a disease
  – HLA-B8 DR3 increases the risk of autoimmune disease

Exposure to causative agent

▌ Increased exposure to an infectious agent, carcinogen or other agent may be a function of geographical location, immediate personal contacts, work environment or personal habits such as diet, alcohol or smoking

Availability of healthcare

▌ Availability and utilisation of healthcare resources impacts upon prevention of disease (e.g. vaccination) and the stage at which a disease presents; this may have a large impact on outcome

Social and cultural beliefs

▌ The response to disease is modified by an individual's perceptions of illness and his or her society's approach to disease management

Definitions in epidemiology
Incidence

▌ Number of new cases arising during a defined period of time
  – 300 per year

Prevalence

▌ Total number of cases in a population per unit time

Prevalence rate

▌ Prevalence per unit population

Mortality

▌ Death rate per unit time

Mortality rate

▌ Death rate per unit population per unit time

Age-standardised mortality

▌ Correction of the mortality rate for a disease for age

Standardised mortality ratio

▌ Ratio of deaths observed in a cohort to the number expected across the whole population.
▌ E.g. the mortality in any specific age range in smokers is higher than that for the population as a whole

AUDIT AND GOVERNANCE

▌ Audit is a method of monitoring performance and standards in healthcare
▌ Governance is the mechanism by which standards are maintained

Stages of audit

▌ Describe the variable to be audited
▌ Choose an appropriate standard to be used as a benchmark for performance
▌ Collect the data on local performance
▌ Compare local results with the standard
▌ Identify ways of improving local performance
▌ Repeat audit after implementation of the new protocols in order to assess their effect

Rules

▌ Audit should be non-confrontational and non-judgemental
▌ Individuals should not be openly targeted
▌ However, an individual doctor who is under-performing should be encouraged to improve practice and supported in doing so

Governance

▌ The means by which organisations ensure the provision of quality clinical care by making individuals accountable for setting, maintaining and monitoring performance standards

▌ Involves individuals and groups of healthcare workers in identifying best practice and how it may be achieved

SELF ASSESSMENT QUESTIONS

Best one of five questions

1. A study of a pulse rate in an adult population of 500 people is carried out. Which one of the following would be most appropriate method of describing the dataset that results?
   A. Mean and standard deviation
   B. Mode and range
   C. Median and interquartile range
   D. Mean and Standard Error
   E. Median and 95% confidence intervals

2. A clinical trial of a new drug is carried out and an 'intention to treat' analysis performed. What is the best description of this form of analysis?
   A. All patients who completed the trial are included
   B. All patients who were considered for the trial were included
   C. All patients who were randomised in the trial were included
   D. All patients who took the drug rather than placebo were included
   E. All patients who dropped out of the study were excluded from the analysis

3. A study looking at 1-year survival in patients randomised to one of two forms of drug treatment was carried out. What would be the most appropriate analysis tool to compare the treatments?
   A. Student T test

   B. Mann–Whitney test
   C. Paired T test
   D. Chi squared test
   E. Regression analysis

4. Which one of the following is the best definition of 'population screening'?
   A. Investigation of symptomatic patients for the underlying cause
   B. Assessment of a patient with a previous diagnosis for recurrence of the disease
   C. Assessment of patients with a disease for evidence of an associated condition
   D. Assessment of asymptomatic patients for a disease
   E. Random selection of a sample from a population for inclusion in a trial

5. Which one of the following defines prevalence?
   A. Number of patients with a disease seen in the hospital setting
   B. Number of patients with a disease expressed as a proportion of the total population
   C. Number of new patients presenting each year with a disease
   D. Number of new cases of the disease per 100 000 people per year
   E. Total number of cases within the total population per year

4. Clinical pharmacology
1. FTFTF
2. TFFTF
3. TTTTT
4. TTFFT
5. TTFTT
6. TTFTF

5. Radiology
1. TTFTT
2. TFFTT
3. C
4. B
5. C
6. D
7. C
8. B

6. Clinical chemistry
1. D
2. C
3. C
4. E
5. A
6. E
7. A
8. C
9. A

7. Infectious diseases
1. TFTTT
2. TFTFF

3. TFTFF
4. TTFTF
5. TTTTF
6. TFTTT
7. TFTTT
8. TFTFF
9. TTFTF
10. TFTTF
11. TFTFF
12. TFTTT
13. TFTTT
14. TTFFT
15. TTTFT
16. FFTTF
17. TTTTT
18. FTTFF
19. TFFTF
20. TTTFF
21. D
22. A
23. E
24. A
25. B
26. C
27. C
28. D
29. E

8. Respiratory medicine
1. A
2. B
3. A

4. D
5. E
6. A
7. A
8. E
9. B
10. A
11. B
12. B
13. A
14. B
15. B

9. Cardiology
1. C
2. E
3. B
4. B
5. E
6. A
7. B
8. C
9. A
10. D
11. B
12. B
13. E
14. A
15. A

10. Gastroenterology
1. E
2. A

3. D
4. E
5. A
6. C
7. A
8. C
9. C
10. D
11. D
12. B
13. A
14. A
15. D
16. C
17. B
18. B
19. E
20. D
21. B
22. B
23. A
24. C
25. A
26. D
27. B
28. FTTFF
29. FFTTT
30. TTFTT
31. FTTFF
32. TTTFT
33. TTTFF
34. FTTFF
35. TTFFT
36. TTTFT
37. TTFTT
38. TFTFF
39. TTFTF
40. TFFTT

11. Rheumatology
1. B
2. D
3. B
4. D
5. E

6. C
7. C
8. B
9. D
10. E
11. A
12. D

12. Dermatology
1. E
2. C
3. C
4. C
5. B
6. D
7. C
8. B
9. C
10. C

13. Endocrinology
1. C
2. A
3. C
4. C
5. E
6. C
7. B
8. E
9. E
10. B
11. E
12. E
13. C
14. B
15. A
16. C
17. D
18. E
19. C

14. Renal medicine
1. B
2. A

3. D
4. A
5. E
6. E
7. B
8. D
9. B
10. D
11. B
12. B
13. E
14. A

15. Haematology
1. FTTFF
2. TTFTF
3. TFTTT
4. TFTTF
5. TFFFT
6. TTTTT
7. B
8. C
9. B
10. C

16. Oncology
1. TTTTT
2. FTFFT
3. TFTTF
4. FFTFF
5. FTTFF
6. FFTTF
7. C
8. D
9. D
10. B
11. C
12. D

17. Neurology
1. B
2. D
3. D
4. B

5. D

6. A

7. E

8. E

9. E

10. B

11. D

12. E

13. D

14. E

15. D

16. B

17. A

18. E

18. Psychological medicine

1. E

2. C

3. B

4. C

5. B

6. D

7. E

8. C

9. E

10. C

11. C

12. B

13. A

14. E

15. C

19. Statistics

1. A

2. C

3. D

4. D

5. D

5. Radiology
1. **I.** F. PA chest is the classical test but CT is more accurate.
   II. I.
   III. K. Much more sensitive than CT for liver lesions.
   IV. D. 'Pepperpot' skull lytic lesions are seen.

6. Clinical chemistry
1. **I.** C. Confusion is non-specific. Oedema suggests right heart failure. Hypokalaemia is an unwanted effect of loop diuretics. Renal failure could be secondary to heart failure or unwanted effect of diuretics.
   II. I. Hypokalaemia, hypomagnesaemia, dehydration and normal anion gap metabolic acidosis all result from electrolyte and water losses from high ileostomy outputs.
   III. D. Hypoxia and low PCO_2 suggests respiratory problem, fever suggests infection. Low sodium is a result of syndrome of inappropriate ADH (SIADH) and is associated with pneumonia.
2. **I.** H. Hypercapnia and hypoxia suggest type II respiratory failure.
   II. F. Metabolic acidosis with respiratory compensation (low PCO_2) in a patient with diabetes who is unwell and vomiting is very suggestive of diabetic ketoacidosis.
   III. C. Metabolic acidosis with high anion gap is compatible with aspirin overdose.
3. **I.** A. All three are markers of acute cardiac muscle damage.
   II. D. Lymphadenopathy and an elevated LDH give the diagnosis.
   III. E. Normal LFTs with a low Hb and elevated bilirubin point to this answer.

7. Infectious Disease
1. **I.** E. There is evidence of immunocompromise and/or reactivated TB (chest X-ray, lymphadenopathy, fever).
   II. J. Rust-coloured sputum and peri-oral HSV are associated with *Strep. pneumoniae*.
   III. F. Hepatosplenomegaly, jaundice, a fever and low platelets are all characteristic of malaria.

2. I. L. Liver ultrasound would demonstrate cholecystitis (thickened inflamed gallbladder) and cholangitis (gas in biliary tree, stones or an obstructed biliary tree). CT would be the second choice.

    II. B. The clinical picture is that of malaria.

    III. G. The data suggest infective endocarditis. Multiple sets of blood cultures are needed to detect the organism and derive the antibiotic sensitivities.

8. Respiratory medicine

1. I. B. Eczema suggests atopy in a young woman. Spirometry results suggest an obstructive defect. These, together with history, make asthma very likely.

    II. A. Breathlessness with clubbing and weight loss strongly suggest lung cancer, especially with progressive symptoms.

    III. H. Normal chest X-ray and pulmonary function tests exclude many of the answers. NSAIDs (e.g. ibuprofen) cause GI ulceration and iron deficiency particularly in elderly patients.

2. I. A. *Strep. pneunomiae* is the commonest cause of pneumonia and is associated with rusty coloured sputum.

    II. E. The marked hypoxia with normal chest X-ray suggests pneumocystis pneumonia in this immunocompromised patient.

    III. F. *Staph. aureus* pneumonia cavitates and is associated with flu outbreaks.

3. I. F. The clue is the fact that she gets better when she is away from the farm; extrinsic allergic alveolitis symptoms are worst at the time of antigen exposure.

    II. A. Cough and bilateral lymphadenopathy is a common presentation of sarcoid.

    III. H. His exposure to asbestos, the presence of chest pain and the chest X-ray findings make mesothelioma likely.

9. Cardiology

1. I. D. The presence of different blood pressures in each arm, interscapular pain and Marfans point to a dissected thoracic aorta.

    II. B. This is exercise-induced angina in a patient with risk factors (diabetes mellitus and smoking).

    III. A. The age and the relationship to food are suggestive of a gastrointestinal rather than cardiac cause.

2. I. B. The right heart failure and cardiomegaly in a drinker suggest alcoholic cardiomyopathy.

    II. C. Deep vein thrombosis with a pulmonary embolus – recent travel with a swollen leg and breathlessness.

    III. C. The history of diabetes and the presence of an ulcerated area could be cellulites or vascular insufficiency. The history favours the former.

3. I. B. The rate of 160 bpm and no 'p' waves in a smoker suggest AF.
   II. I. The tachycardia is due to the β-agonist (it also causes tremor). If the patient was not on inhalers consider thyrotoxicosis.
   III. D. The symptoms are all due to anxiety-related hyperventilation – shortness of breath and tingling of the fingers and mouth.

10. Gastroenterology

1. I. D. Autonomic neuropathy due to diabetes mellitus links the symptoms.
   II. H. The mucus and low potassium suggest a tubulo-villous adenoma. The mucus is very potassium rich and can be profuse.
   III. G. Ulcerative colitis (anaemia, fever and diarrhoea) all point to severe disease.
2. I. E. The risk factors of diabetes and heart disease, combined with pain and diarrhoea after food, suggest mesenteric ischaemia.
   II. G. Ulcers, weight loss and anaemia, plus erythema nodosum, all point to inflammatory bowel disease and therefore Crohn's in this question.
   III. H. Irritable bowel – the alternating bowel habit, bloating and left iliac fossa pain are suggestive and the weight gain discounts other pathologies.
3. I. B. Growth failure with GI symptoms points towards coeliac disease, Crohn's or cystic fibrosis. The latter is unlikely to present as late as this.
   II. A. Pernicious anaemia – the low vitamin B_{12} and the history of autoimmune thyroid disease point to this.
   III. E. The history suggests chronic pancreatitis – steatorrhoa and chronic alcoholism.
4. I. I. NSAIDs markedly increase the risk of gastric ulceration.
   II. H. The change in bowel habit and weight loss suggest that a carcinoma is the most important diagnosis to rule out.
   III. J. Bright red rectal bleeding suggests a rectal or anal cause, and in this age group haemorrhoids are the most likely.

11. Rheumatology

1. I. D. Syndesmophytes are suggestive of ankylosing spondilytis and the ESR and HLA status support this.
   II. B. Osteoarthritis is a common cause of backpain. Normal bloods and no erosions on X-ray make the other diagnoses unlikely.
   III. A. Recent wrist fracture in a post-menopausal woman with normal bloods is highly suggestive of osteoporosis. She may have had steroids for her asthma, making osteoporosis more likely.
2. I. D. Elevated urate suggests gout. The distribution of the joint symptoms is compatible with gout.
   II. F. Rash, joint pains and raised inflammatory markers with a positive ANA is strongly suggestive of SLE.
   III. B. Heberden's nodes with normal ESR suggests osteoarthritis.

3. **I.** H. Recurrent miscarriages are the key here.

   II. C. The MCP joint erosions and a systemic illness point to rheumatoid.

   III. A. Anti-entromere antibodies are associated with systemic sclerosis.

12. Dermatology

1. **I.** I. Raised, purple, painful red areas on the legs suggest erythema nodosum which is associated with Crohn's disease.

   II. A. History of atopy. Distribution suggests eczema (flexoral).

   III. F. Yellow crusts strongly suggests *Staph. aureus* infection.

2. **I.** F. An ulcer which is rapidly increasing in size in a patient with Crohn's disease is highly suggestive of pyoderma gangrenosum.

   II. A. The pigmentation and brown colour suggest venous ulceration.

   III. B. Being a gardener suggests UV exposure. The appearance and hard node suggests SCC rather than malignant melanoma.

3. **I.** G. Infection with *Corynebacterium minutissimum*.

   II. F. Jaundice and itching = biliary obstruction.

   III. A. Iron deficiency is associates with itching.

13. Endocrinology

1. **I.** D. She has multiple endocrine neoplasia type I (a parathyroid adenoma causing hyperparathyroidism, associated with a pancreatic tumour). The high calcium resulting from this is causing the constipation and polyuria.

   II. B. She has Sheehan's syndrome – a pituitary infarction following a post-partum haemorrhage – leading to diabetes insipidus. This is rare.

   III. A. There is a metabolic acidosis (low bicarbonate), thirst, polyuria and weight loss – classical early onset diabetes mellitus.

2. **I.** A. She has autoimmune disease already so her risk of a further autoimmune disease is increased. Anxiety, palpitations, diarrhoea and weight loss are all pointing towards thyrotoxicosis.

   II. E. The palmar pigmentation, abdominal pain and postural hypotension suggest Addison's disease (in this case due to adrenal tuberculosis suggested by sweats, weight loss and foreign travel).

   III. B. 50% of coeliac disease presents with iron deficiency. Weight loss and abdominal pain support this. The southern Irish origins increase the risk of coeliac.

14. Renal medicine

1. **I.** C. The history of gout increases the risk of renal stones. The colicky pain and sudden onset in the absence of indicators of infection support this.

   II. H. The chest signs point to a pneumonia. The urinary abnormalities may be due to an atypical pneumonia (e.g. mycoplasma or legionella).

   III. E. There is an association between polycystic kidney disease and berry aneurysms that result in subarachnoid haemorrhage. The pain is probably due to bleeding into one of the renal cysts.

2. I. A. The presence of liver cirrhosis with new acute renal failure favours hepatorenal syndrome as the cause.
    II. F. Haemolytic-uraemic syndrome results from *E. coli* O157 and occurs after food poisoning with this organism. The anaemia and thrombocytopenia are as a result of the haemolysis.
    III. I. The mass in his pelvis is his bladder. This is a classical presentation of acute retention due to prostatic enlargement.

15. Haematology
1. I. A.
    II. D. Sickle results in sickled red cells and regional hypoxia causing severe pain.
    III. B. Although both B_{12} and folic acid deficiency cause macrocytosis, only B_{12} requires the stomach to be present to be absorbed.
2. I. I.
    II. J.
    III. H. Both reticulocytes and platelets increase after blood loss but platelets do not have nucleii.
3. I. C. O 44%, A 45%, B 8%, AB 3%.
    II. A.
    III. F. The mother must be RhD negative. A first RhD positive etus induces anti-D antibodies. The second suffers the syndrome.

17. Neurology
1. I. C. The distal progressive weakness and areflexia are typical of Guillain-Barré. The history of a recent GI infection supports this.
    II. A. The smoking and hypertension are key risk factors for ischaemic stroke. This is a non-dominant side event with dysphasia.
    III. H. The shuffling gait, micrographia and resting tremor all point to Parkinson's.
2. I. F. The rash, photophobia and fever all suggest meningitis (probably meningococcal).
    II. A. The combination of abdominal symptoms and unilateral headache, probably initiated by alcohol, points to migraine.
    III. D. The retinal changes suggest malignant hypertension, and are not features of diabetic retinopathy.
3. I. G. All the elements are here for a benzodiazepine overdose, using drugs prescribed by the GP. She could be either ketoacidotic or hypoglycaemic but the history points to deliberate self-harm due to reactive depression.
    II. I. Septicaemia due to urinary sepsis.
    III. E. Hypotension, bradycardia and, in particular, J waves on the ECG all point to hypothermia.

18. Psychological medicine

1. **I.** F. The pattern of memory loss is compatible with early dementia.

   II. D. She has first rank symptoms of schizophrenia. Her ethnicity increases the risk of this disease.

   III. H. High MCV suggests alcohol excess. Visual hallucinations, sweating and tachycardia occur in alcohol withdrawal syndrome.

2. **I.** D. Persecutory ideation and thought broadcasting suggest schizophrenia.

   II. I. Paranoia and agitation with a history of drug addiction points to amphetamines.

   III. B. Sleep loss, increased libido and spending beyond one's means are suggestive of mania.

3. **I.** B. Tricyclics cause weight gain and so would be relatively contraindicated. SSRIs are useful in reactive depression.

   II. G. Anxiety disorders are usually effectively treated with CBT.

   III. H. Carbemazepine is a useful second-line drug in bipolar disorders.

Appendix C

Normal reference ranges
Normal values for laboratory tests

These may vary from hospital to hospital.

Test	Abbreviation	Normal range	Units
Full blood count			
Haemoglobin	Hb	Males 13.5–17.7	g/dL
		Females 11.5–16.5	g/dL
Mean corpuscular volume	MCV	80–96	fL
Mean corpuscular haemoglobin	MCH	27–33	pg
Mean corpuscular haemoglobin concentration	MCHC	32–36	g/dL
Reticulocyte count	retics	0.5–2.5%	
Red cell count	RCC	Males: 4.5–6	$\times 10^{12}$/L
		Females: 3.9–5.0	$\times 10^{12}$/L
White cell count	WCC	4–11	$\times 10^{9}$/L
Basophils		0.01–0.1	$\times 10^{9}$/L
Eosinophils		0.04–0.4	$\times 10^{9}$/L
Lymphocytes		1.5–4.0	$\times 10^{9}$/L
Monocytes		0.2–0.8	$\times 10^{9}$/L
Neutrophils		2.0–7.5	$\times 10^{9}$/L
Platelets		150–400	$\times 10^{9}$/L
Haematinics			
Serum B_{12}	B_{12}	160–925	ng/L
Serum folate		2.9–18	µg/L
Ferritin	Fe	Male: 20–260	µg/L
		Female: 6–110	µg/L
Iron		13–32	mmol/L
Total iron binding capacity	TIBC	42–80	mmol/L
Other haematology			
Erythrocyte sedimentation rate	ESR	<20	mm/hour

table continues

Test	Abbreviation	Normal range	Units
Coagulation			
Bleeding time		3–9	minutes
Active partial thromboplastin time	APTT	23–31	seconds
Prothrombin time	PTPT	12–16	seconds
International normalised ratio	INR	1.0–1.3	
Urea and electrolytes			
Sodium	Na^+	135–146	mmol/L
Potassium	K^+	3.5–5.0	mmol/L
Chloride	Cl^-	95–106	mmol/L
Urea		2.5–6.7	mmol/L
Creatinine		79–118	μmol/L
Liver function tests			
Alanine aminotransferase	ALT	5–40	IU/L
Aspartate aminotransferase	AST	12–40	IU/L
Gamma glutaryl transpeptidase	gT	10–40	IU/L
Alkaline phosphatase	ALP	39–117	IU/L
Bilirubin	Bili	<17	μmol/L
Other biochemistry			
Glucose (fasting)		4.5–5.5	mmol/L
Glycosylated haemoglobin	Hb A_{1c}	3.7–5.1	
Calcium	Ca^{2+}	2.20–2.67	mmol/L
Phosphate	PO_4^{3-}	0.8–1.5	mmol/L
C reactive protein	CRP	<10	mg/L
Urate		0.18–0.42	mmol/L
Lipids			
Cholesterol	Chol	3.5–6.5	mmol/L
HDL cholesterol	HDL	Male: 0.8–1.8	mmol/L
		Female: 1.0–2.3	mmol/L
Triglycerides	Trig	Male: 0.7–2.1	mmol/L
		Female: 0.5–1.7	mmol/L
Arterial blood gases			
Arterial partial oxygen pressure	Pao_2	10–13.3	kPa
Arterial partial carbon dioxide pressure	$Paco_2$	4.8–6.1	kPa
pH	pH	7.35–7.45	
Bicarbonate	HCO_3	24–28	mmol

Appendix D
Bibliography and further reading

Kumar P, Clark M (eds) (2006) *Clinical Medicine*, 6th edn. Edinburgh: W.B. Saunders.

Warrell D, Cox T, Firth JD, Benz EJ (eds) (2003) *Oxford Textbook of Medicine*, 4th edn. Oxford: Oxford University Press.

Hampton J (2003) *The ECG Made Easy*, 6th edn. Edinburgh: Churchill Livingstone.

Corne J, Carroll M, Delany D, Brown I (2002) *Chest X-ray Made Easy*, 2nd edn. Edinburgh: Churchill Livingstone.

Marshall, WJ (2000) *Clinical Chemistry* 4th edn. London: Mosby.

Sackett D, Strauss S, Richardson WS, Rosenberg W, Hayes RB (2000) *Evidence Based Medicine*, 2nd edn. Edinburgh: Churchill Livingstone.

Websites

www.kumarandclark.com – *Clinical Medicine* on line.

www.fleshandbones.com – a general site for medical students and instructors.

www.ncbi.nih.gov/entrez/query.fcgi – Pubmed, a search engine for biomedical research.

Index

Note: entries in **bold** indicate Figures, entries in *Italics* indicate Tables and Boxes, questions are indicated by Q

abdomen
  anatomical regions **250**
  distension 28
  examination 248–249
  pain 28, 55, 152, 262–263, 266, 277,
    279, *321*, 325, 359–360, 374
  X-ray *32*, **84**, *392*
abscesses 95, 98, 102, 136, 266–267, 292
Acanthosis nigricans 341
acarbose 372
ACE inhibitors 53, 106, *115*, 210, 215,
  222, *225*, 396
achalasia 88, **89**, 257
aciclovir 134, 335, 496–497, 515
acid-base disorders 57, 118, *374. See
    also* acidosis; alkalosis
acidosis *115*, 374, 398
  metabolic 54, 118–119, 125Q, 384, *486*
  respiratory 118–125
  See also ketoacidosis
Acquired Immune Deficiency
    Syndrome (AIDS) 55, 146, **147**,
    148, *169*, 499
acromegaly 18, 223, *309*, *322*, 353, *354*,
    367, 509
ACTH *114*, 174, 349–350, 354, 356–357,
    358, 377Q, 492
activated partial thromboplastin time
    431, *432*
acute. *See specific disease or condition*
acyclovir 335
Addison's disease *60*, 110, *115*, 326,
    358, 419–420
adenitis 277
adenocarcinoma 173, 256–257, 259,
    262, 265, 269, 279, 298, 366

adenoviruses *6*, 144
ADH 108, 110, 112, 354, 361–362, *363*
adrenal gland
  adenoma 357–358, *358*, 366
  carcinoma 357
  failure 350, 356, *486*
  hormone abnormalities 356
  hyperplasia 222
adrenalectomy 358
adrenocorticotrophic hormone 114,
    174, 349, 354
AIDS. *See* Acquired Immune
    Deficiency Syndrome
AL amyloidosis 389
alanine aminotransferase 122
albumin 121, 268, *278*, *287*, *288*, 397, 411
alcohol 50, 116, 122, 222, 224, 239, 256,
    276, *277*, *278*, *281*, 286, 314, 337,
    348, 357, 417, *421*, 439, 453, *511*, *531*
  abuse 225, 226Q, 302, *419*, 541,
    541, 545
  addiction 541
  alcoholism 171, 231, 290
  dependence 542, 545, 547
  withdrawal *117*, 291, 487, *529*, 537,
    550Q
Alcoholics Anonymous 545
aldosterone *61*, 108, 112, *114*, *115*, 349,
    364, **365**
alkaline phosphatase 121–122, *287*,
    322, 397, 567
alkalosis *114*
  metatoblic 118–119, 365, *365*
  respiratory 54, 70, *117*, 117–118, 126
allergies 25
allopurinol 53, 124, *294*, 443

α-herpesvirus 144
α-receptor blockers 407
alveoli 161, *166. See also* lung
alveolitis 184–185, *186*
Alzheimer's disease *464, 531*
amantadine 135
amenorrhoea 356, 361, 400–401, 534, 547
amiloride *61, 115,* 180
aminoglycosides 116, 132
amnesia *543,* 546
amniocentesis 468
Amoeba 276, 292
amoxicillin 131, 144, 153, 170, 208, *294,* 393
amphetamines 535, *546,* 537
amphotericin 116, 134
amylase *277,* 278–279
amyloidosis *109,* 389–390, 510, *511,* 512
amyotrophic lateral sclerosis 507
anaemia 145, 148, 163, 169, 174, 183, 221, 232–233, *248,* 258–259, 263–264, 268, 287, 292, *311,* 319, 352, 369, 400–402, 410Q, 413, *421, 422,* 423, 439–442, 444–445, 461, 513
  B$_{12}$ deficiency *419*
  haemolytic 52, 120–121, 143, 169, 248, 280, 317, 415, 422, 424–425, *425,* **426**
  iron deficiency 249, 268–270, *414,* 415–416
  megaloblastic 32, 301Q, 418, 421, *446,* 512
  normochromic normocytic 183, **316,** 317, 319, 415
  pernicious 260, 262, 379Q, 418, *419, 420,* 447Q, 457
  sideroblastic 415, 417
analgesia 278–279, *311,* 335, 342, 394, *422,* 423, 438, *546,* **462,** 462–463, 500–501
anaphylactic reaction 51, 134
androgens 323, *361*
aneurysm 81, *198,* 200, 207, 217, 232, 328, *395,* 403–404, 410Q, 482, 506
angina 14, 24–25, *62, 64, 65,* 204, 207, 210–212, **213,** *214,* 240, 243Q, 302, 342, 344Q, 415
angiography 71, 96, 212, 214, 216, 222, 438, 483, 505–506
angioplasty 101

angiotensin *63,* 108, 183, 364, **365,** 381, 491
  -converting enzyme (ACE) inhibitors *63*
  receptor antagonists *63*
anion exchange resins *66*
ankylosing spondylitis 19, 266, 312, 467
anorexia *61,* 171, 221, 257, 277, 279, 282, *322,* 356, 359–361, *419,* 463, 546, 550
anosmia 515
antacids 29, 45, 116, 119, 256, 273
anthrax 138, *154*
antibiotics 34, *53,* 131, **132,** 150, 155Q, 158Q, 170, 172, 177–178, 180, 232, 259, 265, 266, 269–270, 275, 288, 292, 308, 314, 319, 334–335, 337, *340,* 342, 344Q, 374, 393, 423, 459, 460, 495, *495,* 499
anticholinesterases 513
anticoagulants. *See* blood: anticoagulants
anticonvulsants *419,* 500, *529*
antidepressants 273, **538**
antidiuretic hormone 108, 110, 116, 361, 363, 377Q
antiemetics 460, **461,** 462–463, 501
antimetabolites 459
antiphospholipid syndrome 318, 436
antipsychotics 534
antiretroviral drugs 135, 149
antispasmodics 271, 463
antitrypsin disease *281,* 287
anuria 29, 395, *407*
anxiety *67,* 146, 220, 326, 337, 365, 379Q, 527, 541–542, *542,* 544, 550, 552
aortic
  dissection 210, 229
  regurgitation *196, 198,* 210
  stenosis 63–64, 196, *196, 198,* 201, 204, 210, *221,* 228, 236, 489
  valve 199
aphasia 502–503, *531*
aphonia *543*
apolipoprotein 390
apraxia 291, *296*
arrhythmias. *See* heart: arrhythmias
arteriography 383
arteriovenous malformation (AVM) 506
arterial stenosis. *See also* stenosis: arterial

arthralgia *231*, 232, 321
arthritis 139–140, 144, 153, 230, 268, 308, 313, *321*, 338
asbestos and asbestosis 75, 173, 453, 457
asbestosis 168, 181, *185*
ascites 61, 87, 108, 211, 221, 245, *248*, 252, *252*, 260, 287, *288*, 292, 297Q, 301
aspartate aminotransferase 120–121
aspergillosis 150
Aspergillus fumigatus 169
asphyxia *43*
aspirin 9, 16, 46, 50, 54, 119, 212, *214*, 216, *217*, 227, 231, 268, *315*, 318, 344Q, 398, 424, 429, 434–435, 505, 560–561
asthenia *43*
asthma 26–28, 33, 48, *62*, *67–68*, 150, *162*, *165*, *167*, 168, 175, *176*, 180, 184, 187, 190Q–191Q, *196*, 240, 330Q, 336, 344Q, *446*
ataxia *53*, 57, 115, 454, 488, 493, 497–498, 503, 508, 511, *539*
atrial
  fibrillation *18*, 36, *61*, *65*, 196, 208–209, *221*, 237, 244Q, 245, *351*, 353, 503–505
  flutter 237
  septal defect (ASD) 226, 236
  tachyarrhythmias 236
atrial natriuretic peptide 108
atrioventricular block *64*, **234**
audit and governance 563–564
auscultation of heart sounds 198, *199*
autoimmune
  disease 230, *359*, 419
  thrombocytopenic purpura 446
  thyroid disease 419
autosomal
  disorders *464*, 465
  inheritance **466**
azathioprine 51, 53, 185, 266, 268, 276, 286, *294*, *311*, 317, *320*, 337, 341, *421*, 513
azoles 134

Bacillus 138, 275
bacteria *6*, 254, 382, 384, 460, *494*
  infection 130, 136, 274, 334, 391, 498
  overgrowth *263*, 264, 319, *419*

barium
  enema 71, **90**, **91**, 269, 270
  meal **90**, 259, 266
  swallow 88, **89**, 257, 262
Barrett's oesophagus 256, 297Q, 457
Bartter's syndrome *116*
basophils 411, 566
Behçet's disease *494*
Bell's palsy 474, 514, *515*
benzodiazepines 57, *67*, *291*, 542, *546*, 552
benzylpenicillin 131, 495
bereavement *537*, 540
berylliosis *185*
best answer (best one of five) questions 10–13, 102–103, 125–126, 157–158, 190–192, 297–299, 329–330, 343–344, 448, 469–470, 549–551, 565
β-blockers *62*, *64*, *109*, 212, 214–215, 222, 225, 233, 238
β-lactams 131
bile duct obstruction 121, 122
biliary
  cirrhosis *248*, *250*, 264, 281, 288, 324
  colic 29
  stenting 101
  tree diseases 293
bilirubin 121, 127Q, **280**, *287*, 567
biopsy
  bone marrow 439, 440
  brain 484
  CT-guided 102Q
  directed 101
  endomyocardial 230
  endoscopic 457
  kidney 317, 383, 386, 401
  liver 290
  lymph node 440
  pleural 168
  prostatic 405
bipolar disorder **535**
bisphosphonates 259, 323, 325–326, *327*
bladder
  cancer *162*
  tumour 405
bleeding. *See* haemorrhage
bleeding time 431–432, *432*, 567
blood
  anticoagulants *65*

blood (*contd*)
  coagulopathy 25, 431, *432*, 433–434
  coagulation 247, 428–429, **430**, 431
  components 411
  count 130, 152, 260, 264, 269, 271,
    277, 291–292, 397, 401, *413*, 417,
    422, 423, *437*, 439–442, 445, 495,
    498, 505, 529, 566
  cultures 35, 130, 232, 292, 308, 397,
    485, 494, 498
  erythrocyte sedimentation rate (ESR)
    124, 183, *231*, 232, 268, 317–318,
    320, 331Q, 369, 397, 404, 413, 439,
    445, *482*, 535
  gases 126Q, 167, *167*
  glucose 40, 224, 247, 373–374, *398*,
    484, *495*
  groups 425–426, *427*
  mean corpuscular Hb (MCH) *413*
  mean corpuscular Hb concentration
    (MCHC) *413*
  mean corpuscular volume (MCV)
    413
  packed cell volume (PCV) *413*
  pressure *169*, *196*, 196–197, **223**, 245,
    348, 373, *485*, 504 (*see also*
    hypertension; hypotension)
  products 427
  pulse (*see* pulse)
  red cell count (RCC) *413*
  tests 31Q, 126Q–127Q, 174, 183,
    301Q, 317, 373, 379Q, 410Q,
    426, 551
  transfusions *115*, 129, 147, 149, 423,
    424–427, 428, 433–434, *434*, 444,
    447Q
  white cell count (WCC) *231*, 308,
    413, 442, 448Q, 499, *534*
  white cell scan 98
bone
  density 323, 360
  disease 322
  marrow fibrosis 444
  marrow transplantation 424
  pain 325, 400, 422, 444, 462
  scan 99
borderline personality disorder 537
Borrelia burgdorferi 143
Bouchard's nodes *307*

bowel
  habit 271
  obstruction 463
bradycardia *18*, *53*, *62*, 146, *176*, 189,
    233, 352, *499*
bradykinesia 489
brain
  dysfunction *486*
  failure *43*
  haemorrhage (*see* haemorrhage:
    brain)
  intracranial pressure 233, 484, *485*,
    494, 499, *515*, 522
breast-feeding *66*
breath sounds *166*
breath tests 254, 258
breathlessness 25, 27, 126, 162–163, 169,
    173, 175–177, 181, 184, 186–187,
    192, 192Q, 195, 208–213, *217*, *220*,
    226–227, 239, 353, 415, 437–438
British National Formulary (BNF)
    52, 58
bromocriptine 355
bronchiectasis 150, *163*, 166, 178,
    179, 390
bronchitis 139, *162*, 180, 208
bronchopneumonia **76**, 168, 490
bronchoscopy 140, 166, 174
bronchospasm *62*, *220*, 225, 256
Brucella 138–139
bruising *248*, 285, 287, 357, 390, 441, 444
Budd-Chiari syndrome *252*
bulbar palsy 516
bulimia nervosa 547
bundle branch block 236
burns 108, *278*, 433

cachexia *43*, 123
calcipotriol 338
calcitonin *327*
calcium
  channel blockers 45, *64*, *109*, 212, *225*
  homeostasis 360
  metabolism disorders 325–327
Campylobacter 139, 275, 510
cancer
  in adults 452
  aetiology 453
  basal cell *339*, 343Q, 453, 469

biology 455
bronchial 26, 30–31, 78, **79**, *173*, 173–175, 180, 456–457, 470Q
cervical 454–455, 458
childhood 452
colic in 29, 393
colorectal *6*, 254, 267–269, 273, 299, 455, 458, 470Q, *270*
diagnosis 456–458
epidemiology 452
familial 269
gastric 249, 258, 420, 452, **453**, 454, 457
genetics 454
hepatocellular *250*, 281, 283–284, 287–291, 293, 452–455, 457, 458
kidney 122, *251*, 404
lung 166, 173, 190Q–191Q, 363, 453, 457, 518, 552
metastases **78**, 79, **80**, 339, 356, 455, *456–457*, 481, *482*, *499*
oesophageal 256–257, 264, 297Q, 453, 456–457
palliative care for 462–463
pancreatic *248*, 281, 253, 363, 456
prostate 363, 405
skin 43, 148, 173–174, 257, 297, 339, 341, 343Q, 344–345, *339, 343*, 405, 453, 469
squamous cell 43, 148, 173–174, 257, 297, 339, 341, 344–345, 405, 453
thyroid 352
treatment 458–460
Candida albicans 134, 150, 336, 368, *494*
candidiasis 150
cannabis 533, *546*
carbamazepine 50, 363, 462, 488, 539
carbapenems 132
carbenoxolone *114*
carbimazole *294*, 353
carbon monoxide 187
carbon monoxide poisoning 187
carcinoma. *See* cancer
cardiac. *See* heart
cardiogenic shock *62*, 217
cardiomyopathy 183, 206–207, 209, 220, *221*, 235–236, 289, 390, 508, 514
cardiovascular system examination 195–202
carditis 230, *231*

carotid
  bruit 199–200, 503–504
  pulse 196
carpal tunnel syndrome 18, 390, 509
CAT scans 91
catecholamines 108, 366
catheterisation 34–35, *207*, 208, 210, 229, *407*
cause of death statement 42
cefotaxime 139, 495
cefuroxime 131, 393
cellulitis 136
cephalosporins 131
cerebral
  atrophy 482, 491
  cortex **503**, **504**
  infarction 503
  ischaemia 536
  oedema 55, 225
  tumours 482
cerebrospinal fluid (CSF) 130, 134, 140, 412, 460, 483, *484*, 485, 492, 495–496, 506, 510, 522
cerebrovascular
  accident 25, 92
  disease 96, 224, 502, *502*, 504, 522, *531*
cestodes 276
Chagas disease 151, 229
chemotherapy 174, 257, 262, 269, 339, 391, 399, 405–406, 413, 440, 441–445, 459–460
chest
  leads 33, 202
  pain 15, 24–27, 102Q, 120, *169*, *173*, 181, 187, 193Q, 204, 212–213, 217, *217*, 228, 239, 244Q, 245, *437*, *542*
  X-ray (*see* X-rays: chest)
chickenpox 144
Chlamydia 153, *169*, 313, *340*, 392
chloramphenicol 133
chlorpromazine *294*
chlorpropamide 363
cholangiocarcinoma 253, 281, 295
cholangiopancreatography 253
cholangitis sclerosing 148, *248*, 253, 266, 268, 281, 282, 295
cholecystitis acute 294
Cholera *6*, 139, *154*, 272, 274
cholestasis *248*, *287*, 292, 341

cholesterol 25, 567

chondrocalcinosis *309*

chorea *231*, 318, 490–491, 498

chromosome abnormalities 454, 463–464

chronic obstructive pulmonary disease 17, 27, **75**, *165*, 176

Churg–Strauss syndrome 184, *321*, *446*

Chvostek's sign 327

ciclosporin *115*, 116, 268–269, *294*, *311*, 313, *321*, *322*, 337, 341

cigarette smoking 161, *162*, 405

cimetidine 51, *59*, *294*

ciprofloxacin 133, 153, 264, 393

cirrhosis 108, *163*, 180, *280*, 281, 284, 286, *288*, 288–290, 299

cisplatin 116, 459, *511*

clinical history 24

clinical trials 559

Clostridium 138, 275

clotting factors 411

clubbing. *See* finger clubbing

CMV. *See* cytomegalovirus

CNS abnormalities 535

coagulation. *See* blood: coagulation

coal-worker's pneumoconiosis 180

coarctation of the aorta 196, 223, 228

cocaine *294*, *546*

codeine 462, *546*

coeliac disease *6*, 185, 262–263, *324*, *419*

cognitive/behavioural therapy 539

colitis 268, 274

collagen 305, 328

Colles' fracture 323

colon
  cancer (*see* cancer: colorectal)
  disease 268

colonoscopy 253, 266, 268–270

colostomy 18, 249

coma *43*, 55, 57, 111–112, 151, *176*, 177, 188–189, 286, *296*, 363, *371*, 374, *482*, 484–485, *485*, *487*, 496, 503, 505, 524, 530, *539*

community acquired pneumonia *169*

compulsion 528

computerised tomography (CT) 72, 91, 29–31, 71–72, 91, **94**, **95**, 101, 102Q, 131, 140, 174, 185, 257, 262, 265, 269–270, 278–279, 317, 356, 366,

383, 404, *437*, 438–439, 457, 483–484, *485*, 488, 491, 495–496, 498, 500, 504–506, 513, 531
  abdominal 31, 71, 94–95, 401, 406, 440
  body 94
  chest 14, 31, 71, 166, 183, 440
  head 29–30, 71, 92, **93**, 102, 482, 494, 505, 521, 529
  lung 95, 178
  pneumocolon, 95
  spiral 394

congestive heart failure 25–26

conjunctivitis 133, 139, 145, 151, 153, 156Q, 182, 266, 268, 313–314

connective tissue disease 315

Conn's syndrome *114*, 222, 364, *365*

consciousness disturbed 488–489

constipation 28, *66*, **88**, 273, 291, 352, 360, 401, 463, *534*, *536*, *539*

contrast studies 96

controlled trial 559

convulsions 111–112, 151, 115, *291*, 487, *539*

Coombs' test 424–425, **426**

COPD. *See* lung: chronic obstructive disease in

cor pulmonale 236

cordocentesis 468

coronary angiography 207

coronary artery disease 212, 224, 236

coronary syndrome, acute 213

coroner *42*, 44

correlation and regression 557–558

correlation coefficient 557

corticosteroids 40, *114*, 176–177, 231, *311*, *322*, 348, 367, 492, 513

corticotrophin releasing hormone (CRH) **354**, **357**

cortisol 349–350, 356, *358*, *485*, 535

Corynebacterium 137

cough 26–27, *63*, 140, 168, 171, *173*, 175–176, 178, 181, 184, 186, *220*, 456

COX II inhibitors 259

Coxiella burneti 169–170, 228–231, 277, 384, *494*, 495

crackles 14, 159Q, 164, *166*, 178, 185–186, 199, 221, 277, 422, 437

cranial nerves 472–476, 493, 514, *515*
  I Olfactory 472
  II Optic 472
  III Oculomotor 473
  IV Trochlear (superior oblique muscle) 474
  V Trigeminal 474
  VI Abducens (lateral rectus muscle) 474
  VII Facial 474
  VIII Vestibulocochlear 475
  IX Glossopharyngeal 475
  X Vagus **461**, *475*
  XI Accessory 475
  XII Hypoglossal 476
craniopharyngioma 356
creatine kinase 120, 214
creatinine 383
crest syndrome 319
Creutzfeldt-Jakob disease 497, 522, *531*
Crigler-Najjar syndrome *280*, 281
Crohn's disease 18, 29, **90**, 126Q, *130*, *263*, 265, **267**, 273, 298–299, 314, 344Q, *419*
crossover trials 560
croup 144
cryoglobulinaemia 389
cryoglobulins 384
Cryptococcus neoformans 494
Cryptosporidium 148, 276
CT. *See* computerised tomography
Cushing's syndrome 18, *114*, 222, *317*, *322*, 356–358, 367, 376Q, *513*, *529*, 535–536
cyanosis 163–164, *176*, 177, 195, 227–228, 318, 443
cystic fibrosis 18, *169*, *179*, 287, 367, *464*, 467
cytomegalovirus (CMV) 134, 144, 148–149, *169*, 285, 389

dactylitis 313
data 553
  bias 556, 559
  parametric 556
  randomisation 559
  types 553–559
  See also statistics
D-dimer assay 431

deafness *60*, 145, 325, 361, 464, 475, *515*
death certificates 41
debility *43*
deep venous thrombosis. *See* thrombosis
defaecation 29
degenerative disorders 507
dehydration 106, 123, 314, 339, 359, 362, 374, 393, 422
delayed puberty *347*, 356
deliberate self-harm assessment 38
delirium
delusions 528, *529*, 533, *536*
dementia 148, 289, 291, 421, *482*, 490–491, 493, 497–498, 507, 511, 518, 527, 530, *531*, 532, 537, 541–542, 549
depression 38, 58, *167*, 204, 212–213, 216, 273, *320*, 325, 352, 359, 443, 463, 525, 527, 530, 534–535, *536*, 537–538, 540–544, *542*, 547, 549, 552
depressive illness *537*, 540
dermatitis herpetiformis 263
dermatology 333
dermatomes of spinal roots **481**
descriptional statistics 553, **554**, 555
detoxification 247
dexamethasone 350, *358*, 506
dextrocardia 17, **83**, 198
diabetes 12, 14, 41, 245, *261*, 264, 279, 289, 301–302, *317*, 349, *363*, *400*, *515*, 522, 524
  amyotrophy and 369
  emergencies 373–375
  clinic checkups 373
  eye disease and 25, **370**
  foot disease and 369, *371*
  insipidus 112, 361, 377Q, 464
  ketoacidosis 373–374
  mellitus 25, 40, 43–44, 46, *109*, 126Q, **171**, 212, 293, 301Q–302Q, *322*, 334–336, 341–342, 345Q, *347*, *348*, 355, 357–358, 361, 366–367, **368**, 371, 377Q, *388*, 389, 392, 399, 464, 509, 510, *511*, 512
  type I 46, 378Q
  type II 302Q, 373, 378Q
  WHO classification of 366
dialysis 113, *117*, 398, 402

diamorphine *220, 422*, 462
diarrhoea 6, 26, 28, *59, 61*, 108, 110, *114*,
    116, 119, 134, 148, 150, 170,
    263–266, 268, 275–276, 280, 291,
    299, 301–303, 400
    bloody *269*, 274–275, 301Q, 344Q,
        353, 359, 369, 379Q, 512, *542*
    inflamatory 273
    osmotic 271
    secretory 272, 274
diazepam 67, *486*, 488
digital subtraction angiography 97
digoxin 53, *61, 115*, 116, 209, 222, 238,
    529
diltiazem 50, *53*, 64, *294*
diphtheria *135*, 135–136, 138, *154*, 230
disease. *See specific disease*
diseases notifiable under the Public
    Health (Infectious Diseases)
    Regulations (1988) *154*
disseminated intravascular coagulation
    (DIC) 433
dissociative (conversion) disorder 543
diuretics 29, 45, 51, 53, *53, 60–61*, 62–63,
    67, 106, 108–110, *114*, 116, *117*, 119,
    125Q, 177, 209–210, 222, *225*, 288,
    291, 314–315, *326*, 342, 547
diverticulitis 271
dizziness 25, 235, 240, 260, *542*
DNA 133–134, 144, 147, 149, 180, 268,
    282–283, 317, 384, 454, 459, 464, 468
domperidone 460
dopamine 533–534
Down's syndrome 226, 463, 467–468
drain insertion 101
dress code 3
Dressler's syndrome 217, 228–229
drug(s)
    absorption 48
    abuse 545
    addiction 541
    adverse effects 51–52
    allergies 40
    antiviral 134–135
    cholestasis and *294*
    distribution 48
    elimination kinetics 49
    excretion 49
    groups, common 58
    half-life 49
    hepatitis from *294*
    hypersensitivity 51–52
    interactions 52–53, *53*
    lipid-modulating 66
    metabolism 49–50
    poisoning 54
    prescriptions 41, 68–69
    reactions, adverse 51
    -receptor interactions 46–47
    routes of administration 47
    sympathomimetic 233
    $t_{\{1/2\}}$ 49
    toxicity 116
    volume of distribution (VD) 48
    withdrawal *529*
Duchenne muscular dystrophy *464, 513*
Duckett Jones diagnostic *231*
Dupuytren's contractures *248*, 249, 287
DVT. *See* thrombosis
dynamic scintigraphy 383
dysarthria 57, 488, 503, 507–508,
    518, 539
dysentery *154*, 276
dyspepsia *59, 67*, 258
dysphagia 174, 256–258, 416, 456, 493,
    503, 507, *515*, 516, *542*
dysphasia 503, **503**
dyspnoea 226, 428
dystonia 327
dystrophia myotonica 514
dysuria 153, 392

E. coli. See Escherichia coli
eating disorders 546
EBV. *See* Epstein-Barr virus
ECG. *See* electrocardiogram
echocardiogram. *See* echocardiography
echocardiography 206, 208–209, 222,
    224, 229–230, 232, 438, 505
eclampsia 124, 292
ecstasy *546*
eczema 192Q, 333, 336, 338, 343Q,
    446, 437
ED$_{50}$ 47
Ehlers–Danlos syndrome 328
Eisenmenger's syndrome 226, 227
electrocardiogram 5, 16, 33–34, 113, 115,
    177, 202, 202–204, **204, 206**, 208, 210,

212, **213**, 214, **215**, **216**, *216, 217, 220,*
222, 224, 229–230, 233, **234–239**,
239–241, 246, *398,* 399, *437,* 438, *485,*
505, 524, 529–530, *539*
electroconvulsive therapy (ECT) 538
electroencephalography (EEG) 483
electrolyte balance 105–106
electromyelography (EMG) 483
embolism *65,* 101, 217, 236, 435–437,
503–504
emphysema *162,* 168, 198, 328
empyema *163,* 170
enalapril *63,* 225, *294*
encephalitis *154,* 355, *486, 487,* 489
encephalomyelitis 146
endocarditis *130,* 136–137, 139, *163,*
195, 209, 211, 227, 231, 244Q, 389,
417, 498, *546*
endocrine
disorders 347, *348*
neoplasia 366
tumours *347*
endocrinology 347, *347–348*
endoscopy 166, 253, 256–259, *261,*
262–263, 287, 301Q
Entamoeba histolytica 276, 292
enterobacteria 139
Enterococcus faecalis 231, 292, 391
enterocolitis 136, 275
enteroscopy 254
enzyme induction/inhibition 45, 50–51
eosinophilia 150, *446*
eosinophils 411, 566
epidemiology 562–563
epilepsy 39, 291, 483–484, *486,* 493, *529*
epileptic seizures 484, *487*
Epstein-Barr virus *130,* 145, 156Q, *250,*
285, 297Q, *340,* 384, 389, 440, 454,
494, 495
erectile dysfunction *60, 61, 62, 63, 66,*
225, 354, 368–369, 401, 512, *536*
erythema
marginatum 230, *231*
multiforme 144, *340, 340,* 343Q
nodosum 150, 182, 266, 268, *321,* 339,
340, 343Q
erythocyte sedimentation rate 413
erythroderma 338, 344
erythromycin 50, 133, 139, 143, *294*

erythropoiesis 413, 417, 423
erythropoietin 381, 402
Escherichia coli 139, 272, 274, 292, 391
ethanol poisoning 58
evidence-based medicine 560
examination techniques 4. *See also*
specific organs or procedures
exam types
best answer 10–13. *See also* best
answer (best one of five) questions
clinical 3, 17–19
essay 16–17
extended matching 11–14. *See also*
extended matching questions
multiple choice 2, 9. *See also* multiple
choice questions
negative marking in 10
short answer 13–14. *See also* short
answer questions
true or false 10
viva voce 4
written 1, 9
See also self-assessment questions
exam tips and tactics 10, 13–14,
16–17, 23
excretion urography 382, 392, 394–395,
404–405
exercise 25, 27, *115,* 120–121, 175, 204,
206, 207, 210, 212, 216, 224, 238,
311, 315, 322, 323, 372, 537, 544, 547
exhaustion 43, *62, 63*
experimental design, errors in 556
extended matching questions 103,
126–127, 158–159, 192–193,
244–246, 301–303, 330–331,
344–345, 378–379, 409–410,
448–449, 523–524, 551–552
extracellular fluid volume 106, **107, 108**

faecal occult blood 255, 270, 458
faintness 25
Fallot's tetralogy 227
familial amyloidosis 389–390
Fanconi's syndrome *324*
fatigue 43, *62, 63*
ferritin 12, 289, 416–417
fetal rhesus D syndrome 427
fever 27, 112, *130,* 146–147, 150, 171,
182, 186, 228, 230, *231,* 233, 268,

275–276, 292, *320*, 366, 392, 439, 494, 496, 498
fibrates *66*
fibrillation
    atrial *18*, 36, *61*, *65*, 196, 208–209, *221*, 237, **238**, 245Q, *351*, 353, 503–505
    ventricular **219**, 242, **242**
fibrin 385, **430**
fibrin degradation products (FDPs) 431
fibrinogen 390, 411, 428
fibrinolysis 429
fibrosis 163, *165*, *166*, 172, *294*
filariasis 152
finger clubbing *163*, 163, 173, 178, 180, 185, 190Q, 195, 227, 232, *248*, 249
fistulae 116, 266
5HT agonists and antagonists 501
fluid
    balance 105–106
    requirements 106
    thrill 252
folate deficiency 414, 417, 421, 488
follicle stimulating hormone (FSH) 46, 349, 354, *354*, 361
Friedreich's ataxia 18, *464*, 508
FSH. *See* follicle stimulating hormone
fugue *543*
fulminant hepatic failure 286
fungal disease 150
fungi *494*, 498

gait 479, *543*
gallop rhythm 220–221, 437
gallstones 28, *66*, 84, 87, **95**, 180, *248*, 267, 276, *277*, 278–279, 281, *293*, 293–295, 423
γ-aminobutyric (GABA) 67, 491
gamma glutamyl transpeptidase 122
ganciclovir 134
ganglion blockers *109*
gastrectomy *419*
gastritis 258, 260
gastroenteritis 144
gastrointestinal
    abnormalities 84–88
    infections 273
    motility 273
gastro-oesophageal reflux 24, 28–29, 255, 256–257, 297Q

gastroscopy 253
Gaucher's disease *251*
genetic(s)
    defects 464
    diagnosis 131
    human 463–468
    imprinting 465
    predisposition 266, 268, 562
    screening and counselling 467
gentamicin *114*, 133, 138, 208, 393, 398, *515*
german measles 145
giardia *263*, 276
Gilbert's syndrome 122, *248*, *280*, 281
Glasgow coma scale *485–486*
glaucoma *64*
gliclazide 46, 372
glioma 356, *515*
glomerulonephritis 149, 184, 222, *321*, 384, 387, *388*, 388–389, *400*
glomerulosclerosis 369
glutamyltranspeptidase 121
glyceryl trinitrate 25, 212
glycoproteins 305, 412
goblet cell 267
goitre 351, 353
gonococcal infection *395*
gonorrhoea 153
Goodpasture's syndrome 184, 387, *388*, 408Q
gout 29, 51, *60*, 124, 314, *315*, 401, 409Q, 443, 444
governance 563–564
gram-negative baccilus and cocci 137–138
gram-positive cocci 136
Graves' disease 348, 351–353, 376Q
Grey-Turner sign 277
grief reaction *537*
growth axis 355
growth hormone 353–354, *354*, 356
growth hormone releasing hormone **354**
Guillain-Barré syndrome 275, 510, 512
gynaecomastia *61*

H$_2$ breath test 254
H$_2$-receptor antagonists 59
haematemesis 258, 260, *261*

haematology. *See specific blood component*

haematoma 506–507, *531*

haematuria 29, 31, 102, 153, 158Q, 225, 232, 385, 387, *388*, 392–394, 403–405, *434*

haemochromatosis *250*, 281, 286, *309*, 356, 367, *464*

haemodialysis 55, 116, *419*, 402

haemofiltration 402

haemoglobin (Hb) 121, 127Q, 177, 187, 260, 268, 345Q, 372–373, *413*, 413–414, 421–423, 442–443, 447Q, 566–567

haemoglobinuria 424–425, 428

haemolysis 130, 151–152, 248, 292, 391, 414–415, *419*, 422–426, 428, 442–443

haemolytic anaemia. *See* anaemia: haemolytic

haemolytic uraemic syndrome (HUS) 391, 397, *446*

haemophilia *309*, 431, *432*, *464*, 467

haemophilus influenzae 135–136, 154, 169, 308, 423, 494

haemopoiesis **412**

haemoptysis 25, 27, 171, *173*, 178, 180, 184, 208, 387, 437

haemorrhage 30, 108, 110, 123, 168, 184, 225, 259–260, 262, 271, 286, 291, 317, *320*, 328, *359*, 361, 443, 504

  brain 16, 42–43, 92, **93,** 96, 101, 379Q, 403, 410Q, 433, 446, 463, 482–483, *486, 494, 502,* 501–502, 505–506, *519, 529*

  gastrointestinal 259, *261*

  splinter 195, 232

haemorrhagic colitis 274

hallucinations 115, 129, 187, *291*, 463, *487*, 490, 528–529, 532–533, *536, 546,* 551–552

haloperidol *294*

hands, examination of 306–308

Hashimoto's thyroiditis 352

hay fever 336

headache 59, *61, 64, 66*, 138, 143–147, 151, 174, 187, 224, *320*, 354, 365, 415, *445*, 494, 496, 498, *499*, 505–507, 523–524, *542*

migraine 318, 500–501

  tension 500

heart

  arrest *43*

  arrhythmias *53*, 57, *61–62*, 65, 112–113, 144, 216, *220*, 230, 233, 240, 319, 365, 489, 512, *534, 539*

  auscultation *199*

  axis **205**

  block 62, 65

  catheterization 207

  disease, congenital 207, 225, 236

  disease, valvular 208, 318, 503

  drugs *61–62*

  enlarged 221

  enzymes 214, 230

  failure 25–26, *43*, 60, *61*, 62, 64, 83, 106, 108, 111, *114*, 122–123, 185, 207, 209, 214, 217, 219–221, *221, 227*, 230–233, 238, 265, 353, 355, 396, 401, 415, 536–537

  fibrillation (*see* fibrillation)

  filling 200, 221

  glycosides *61*

  infarction 62, 63, 65, *114*, 120–121, 214, **215**, 236, *436*

  infection (*see* mycocarditis)

  inflammatory and infective diseases of 228

  ischaemic disease of *12*, 25–27, 97, *162*, 204, 209, 212–220, *221*, 235–236, 369, 502

  lesions 79

  markers 120

  monitoring *214, 217, 486*

  murmur 17, 157Q, 159Q, 198, *199*, **201**, 208–211, 226–228, 230, 232, 415

  output 219, *221*, 399

  pulmonary valve stenosis in 265

  rupture 217

  septal defects 217, 226, 236

  shunts *221*, 226–228

  sounds 17, **200**, 209–211

  tachyarrhythmias 236, 240

  transplant 222

  troponins 120

  valves 65, 80, *197*, 201, 206–207, 209, 211, 221–222, 231–232, 250, 265

  See also cyanosis

Index

Heberden's nodes *307*, *310*
Helicobacter pylori *59*, 139, 254, 258–260, 262, 297Q, 454
HELLP syndrome 292
helminths 276
hemiparesis 18, 502–503
Henoch-Schönlein purpura 387
heparin *65*, *115*, *214*, *269*, 318, *322*, 374–375, 431, 435–436, *437*, 438, 510
hepatic. *See* liver
hepatitis 120–122, 124, 144, 153, 249, *277*, *280*, *287*, 289, 292, 301, 384, 389, 453
  alcoholic 290
  autoimmune 185, 264, 281, 285–286
  B 131, 135–136, 282–283, **283**, **284**, 286, 293, 300Q, 384, *388*, 401, 457, *546*
  C 131, 135, 185, 264, *281*, **284**, 285, 293, *301Q*, 321, 469Q
  chronic 135, *281*, 284, **285**, 290, *294*, 469Q
  viral 35, 130, *154*, 156Q, *248*, *250*–251, 281–282, 452, 454
hepatojugular reflux *197*
hepatomegaly 12, 151–152, 177, *248*, *250*, 265, 282, 292, 297Q, 390, 403, 439
hepatorenal failure *43*
hepatosplenomegaly 18, 129, 138, 143, 151, 153, 183, *251*, 288–289, 390–391, 442
hereditary haemochromatosis 289
hernia **83**, 83, 249, 255, 256
hernial orifices 253
Herpes simplex 134, 144, 335, *494*, 495
Herpes zoster 335, 496
hirsutism 357
histoplasmosis 150
HIV. *See* human immunodeficiency virus
Hodgkin's disease 438–439, *439*, 446
homocystinuria *419*
honeycomb lung 183–184, *185*
hookworm 276, *446*
hormones 46, 272, 347, 349. *See also* endocrinology
Horner's syndrome 174, 501, 518, 520
Howell-Jolly bodies 264
human chorionic gonadotrophin (HCG) *348*, 406, 458, 467

human immunodeficiency virus (HIV) 35, 131, *141*, 146, **147**, 148–149, 154, 156Q, 157Q–158Q, 171–172, *179*, 192Q, *340*, 341, 384, 428, 440, *494*, 498, 510, *531*, *546*
human papilloma virus (HPV) 154
Huntington's disease 490, 521, *531*
hydralazine 52, 316
hydrocephalus 482, 498, 482, *531*
hydroxychloroquine *311*, 341
hyperaldosteronism *116*, *326*, *347*, *360*, 364, *365*
hyperbilirubinaemia *280*, 300
hypercalcaemia 6, 182, 259, 277, 325, *326*, 360, 362, 393, 445
hypercalciuria 116, 393
hypercapnia 68
hypercholesterolaemia *66*
hypercortisolaemia 535
hyperglycaemia 110, 366, 367, 373–375, *486*
hyperkalaemia *61*, *63*, 113, 115, 125Q, 236, *398*
hyperlipidaemia *66*, 212, 277, 293, 401, 502
hypermagnesaemia 116–117
hypernatraemia 111, *486*
hyperoxaluria 393
hyperparathyroidism *117*, 119, *315*, *322*, *326*, 349, 359, *360*, 401, 536
hyperphosphataemia, *117*
hyperprolactinaemia 361, 401
hyperpyrexia 54, *546*
hyperreflexia 57, 115, 146
hypersplenism 151, *446*
hypertension 5, 25, *60*, *62*, *63*, *64*, 96, 192Q, *198*, 208, 210, 212, 220, *221*, **223**, 228, 236, 243Q, 252, 287, *315*, *317*, *320*, 341–342, *348*, 355, 357, 364–365, 369, 383, *400*, 401, 403–404, 467, 502, 505–506, 560
  essential 222
  malignant 225, 310
  portal 153, *251*, *252*, 260, *288*
  pulmonary 185, 209, 211, 226–227, 319
  secondary 222, 224, *225*
  therapy for 505
  See also hypotension
hyperthermia 534

hyperthyroidism *18*, 36, 273, *351*, 352, 367, 535, 542. *See also* thyroid gland
hypertrichosis 488
hyperuricaemia 314, *315*, 393
hyperventilation 54, 374
hypoalbuminaemia 83, 108, 111, *252*, 339
hypoadrenalism primary 359
hypocalcaemia 273, 278, 326, *327*, 330Q, 359–360, *531*
hypochondriasis 536, 544
hypoglycaemia 58, 152, 286, *371*, 373, *486*, 489, 529, 542
hypokalaemia *60*, *62*, 112, *114*, 225, 362
hypomagnesaemia 115–116
hyponatraemia *60*, *61*, 110–111, 174, 363, *486*, 487
hypoparathyroidism *327*, 360, *360*
hypophosphataemia 117
hypophysectomy 355
hypopituitarism 355, 361, 415
hyporeflexia 116
hyposplenism 264, 423
hypotension 53, 57, *60*, *62*, *63*, *64*, 109, 113, 129, *176*, 189, 214, *220*, 225, *225*, 260, *269*, 303, 359, 396, 402, 428, *437*, 512, *534*, *539*
    postural *60*, *64*, 109, *109*, 369, 379Q
    See also hypertension
hypothalamic
    -anterior pituitary axis *354*, **354,** 356
    -pituitary-adrenal axis **357**
    -posterior pituitary axis *363*
hypothermia 233, 277, 339, *486*
hypothyroidism *18*, 36–37, 46, 110, 122, 233, 273, 302, *315*, *351*, 352, 356, 376Q, 414–415, *421*, *482*, *486*, 509, 525, *531*, 536, *539*. *See also* thyroid gland
hypovolaemia 109–110, 396, 399
hypoxaemia *68*

IgG antibodies 513
ileostomy *18*, 108, *114*, 119, 249
imaging methods 71
immunological diagnosis 130
impetigo 136
incontinence 407, *487*, 493, 518
infarction. *See* heart: infarction

infections
    acute 282, 284
    anaerobic 133
    bacterial 136–139, 148, 230, 274, 334, 391, 448
    chest *18*, 77, *173*, 178, 180
    chronic 283, **283**, 285, 417
    fetal 145
    fungal 335–336, *340*, 389, 460
    HIV (*see* human immunodeficiency virus)
    respiratory 25–26, 176, 387, 391
    urinary 29, 130, 369, 391–394, 406, 410Q
    viral 130, 144–146, 335, 389, 446, 492, 514
    See also specific organ and specific disease-causing organism
infertility 356
inflammatory bowel disease 6, *163*, 265, 314, *323*, *340*, 390, *436*
inflammatory disease 28, *419*
infliximab 266, *269*, *311*, 313
influenza 135–136, 146, *169*, 229, 496
inheritance
    autosomal dominant **465**
    multifactorial 466
    X-linked recessive **467**
insomnia *67*, 400, *536*, 544
insulin 40–41, 46, *114*, *117*, 149, 341, *354*, **355**, 366–367, 371–375, *398*
    prolonged acting 372
    soluble 372
    treatment *372*, 373
    See also diabetes
interferon 135, 404, 442, 459, 492
intravenous replacement fluids 105
iodine *348*
iron
    absorption **416**
    deficiency 249, 263, 269, 301, 379Q, 415–416
    metabolism 415
irritability 115, 353, 540, *542*
irritable bowel syndrome 271, 299, 525
ischaemic heart disease. *See* heart: ischaemic disease of
isoniazid 51, *141*, 172, *281*, 286, *294*, 316, 417, *511*

Janeway lesions 232
jaundice *12*, 29, 55, 143, 146, 159Q,
  248, 248–249, 279–280, *280*, 282,
  285–288, *288*, 294–295, 297Q, 300,
  415, 420, 424, 456, *534*
joint
  examination 306
  fibrocartilaginous 306
  pain 308, *309*, 325, 387
  synovial 305, **305**
jugular vein
  pressure *197*
  pulse (JVP) 164, 177, 197, *197*, *198*,
    211, *220*, 221, 229, 235, 437

kala-azar 150, *250*, *251*
Kallmann's syndrome 355
Kaposi's sarcoma 145, 148
Kartagener's syndrome *179*
Kayser-Fleischer rings 290
Kernig's sign 494, 506
ketoacidosis 41, *114*, *115*, 116, *117*, 119,
  277, 368, *372*, 378Q
ketonuria 374
kidney
  acute tubular necrosis in 110, 112,
    396, 409Q
  autosomal dominant polycystic
    disease of 403
  calculi in **88**, 360, 382, 393, 408Q
  disease *114*, 123, 148, 224, 289, *324*,
    369, 390, 393, 423
  enlarged *251*
  examination 251, 381–382
  failure 43, 58, *59–60*, 106, 108, 111,
    115–116, *117*, 119–121, 143, 152, 225,
    259, 277–278, 315, 319, *320*, 322, *324*,
    327, 341, 359, 369, 383–387, *388*, 389,
    391, 395, 397–404, 409Q–410Q, 415,
    428, 463, 524, *529*, *546*
  functions 381
  impairment *64*, *66*
  polycystic 392
  stones 28–30, 88, 95–96, 267, 325,
    393, *394*, 404
  tests 123–124, 382–384
  transplantation 403
  tuberculosis 393
  tubular acidosis 114, *115*, 185, 362, 393

Klebsiella 170, 277, 391
Klinefelter's syndrome 464
koilonychia 249, 415–416
Korsakoff's syndrome 291
Kussmaul's sign 229
kwashiorkor 123, 263
kyphosis 323

lactate dehydrogenase (LDH) 121,
  127Q, 214, *278*
Lambert-Eaton myasthenic-myopathic
  syndrome 514
Langerhan's histiocytosis 356
laxatives *6*, 273
LD$_{50}$, 46–47
Legionella pneumophila 169
leishmaniasis 150–151
leprosy 141, *340*, 510
Leptospira interrogans 143
leptospirosis 143, *154*
leucocyte alkaline phosphatase 443
leucocytosis 292, *422*, 423
leuconychia 248–249
leucopenia 51, 145, 317, *534*
leukaemia *114*, *115*, 124, *130*, *251*,
  315, 340, *425*, 440–441, *446*,
  452, *452*
  acute myeloid (AML) 441, *441*, 454
  acute lymphoblastic 438
  acute promyelocytic 454
  chronic *250*, 442
  chronic lymphocytic (CLL) 442
  chronic myeloid (CML) 442, 438
  hairy cell 443
leutinizing hormone (LH) 46, *354*, *361*
levodopa 490
life support algorithm **219**
limb leads for ECG 33, 202
lipoatrophy 373
listeria 138, 494
lithotripsy 394
livedo reticularis 318, 320
liver
  abscess 292
  biochemistry 121, **283**
  cysts **96**, 103Q, 403–404
  disease 18, 32, 58, *59*, *61*, 64, *65*,
    66, *67*, 120–121, 245, 248, *250*,

251, *252*, 260, *261*, 282–285, *288*,
290–293, *322*, 340–341, 414, *421*,
425, 433
  drugs for 295–296
  encephalopathy 291–292, *296*, 483
  examination 250
  failure *43*, *60*, 111, *114*, 123, 292, *531*
  function tests 121, 278, *287*, 291–292,
    567
  malignancy 122, 270, 281, 293 (*see
    also* cancer: hepatocellular)
  steatosis 293
  ultrasound **95**
lockjaw 138
Lown-Ganong-Levine syndrome 239
lumbar puncture (lp) 483–484, 494,
  499, 506
lung
  cancer (*see* cancer: lung)
  chronic obstructive disease in
    (COPD) 26, 28, 75, *162*, 165, *167*,
    169, 172, 176, 187, 191Q
  diseases *165*, 180
  embolus 27, 72, 83, 95, 98, **98**, 120,
    166, 221, 236, 431, *437*
  fibrosis 17, 28, 52, 180, 182–183,
    184, 319
  function 167, 175
  infection 26, 168
  inflammation 182
  interstitial disease 166
  metastases **78**, **80**
  oedema 25–26, 30, 55, *60*, 76, **81**, **82**,
    108, *166*, 180, 200, 220, 398, 400
lupus 52, 182, 318, 341
lutinizing hormone releasing hormone
  (LHRH) 354, *354*, **354**, *361*, 406
Lyme disease 143, **143**
lymphadenopathy 78, **79**, 129, 138,
  142–143, 145, 147, 151, 158Q, 164,
  182, 193Q, 249, 279, 439–440, 442,
  445, 456
lymphocytes 155Q, 411, 438, 442,
  448Q, 566
lymphocytosis 130
lymphoma 79, 121–122, 124, 130, 148,
  251, 259, 262, *263*, 265, 298, *326*,
  340, 341, 356, *425*, 439, *452*, 499
  bowel 263–264

  Burkitt's 145, 440, 454–455
  Non-Hodgkin's 438, 440
lysosyme 390

macrocytosis 418, *421*, 448Q
macrolides 133
magnesium 114. *See also*
  hypermagnesaemia;
  hypomagnesaemia
magnesium sulphate 176, 271, 273
magnetic resonance imaging (MRI) 72,
  96, **97**, 269, 279, *311*, 317, 356, 366,
  383, 404, 482, *485*, 488, 491–492,
  498, 500, 504, 513, 519–520, 531,
  535
malabsorption *263*, 276, 302, 419
malaria 130, 151, *152*, *154*, 156, *248*,
  250, *251*, *388*, 389, 401, 425
malathion 336
malignancy. *See* cancer
Mallory-Weiss tear 260
malnutrition 116, 267, 277, *288*
mania 526, 534–535, *536*, *539*, 549, 552
Marfan's syndrome 210, 245, 328, *464*
maternity blues 540
measles *135*, 136, 146, *154*, 158Q, 384,
  388, 496
Meckel's diverticulum 90
medical
  emergencies 1, 23
  finals 1, 9
  imaging 71
melaena 258, 259–260, *261*, 303
meningioma 356, *499*, *519*
meningitis 136–140, *141*, 142, 145, 148,
  150, *154*, 355, 363, 483, *494*,
  494–495, *495*, 497, 501, *515*
meningococcus *135*, 136, 495
meningoencephalitis 144, 151, 183
menopause *309*, 314, *322*
menstruation
  cycle 349
  disorders *347*
  disturbance 352, 357, 359
Mental Health Act 548, *548*, 550
mental state examination 37, 472, 526
mesothelioma *163*, 181, 453
metastases. *See* cancer: metastases
metformin 372

methadone 545, *546*

methotrexate 266, 459

methyldopa 52, *281*, *294*, 316, 424, *425*

metoclopramide *217*, 460

metronidazole 133, 264, *511*

microalbuminuria 369

microaneurysms *320*, 505

microbiology request forms 35

migraine 318, 500–501. *See also* headache

miliary shadows 78

mineralocorticoids 108, *114*, 358

miscarriage 318, 331Q

mitral

  regurgitation *198*, 209

  stenosis *198*, 208

  valve 195, 198, 209, 220

mode of death *43*

molluscum contagiosum 145, 148

monobactams 132

monocytes 411, 566

mononeuritis multiplex 369, 510

mononeuropathies 508–509

mononucleosis 145, *425*

mood 527, 534, **537**

morphine 41, 49, 462, *546*

mortality

  age-standardised *452*

  causes of **451**

  employment-related 44

motor function 476

motor neurone disease 507, *515*, 516, 518

MRI. *See* magnetic resonance imaging

multiple choice questions 70, 102–103, 155–158, 243–244, 299–301, 408–409, 447, 469–470, 521–523

multiple sclerosis 409Q, 482, 491, 521, 536

mumps *135*, 146, *154*, 277, 384, 495

murmur. *See* heart: murmur

muscle

  disease 512

  strength 476, *477*

  tone 476, 485

musculoskeletal system examination 306

myalgia 143, 169

myasthenia gravis 512, *513*, 516

mycobacterial disease 139

Mycobacterium 139–142, 148, 155, 170, 494

  leprae 141

  tuberculosis 139, 155Q, 170, *494*

  (*see also* turberculosis)

mycoplasma 169, 340, 425

myelodysplasia 415, 417, 444

myelofibrosis *251*, 442, 444

myelography 483, 519

myeloma 103, *117*, 124, *324*, *326*, 340, 390–391, 438, 445, *446*, 460, 481, *519*

myeloproliferative disorders 443

myocardial. *See* heart

myocarditis 120, 138, 144–146, 169, 229

myoclonus 498

myopathies *513*

myositis *66*

myotonic dystrophy 465, *513*

N-acetylcysteine (NAC) treatment regime *56*

naproxen *67*, 462

narcosis 116

nausea 25, 28, 54, 55, *59*, *60*, *61*, 187, 213, 258–262, 266, 276–277, 282, 358, 363, 374, 400, 460, 463, 490, 501. *See also* vomiting

Neisseria 137, 153, 308, *494*, 495

nematodes 152, 276

neoplasms 78

nephrectomy 404

nephropathy, reflux 109, *400*

nephrotic syndrome 108, *114*, 123, *252*, *288*, 383, 385, **386**, 387, *388*, 390, 408Q, *436*

nerve compression 509

nerve conduction studies 483, 510

nervous system

  examination 471–478

  infection and inflammation of 494

neurofibromatosis *185*, *464*, 510

neuroleptic drugs 532–534

neurological investigations 480

neuropathy, autonomic 6, 148, 369, 390, 508, 510, 512

neuroses 541

neurosyphilis 142, 497

neutropenia 130, 148, 460

neutrophilia 130

neutrophils 277, 411, 566
nicotinic acid *511, 529*
nifedipine 64, *294*
nitrates *64, 109*
nitrofurantoin *294*, 393
nitroimidazoles 133
nocturia 224, 362, 400
non-alcoholic steatohepatitis (NASH) 287, 293
non-steroidal anti-inflammatory drugs (NSAIDs) *67*, 108– 109, *115*, 175, 223, 258–260, *261*, *294*, *311*, 312–315, 317, 394, 399, 462–463
noradrenaline 538
Norwalk virus 274
notifiable diseases 154
nuclear
    imaging 207
    medicine 72, 98
nystagmus 57, 291, 488, 493, 508, 511, *515*
nystatin 134, 150

obesity *18*, 222, 256, 293, *436*, 509
objective structured clinical examinations 9, 21–44, 308
obsessive compulsive disorders 527, 542
obstructive airways disease *62*, 175
obstructive sleep apnoea 177, 191Q
occupational therapy 492, 505
oedema *64*, 108, 211, 220
oesophagus
    cancer (*see* cancer: oesophageal)
    disease 255
    tumour 103Q
oesophagitis 150
oestrogen 108, *294*, 349, *361*, 454, 459
oncogenes 455
operation scars 249
ophthalmoplegia 18, 353
ophthalmoscope 3, 471
ophthalmoscopy 149
oral contraceptives 27, 46, *53*, 192Q, 223, 316, *340, 348, 437*, 502, 535
orthomyxovirus 146
orthopnoea 26, 208, 220
OSCEs. *See* objective structured clinical examinations

Osler's nodes 232
osteoarthritis 19, 306, *307*, 309, *309*, 329Q
osteomalacia 122, 264, *322, 323, 324*, 327, 330Q, 359, 401, 488
osteomyelitis 133, 136, 140, *141*, 390, 417
osteoporosis 52, *317*, 322, 322–323, 329Q, 330Q, *347, 360*, 360, 401
ovaries, tumours of 277
oxyhaemoglobin 167, 187
oxytocin 110, *354*

pacemaker 195, 222, 233, 235–236, 238
Paget's disease 19, 122, *221*, 322, 324, 481
palmar erythema *248*, 249, 287
pancreas 12, 96, 247, 276, 345Q, 367. *See also* cancer: pancreatic
pancreatitis chronic 84, 87, 95, 106, 116, 276, *277, 278*, 278, 295, 300, *327*, 367, 401
panic attacks 365, 552
papilloedema 472, 498, *499*, 506
papillomavirus 454
paracetamol *54*, 55, 286, *294*, **295**, 462, 501, 530
paraesthesiae 326, 360, 400
paramyxovirus 146
paraplegia 421
parasites *6*, 130, 384, *446*. *See also specific parasite*
parathormone 325
parathyroid hormone 327
parathyroid glands 359
paratuberculosis 275
paratyphoid fever *154*
Parkinson's disease 18, 35, 489, 521, *531*, 534, 536
Pataú's syndrome 464
Paterson-Kelly syndrome 416
patient
    communication with 39
    exam *18*
    dignity 4
    management of 14
penicillin 52, 131, 136–138, 142–144, *186, 294*, 424, 497
peptic ulcer 59, 67, *67, 67*, 258, 325

percutaneous nephrolithotomy 394
perforation 31, 259, 271, 277, *546*
  bowel 31
  gallbladder 31
pericardial effusion *197*, 198, 207,
  229, 230
pericarditis 140, 145, 169, *197*, 217, *221*,
  228–229, 236, 244Q, 319, 398, 401
peristalsis 249
peritonitis **87**, 140, 288, 292
permethrin 336
peroneal muscular atrophy (Charcot-
  Marie-Tooth disease) 512
persistent ductus arteriosus 227
pertussis *135*, 136
PET. *See* positron emission topography
petechiae 232
Peyer's patches 247
phaeochromocytoma 222, 364, 367, 542
pharmacodynamics 45–53
pharmacogenetics 51, 53
pharmacokinetics 45, 47–48
phenoxybenzamine 47, 366
phenytoin 49–50, *59*, 294, *419*, *486*, 488,
  491, *511*
physiotherapy 490, 492, 505
picoRNAviruses 145
pituitary
  adenoma 357
  disorders 353
  lesions 482
  tumour 353
pituitary-adrenal axis *358*
placental abruption 433
plague *154*
plasma
  osmolality 110
  proteins 53, 411
  See also blood
plasminogen 429
Plasmodium 151, 384
platelet 411, 434, 442, 445, 448Q, 566
  adhesion 428
  aggregation 385
  count *413*, 444, 484
  disorders *432*, 445
  prostaglandin 429
pleural effusions 82
pleurisy 27, 183

pneumococcus 136, 495
Pneumocystis carinii 133, 149, 169
pneumonia 25–27, 31–30, **76**, **78**, 82,
  136–137, 139, 146, 149–150,
  157Q–158Q, *162*, *165*, *167*, 168, *169*,
  170, 172, *179*, 190Q, 192Q, 236, 363,
  371, 374, 498
  atypical 26, 133
  lobar 77, 168
pneumothorax 27–28, 30–31, 72, **73**, **74**,
  102Q, *165*, *176*, 180, 186–187, **188**,
  191Q, 198, *220*, 328
poisoning
  antidotes for *54*
  aspirin 54
  carbon monoxide 187
  ethanol 58
  food 136, *154*
  lead 229, *531*
  mercury *531*
  opiate 57
  paracetamol 55
poliomyelitis *135*, 136, 145, *154*,
  229, 516
poliovirus 145
polyarthritis *231*, 309, *321*
polycystic kidney disease 222, *251*, *400*
polycythaemia 227, 341, 404, *436*, 443
polyenes 134
polymyalgia rheumatica 40, 320,
  329Q, 417
polymyositis 120, *513*
polyneuropathies 183, 342, 368, 389,
  482, 488, 510–511, *511*
polypectomy 254
polyuria 109, 239, 325, 354, 362, 368,
  382, 395, *539*
porphyria *511*, 537
positron emission topography (PET)
  98, **99**, 166, 174, 257, 457, 483, 535
post-mortem examination 41
postpartum psychosis 540
potassium 112
  diuretics and *61*, *62*, 113
  restriction 398, 401
  uptake **113**
poxvirus 145
prednisolone 40, 231, 266, 268
pre-eclampsia 224, 397

pregnancy 58, *63*, *65*, *66*, *67*, 122–123, 133, 224, 233, 256, *277*, 285–286, 415–416, *419*, *421*, 421, 509, 535
prion disease 497–498
proctoscopy 254, 266
progesterone 349
prolactin *354*, 356
propranolol *62*
propylthiouracil *294*, 353
prostaglandins 381
prostate
  benign enlargement of 406
  cancer 363, 405
  diseases 406
  obstruction *395*
prostate-specific antigen (PSA) 406–407, 458
protease inhibitors 149
proteinuria 224–225, 369, 373, 385
proteoglycans 305
proteus mirabilis 391
prothrombin time 121, *287*, 430, *432*, 567
proton pump inhibitors *59*, 256
protozoal disease 150, 276. *See also Cryptosporidium*; giardia
pruritus *66*, 341, 401
PSA. *See* prostate-specific antigen
pseudobulbar palsy 518
pseudodementia *531*, *536*, *543*
pseudohyponatraemia 111
Pseudomonas 133, 169
Pseudoxanthoma elasticum 328
psoriasis 337, 338, 343Q
  arthritis and 313
  chronic plaque 338
  flexoral 338
  guttate 338
psychiatric
  history 525
  law 548
  problems 525
psychogenic polydipsia 110
psychosis 327, 357, *541*, *543*, 546
psychotherapy 539, 543, 547
ptosis 472, 497, 513–514, *515*, 518
puberty *348*, 351
puerperal affective disorders 540
pulmonary. *See* lung

pulse
  collapsing *196*, 211
  jugular **197**, *198*
  oximetry 167, *176*
  radial 34, 195, *196*
pulsus paradoxus 167, *196*, *197*, 229
purgatives 116, 271
pyelonephritis 28, 369, 392–393, 408Q
pyloric stenosis 84, 467
pyoderma gangrenosum 266, **267**, 340
pyrexia 159Q, 232, 266, 487, 409Q–410Q, 523Q–524Q
pyridoxine (B$_6$) *511*

question types. *See* exams types
quinolones 133

rabies 146, *154*, 496
radiofemoral delay 196, 224, 228
radioiodine 352–353
radiology 29, 71, 101, 166, 392, 401
radiotherapy 168, 174, 257, 262, 339, 355, 360, 405–406, 440, 444–445, 459–460, 462–463, 500
raloxifene 323
Ramsay Hunt syndrome 496, 515
ranitidine 46, *59*, 256, *294*
Ransom's criteria 561
Raynaud's phenomenon **316**, 318–319, 389
receptor agonists and antagonists 46
red blood cell. *See* blood
referral decisions *42*
regression 558
Reiter's syndrome 153, 275, 313
renal. *See* kidney
renin 108, 365, 381
respiratory acidosis 118–125
respiratory alkalosis. *See* alkalosis: respiratory
respiratory depression 57–58, *486*, *499*, *546*
respiratory system examination 162–166
results stations, interpretation of 29–30
reticulocytes 413, 415, 566
reticulocytosis *421*
retinal changes 224
retinopathy 224, 368, 369

rhabdomyolysis *115, 117,* 397
rhabdovirus 146
rhesus disease 424
rheumatic fever 137, 208–210, 230, *231,* 244Q, 491
rheumatoid arthritis 5, 14, 19, 83, 183, **184,** 306, *307,* 309, *309, 310,* **312,** *322,* 329Q, 340, 390, 417, 509, 513
rheumatoid factor 183, 319
rheumatology 305
rhinitis allergic 336, *446*
ribavirin 135
rickets 323, *324,* 401, 465
rifampicin 50, *141,* 172, *294,* 495
Rinne's test 475
risk 560–561
RNA viruses 145–146, 282, 284
Romberg's test 479
rosiglitazone 372
rotavirus *6,* 274
Roth spots 232
roundworm 276
rubella *135,* 136, 145–146, *154,* 225, 229, 156Q

Sacoptes scabiei 336
sacroiliitis 266
salicylates 124, *294*
Salmonella 6, 133, 139, 274, 313
sarcoidosis *130,* 168, *185,* 356, *446, 494,* 510
Schilling test 418, 420
Schistosoma 153, 384, 454
schistosomiasis 153, 251, *395, 400*
schizophrenia 526–527, 532, 535, 537, 542, 549
scintigraphy **100,** 383, 533
sclerosis, systemic 19, 183, *185,* 318
scorpion bites 277
screening 149, 254–255, 270, 404, 467, 491, 561
seizures 484, 487, *487*
self-assessment questions 70, 102–103, 125–127, 155–159, 190–193, 243–246, 297–303, 329–331, 343–345, 376–379, 408–410, 447–449, 469–470, 521–524, 549–552
sensation 479–480

sepsis 278, 291
septic shock
septicaemia 109, 129, 137–138, *359,* 433, 494
serotonin 265, 271, 428, 533, 538, 542
serum
    biochemistry 397, *485,* 488
    immunoglobulins 442
    urea and creatinine 224, 383
sex hormone and reproductive disorders 361
sex-linked inheritance 465
sexual abuse 535
sexually transmitted disease 153, 157Q. *See also specific disease*
Sheehan's syndrome 355, 361
Shigella 139, 273, 275, 313
shingles 335, 496
shock *43,* 106, 123, 433, 437
short answer questions 13–14, 379
shortness of breath. *See* breathlessness
Shy-Drager syndrome *109*
sickle cell disease 109–110, 145, *309,* 342, 392, 415, 421, *422,* 424, *464,* 467
sigmoid volvulus 30
sigmoidoscopy 254
sinus
    arrhythmia 233
    bradycardia 233
    node disease 233
skin examination 333
    cancer (*see* cancer: skin)
    lesions 142, 313, *321, 334*
sleep disturbance *62*
sleeping sickness 151
small bowel disorders 30, **85,** 262
smallpox 145, *154,* 600
small round structured viruses (SRSV) 274
smoking 25–27, 161–162, *162,* 173, 176–177, 181, 212, 256, 262, *322, 323,* 342, 405, *436, 437,* 452–453, 469Q, 502, 562
sodium nitroprusside 225
somatoform disorders 544
speech therapy 492, 505
spherocytosis 424
spider naevi *248,* 249, 260, 287

spinal cord
   compression 174, 483, *519*
   disease 518
spirochaetes 142
spirometry 167, 177, 181, 183, 185–186
spironolactone *61*, *115*, 288
spleen examination 251
splenectomy 444
splenomegaly 150–151, 159Q, 232, *248*,
      251, 260, 287, 390, 424, 439, 442–444
spondarthropathies, seronegative 312
spondylosis 481
squamous cell carcinoma 43, 339, 453
staphylococcal infection **137**
Staphylococcus 136, 384, 391, 498
   aureus 6, 133, *169*, 170, 231, 274, 292,
      308, 334, *494*
statins *66*
station
   types 21–23
   example 24–44
   practical procedure 32
statistics
   Chi squared 557
   comparative 556
   confidence intervals 557
   descriptional 553, **554**, 555
   distributions **554, 555,** 555
   hypotheses and 556
   non-parametric 557
   parametric 557
   regression 558, **558**
   See also data
status epilepticus *486*
steatohepatitis, non-alcoholic 287, 293
steatorrhoea 180, 263–265, 279
stem cell 412, 440–441, 460
   defects 444
   proliferation 444
stenosis
   aortic *63, 64*, 196, *196, 198*, 201, 204,
      210, *221*, 228, 236, 243Q, 489
   arterial 101, 102Q, 111, 396, 503
   mitral *198*, 199, 201, 208, 243Q
stents 213, 257, 395, 408
steroids 178, 183, 185–186, 223, 247,
      259, 266, 268, 277, 286, 317, *320*,
      321, 443, 445, 463, 535, 537
stethoscope 3, 34, 164, 196, 201

Stevens-Johnson syndrome 340
Stokes-Adams attacks 235
stomatitis 144, 415–416, 420
stones. *See specific type*
stool tests 254–255
streptococcal infection *340*
streptococcus 136, *169*, 231, 308, 384,
      494, 498
streptokinase *217*, 435
stress management 539
stroke 25, **92**, 369, 474, 502–503, 505,
      518, 525, 532, 560–561
succinylcholine *115*
sudden cardiac death 217
suicide 38–39, *42*, 540–541, *541*, 544, 549
sulphonamides 51, 133, *294*
surgery 25, 27, 178, 258, 262, *348*, 356,
      432, *437*, 505, 521
   bowel 266–267, 302
   brain 500, 505
   cardiac 80, 209–211, 222, 229, 232, 235
   ENT 178
   gastric 258, 261–262
   hernia 255
   lung 17, 174, 177, 187, **188**
   oesophageal 257
   joint *311*, 325
   trauma 6
sweating 25, 54, 213, 217, 365, *371*
Sydenham's chorea 230, 491
sympathomimetic drugs 233
synacthen test 349, *354*, *358*
syncope *43*, 235, 239–240, 438, 489
syndrome of inappropriate ADH
      secretion (SIADH) 116, 363, 377Q
syphilis 142, 154, 355, *494*, 505, *531*
syringobulbia 519
syringomyelia 518–519
systemic lupus erythematosus 183,
      315, **316**, 341, 384, 417, 491

tabes dorsalis **142**, 497
tachycardia *18*, 55, 57, *63, 64*, 109, *176*,
      189, 206, 214, 129, 219, 221, 233, 238,
      239, 240, 240, **241,** 244Q, 246, 260,
      268, *269*, 303, 353, 365, 415, *437*, 534
tachypnoea 176, 186, 189, *220*, 437
tapeworms 153, 276
taxanes 459

Tay-Sachs disease 467
tendon reflexes 477, *478*
tests. *See* exam types
tetanus 135–136, *154*
tetracycline 133, 154, 264, 274
thalassaemia 415, 423–424, 467
thiamin (B$_1$) 291, 511, *511*, *529*, *531*
thiazide diuretics *60*
thirst axis 112, **362**
threadworm 276
thrombin time 431
thrombocythaemia 65, 130, 145, 148,
    152, 317–318, 391, 410Q, 440–441,
    433, 444, 446, *446*, 461
thrombocytosis 446
thromboembolism *65*, 510
thrombolysis 214, 217, *437*, 438, 505
thrombosis 28, *65*, 96, 212, 217, *252*, *288*,
    292, 318, 342, 374, 425, 434–436,
    443–444, *436*, *437*, 502, *515*, 546
thrombotic thrombocytopenic
    purpura 391
thyroid gland
    adenoma 352, 366
    biochemistry *351*
    carcinoma 352
    cyst 352
    disease 264, 341, *347*, 513
    disorders 350
    examination of 36, *351*
    function tests 246, *485*, 529, 531
    See also hyperthyroidism
thyroid stimulating hormone **350**, **354**
thyrotoxicosis 6, *62*, 130, 221, 233, 236,
    299, *326*, 361, 491
thyrotrophin releasing hormone **350**,
    354
tinea
    capitis 335
    corporis 335
    cruris 335
    pedis 335
Tinel's sign 509
tinnitus 54, *60*, 443
TNM classification *270*, *457*
tonsillitis 137
torsades de pointes 241
toxic megacolon 30, 86, **87**, 267–268, *269*
toxic shock syndrome 136

toxocara 152
Toxoplasma gondii 151, 229
toxoplasmosis 151
transfusions, blood 147, 149, 423–424,
    428, 433–434, 447Q
trauma 6, 276, *309*, 342, 356, 367, 433,
    487, *529*
trematodes 153
tremor *18*, 36, 115, *291*, *351*, 353, 365,
    371, 489, 497, *539*, *543*
Treponema pallidum 142, 384, 494
triazoles 134
tricyclic antidepressants 57, *109*, 110,
    538, *539*
Tropheryma whippeii 264
tropical sprue *263*
Trousseau's sign 327
trypanosomiasis 151
tuberculosis 140–141, 150, *154*, 168,
    172, *179*, 190Q, *326*, 340, 359, 363,
    371, 390, 392, *395*, 400, 417, 481,
    482, 495
    AIDS and *147*
    apical 31
    drugs *141*
    fever and *130*
    manifestations **140**, **171**, *252*
    military **78**
    peritoneal *288*
    pulmonary 76–77, **77**, **78**, **79**, *185*
    renal 393
    surgery 17
    vaccination *135*
    See also Mycobacterium: tuberculosis
tumour(s)
    gastric 261
    intracranial *499*
    ovarian *277*
    stromal 261
    markers 458
    necrosis factor 412
    pituitary 356
    screening 458
    staging 457
    suppressors 454
    testicular 406
    urogenital tract and prostate 404
Turner's syndrome 226, 228, 361, 464
typhimurium 274

typhoid fever *154*
typhus fever *154*

ulcers 260, 261, *371*
  bleeding 253
  peptic *59*, 67, *67*, 258, 325
ulcerative colitis **87**, *130*, 185, 267, 273, *281*
ulcerative jejunitis 264
ultrasound 72, 95, 206, 278–279, 284, 287, 289–290, 292, 342, 395, 397, 403–404, 436, 467, 505
  renal tract 96, 382, 401
  liver 95
  pancreas 95
  vascular tree 96
unconsciousness 484
uraemia *43*, 395–398, 408Q, *486*, *511*, *531*
urea 123, 126Q, 169, 254, 260, 277, *278*, 291, 314, 319, 325, 327, 395, 397, 400, 402, *422*, 529, 567
urinalysis 224, 232, 373, 382, 397, 400, 409Q, *482*
urinary tract
  infection 29, 369, 391, 394, 406, 408Q
  obstruction *114*, 394, *395*, 397
urine
  Bence Jones proteins 401
  collections 349
urograms 97

vaccination and vaccines 129, *135*, 135–136, 139, 177, 283, 423, 495
vagal inhibition *43*
valciclovir 335
valproate 50, 539
valve. *See* heart: valves
valvotomy 195, 209
vancomycin 134
varicella zoster virus (VZV) 144, 384, 495–496
vasculitis 83, 184, 319, 341, 389, 396, *400*, *482*, 510
vasovagal attack *43*
vegan diet *419*
venesection 289, 443
ventricle. *See* heart
verapamil 53, *64*, 238, *294*
vertebral crush fractures 323

vertebrobasilar system 502
vertigo 443, 489, 493, 503, *515*
vibrio cholerae 139, 274
villous atrophy *263*
vincristine 459, *511*
viral haemorrhagic fever *154*
viruses and viral infection 6, 130, 274, *281*, 384, 446, *494*. *See also specific virus or disease*
visual evoked potentials (VEP) 483
visual field defects 517
visual loss 502–503
vitamin
  A *326*
  B$_{12}$ 32, *114*, 247, 264, 267, 302, **418**, **420**, 421, 447Q, 482, *511*, *529*, 531, *531*
  D 29, 40, 116, *117*, 323, *324*, *326*, *327*, 327, 333, 338, 381, 465
  fat-soluble 289
  deficiency *432*, 433, *511*, *529*, *531*
vitiligo 420
vomiting 28–29, 54–58, *61*, 102Q, 108, 110, *114*, *117*, 119, 125Q–126Q, 187, 213, *217*, 258, 260, 262, 266, 274–277, 291–294, 358, 374, 393, 400, 409Q, 460, 463, 490, 494, 498, *499*, 501, 503, 506, 523, 547. *See also* nausea
von Willebrand
  disease *432*, *464*
  factor **429**

Waldenström's macroglobulinaemia 390, 445
warfarin 50, *53*, *59*, 61, *65*, *67*, 238, 318, 430–431, 433–434, *434*, 436, 448Q
water
  deprivation test *363*, *364*
  distribution 105
  homeostasis and 108, 247
  total body 105
Weber's test 475
Wegener's granulomatosis 183, *321*, *388*, 389
weight loss 148, 163, 178, 224, 248, 257–258, 262–263, 269, 279, *293*, *311*, 320, 323, 353, 365, 368, 404, 439, 442, 444, *536*

Wernicke-Korsakoff syndrome 291, 511, 529
Whipple's disease 263, 264, *531*
whooping cough *154*
Wilson's disease *281*, 286, 289, *464*
wireless capsule 254
Wiskott-Aldrich syndrome *464*
Wolff-Parkinson-White syndrome 239

X-linked disorders *464*, 465
X-rays 21, 29–30, 71, *311*, 312–313, 323, 325, 327, 330, 330Q–331Q, 382
  abdominal *32*, **84**, *392*
  chest 5–6, 30, **30**, 72, **73**, 102Q, 157Q–158Q, 166, 170, 172–175, *176*, 177–178, 181, *182*, 183–187, 192Q, 193, 193Q, 202, 208–209, 220–221, 224, 229–230, 259, *269*, 319, 325, 358, 406, 422, 437–440, 457, 482, 488, 494–495, 505, 513, 519, 529–531
  pituitary fossa 481
  spinal 481

yellow fever 145, *154*, 285
Yersina enterocolitica 139, 155Q, 275, 313, *340*

Zollinger-Ellison syndrome 259, *263*, 279, 378Q